P9-CKP-943

2018
Nelson's Pediatric Antimicrobial Therapy

24th Edition

John S. Bradley, MD
Editor in Chief

John D. Nelson, MD
Emeritus

Elizabeth D. Barnett, MD
Joseph B. Cantey, MD
David W. Kimberlin, MD
Paul E. Palumbo, MD
Jason Sauberan, PharmD
William J. Steinbach, MD
Contributing Editors

American Academy of Pediatrics

DEDICATED TO THE HEALTH OF ALL CHILDREN®

American Academy of Pediatrics Publishing Staff

Mark Grimes, *Director, Department of Publishing*

Peter Lynch, *Manager, Digital Strategy and Product Development*

Barrett Winston, *Senior Editor, Professional and Clinical Publishing*

Shannan Martin, *Production Manager, Consumer Publications*

Jason Crase, *Manager, Editorial Services*

Mary Lou White, *Chief Product and Services Officer/SVP, Membership, Marketing, and Publishing*

Linda Smessaert, MSIMC, *Senior Marketing Manager, Professional Resources*

Mary Louise Carr, MBA, *Marketing Manager, Clinical Publications*

Published by the American Academy of Pediatrics

345 Park Blvd

Itasca, IL 60143

Telephone: 847/434-4000

Facsimile: 847/434-8000

www.aap.org

The recommendations in this publication do not indicate an exclusive course of treatment or serve as a standard of medical care. Variations, taking into account individual circumstances, may be appropriate. Statements and opinions expressed are those of the authors and not necessarily those of the American Academy of Pediatrics.

Web sites are mentioned for informational purposes only and do not imply an endorsement by the American Academy of Pediatrics. Web site addresses are as current as possible but may change at any time.

Brand names are furnished for identifying purposes only. No endorsement of the manufacturers or products listed is implied.

This publication has been developed by the American Academy of Pediatrics. The authors, editors, and contributors are expert authorities in the field of pediatrics. No commercial involvement of any kind has been solicited or accepted in the development of the content of this publication.

Every effort has been made to ensure that the drug selection and dosages set forth in this text are in accordance with current recommendations and practice at the time of publication. It is the responsibility of the health care professional to check the package insert of each drug for any change in indications or dosage and for added warnings and precautions.

Special discounts are available for bulk purchases of this publication. E-mail our Special Sales Department at aapsales@aap.org for more information.

9-393/1217   1 2 3 4 5 6 7 8 9 10

MA0837

ISSN: 2164-9278 (print)

ISSN: 2164-9286 (electronic)

ISBN: 978-1-61002-109-8

eBook: 978-1-61002-110-4

Editor in Chief

John S. Bradley, MD
Professor of Pediatrics
Chief, Division of Infectious Diseases,
    Department of Pediatrics
University of California, San Diego,
    School of Medicine
Director, Division of Infectious Diseases,
    Rady Children's Hospital San Diego
San Diego, CA

Emeritus

John D. Nelson, MD
Professor Emeritus of Pediatrics
The University of Texas
Southwestern Medical Center at Dallas
Southwestern Medical School
Dallas, TX

Contributing Editors

Elizabeth D. Barnett, MD
Professor of Pediatrics
Boston University School of Medicine
Director, International Clinic and Refugee
    Health Assessment Program,
    Boston Medical Center
GeoSentinel Surveillance Network,
    Boston Medical Center
Boston, MA

Joseph B. Cantey, MD
Assistant Professor of Pediatrics
Divisions of Pediatric Infectious Diseases and
    Neonatology/Perinatal Medicine
University of Texas Health Science Center at
    San Antonio
San Antonio, TX

David W. Kimberlin, MD
Professor of Pediatrics
Codirector, Division of Pediatric
    Infectious Diseases
Sergio Stagno Endowed Chair in
    Pediatric Infectious Diseases
University of Alabama at Birmingham
Birmingham, AL

Paul E. Palumbo, MD
Professor of Pediatrics and Medicine
Geisel School of Medicine at Dartmouth
Director, International Pediatric HIV Program
Dartmouth-Hitchcock Medical Center
Lebanon, NH

Jason Sauberan, PharmD
Assistant Clinical Professor
University of California, San Diego,
    Skaggs School of Pharmacy and
    Pharmaceutical Sciences
Rady Children's Hospital San Diego
San Diego, CA

William J. Steinbach, MD
Professor of Pediatrics
Professor in Molecular Genetics
    and Microbiology
Chief, Division of Pediatric Infectious Diseases
Director, International Pediatric Fungal
    Network
Duke University School of Medicine
Durham, NC

Contents

Introduction

We are very fortunate to be in our 24th edition of *Nelson's Pediatric Antimicrobial Therapy* as we continue to gain momentum in our partnership with the American Academy of Pediatrics (AAP)! Even though it has only been a year since the last revision, there are many important additions, including the approval of a second new antibiotic to treat methicillin-resistant *Staphylococcus aureus* infections and the significant advances in clinical studies for antibiotics to treat the ever-increasing multidrug-resistant gram-negative bacilli that are now in the community (we have a new algorithm to help decide which antibiotic to choose for these pathogens in Chapter 4). All the contributing editors have updated their sections with important new recommendations based on current published data, guidelines, and clinical experience that provide a perspective for interpretation of relevant information unsurpassed in the pediatric infectious diseases community. We are approaching 400 references to support recommendations in Chapter 6, Antimicrobial Therapy According to Clinical Syndromes, alone.

Recognizing the talent in collaborators/colleagues of the editors, and their substantial and ongoing contributions to the quality of the material that is presented in this book, we have created consulting editors, whom we wish to continue to acknowledge each year in this Introduction. We continue to have the opportunity to receive valuable suggestions from Drs Pablo Sanchez and John van den Anker on antimicrobial therapy of the newborn, in support of the work done by JB Cantey and Jason Sauberan on Chapter 5. For those who use the *Nelson's* app, we have a new consulting editor, Dr Howard Smart, to help us create more user-friendly software. Howard is the chief of pediatrics at the Sharp-Rees Stealy multispecialty medical group in San Diego, CA; a graduate of our University of California, San Diego (UCSD) pediatric residency with additional training in pulmonology; and a tech wizard. Howard writes (and sells) his own apps for the iOS platform and actually took parts of the 2017 edition and created his own version of our app! With the support of the AAP and the editors, we plan to incorporate Howard's new enhancements in this 2018 edition. A second consulting editor this year is also part of the San Diego pediatric community, Dr Brian Williams, who trained in medicine and pediatrics during his UCSD residency *and* trained in medicine and pediatrics as a hospitalist. I often see Brian on the wards of our hospital in his role as a hospitalist, taking care of children with infections (among other things), getting advice from *Nelson's*. Brian needs a quick and efficient way to access information, and his advice on organizing information (particularly the search mode of the app) has been invaluable. He is focused, practical, and very collaborative, having come from Wisconsin. You will find many improvements in this 2018 edition based on his suggestions to the AAP and the editors, with many more to come, we hope.

We continue to harmonize the *Nelson's* book with the AAP *Red Book,* and we were given relevant information from the upcoming 2018 edition (easy to understand, given that David Kimberlin is also the editor of the *Red Book*). We are virtually always in sync with explanations that allow the reader to understand the basis for recommendations.

We continue to provide grading of our recommendations—our assessment of how strongly we feel about a recommendation and the strength of the evidence to support our recommendation (noted in the Table).

Strength of Recommendation	Description
A	Strongly recommended
B	Recommended as a good choice
C	One option for therapy that is adequate, perhaps among many other adequate therapies

Level of Evidence	Description
I	Based on well-designed, prospective, randomized, and controlled studies in an appropriate population of children
II	Based on data derived from prospectively collected, small comparative trials, or noncomparative prospective trials, or reasonable retrospective data from clinical trials in children, or data from other populations (eg, adults)
III	Based on case reports, case series, consensus statements, or expert opinion for situations in which sound data do not exist

As we state each year, many of the recommendations by the editors for specific situations have not been systematically evaluated in controlled, prospective, comparative clinical trials. Many of the recommendations may be supported by published data, but the data may never have been presented to or reviewed by the US Food and Drug Administration (FDA) and, therefore, are not in the package label. We all find ourselves in this situation frequently. Many of us are working closely with the FDA to try to narrow the gap in our knowledge of antimicrobial agents between adults and children; the FDA pediatric infectious diseases staff is providing an exceptional effort to shed light on the doses that are safe and effective for neonates, infants, and children, with major efforts to place important new data on safety and efficacy in the antibiotic package labels.

Barrett Winston, our primary AAP editorial contact, has done an amazing job of organizing all the AAP staff, as well as the contributing and consulting editors, to keep us all moving forward with enhancements and upgrades as we now look to the long-term future of the book in partnership with the AAP. Peter Lynch has been working on developing *Nelson's* online, as well as the app, and has shared considerable AAP resources with us. We, of course, continue to appreciate the teamwork of all those at the AAP who make sure this book gets to all the clinicians who may benefit. Thanks to Mark Grimes, Director, Department of Publishing, and our steadfast friends and supporters in the

AAP departments of Publishing and Membership Engagement, Marketing, and Sales—Jeff Mahony, Director, Division of Professional and Consumer Publishing; Linda Smessaert, Senior Marketing Manager, Professional Resources; and the entire staff—who make certain that the considerable information in *Nelson's* makes it to those who are actually caring for children.

We are still very interested to learn from readers/users if there are new chapters or sections you wish for us to develop—and whether you find certain sections particularly helpful, so we don't change or delete them! Please send your suggestions to nelsonabx@aap.org.

We are also incredibly pleased that John Nelson was given an award by the AAP on July 27, 2017, at the AAP PREP:ID course for a lifetime of achievement in education and improving care to children with infectious diseases. We will include a picture of the presentation in the 2018 app when Howard figures out how to attach it!

John S. Bradley, MD

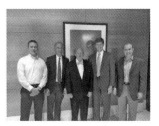

Pictured from left: Jason Sauberan, PharmD; John S. Bradley, MD; John D. Nelson, MD; David W. Kimberlin, MD; and William J. Steinbach, MD.

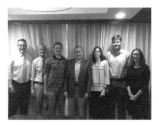

Pictured from left: Mark Grimes; Dr Bradley; Dr Sauberan; Dr Steinbach; Elizabeth D. Barnett, MD; Joseph B. Cantey, MD; and Barrett Winston.

Notable Changes to *2018 Nelson's Pediatric Antimicrobial Therapy,* 24th Edition

Antifungals
- Addition of *Candida auris*
- Specific recommendations about antifungal therapeutic drug levels
- Expanded and new references
- Most current antifungal activity spectrum table
- New coccidioidomycosis guidelines incorporated
- New approaches to mucormycosis included

Antimicrobials
- Antibiotics that are no longer available: cefditoren (Spectracef), ceftibuten (Cedax), penicillin G procaine
- New daptomycin, entecavir, linezolid, and voriconazole dosing
- New mebendazole products (**Warning:** may not yet be commercially available at time of publication)

Drug-Resistant Gram-negative Bacilli and Methicillin-Resistant *Staphylococcus aureus*
- New discussion and algorithm for selection of antibiotics for presumed or documented Gram-negative, multidrug-resistant pathogens
- Updated tables for susceptibility of Gram-positive and Gram-negative pathogens
- Where the newly US Food and Drug Administration–approved pediatric antibiotics for methicillin-resistant *Staphylococcus aureus* (MRSA) (daptomycin and ceftaroline) fit into treatment strategy with increasing clindamycin resistance

References
- Updated references and reviews for therapy of clinically important infections (eg, community-acquired pneumonia in children, endocarditis, MRSA infections)
- Updated references for antibiotic prophylaxis to prevent infection following exposures; surgical prophylaxis

1. Choosing Among Antibiotics Within a Class: Beta-lactams, Macrolides, Aminoglycosides, and Fluoroquinolones

New drugs should be compared with others in the same class regarding (1) antimicrobial spectrum; (2) degree of antibiotic exposure (a function of the pharmacokinetics of the nonprotein-bound drug at the site of infection and the pharmacodynamic properties of the drug); (3) demonstrated efficacy in adequate and well-controlled clinical trials; (4) tolerance, toxicity, and side effects; and (5) cost. If there is no substantial benefit for efficacy or safety for one antimicrobial over another for the isolated or presumed bacterial pathogen(s), one should opt for using an older, more extensively used (with presumably better-defined efficacy and safety), and less expensive drug with the narrowest spectrum of activity.

Beta-lactams

Oral Cephalosporins (cephalexin, cefadroxil, cefaclor, cefprozil, cefuroxime, cefixime, cefdinir, cefpodoxime, cefditoren [tablet only], and ceftibuten). As a class, the oral cephalosporins have the advantage over oral penicillins of somewhat greater spectrum of activity. The serum half-lives of cefpodoxime, ceftibuten, and cefixime are greater than 2 hours. This pharmacokinetic feature accounts for the fact that they may be given in 1 or 2 doses per day for certain indications, particularly otitis media, where the middle ear fluid half-life is likely to be much longer than the serum half-life. For more resistant pathogens, twice daily is preferred (see Chapter 3). The spectrum of activity increases for Gram-negative organisms as one goes from the first-generation cephalosporins (cephalexin and cefadroxil), to the second generation (cefaclor, cefprozil, and cefuroxime) that demonstrates activity against *Haemophilus influenzae* (including beta-lactamase–producing strains), to the third-generation agents (cefdinir, cefixime, cefpodoxime, and ceftibuten) that have enhanced coverage of many enteric Gram-negative bacilli (*Escherichia coli, Klebsiella* spp). However, ceftibuten and cefixime, in particular, have a disadvantage of less activity against *Streptococcus pneumoniae* than the others, particularly against penicillin (beta-lactam) non-susceptible strains. No oral fourth- or fifth-generation cephalosporins (see Parenteral Cephalosporins) currently exist (no activity against *Pseudomonas* or methicillin-resistant *Staphylococcus aureus* [MRSA]). The palatability of generic versions of these products may not have the same better-tasting characteristics as the original products.

Parenteral Cephalosporins. First-generation cephalosporins, such as cefazolin, are used mainly for treatment of Gram-positive infections caused by *S aureus* (excluding MRSA) and group A streptococcus and for surgical prophylaxis; the Gram-negative spectrum is limited but more extensive than ampicillin. Cefazolin is well tolerated on intramuscular or intravenous (IV) injection.

A second-generation cephalosporin (cefuroxime) and the cephamycins (cefoxitin and cefotetan) provide increased activity against many Gram-negative organisms, particularly *Haemophilus* and *E coli*. Cefoxitin has, in addition, activity against approximately 80% of strains of *Bacteroides fragilis* and can be considered for use in place of the more active agents, like metronidazole or carbapenems, when that organism is implicated in nonserious disease.

Third-generation cephalosporins (cefotaxime, ceftriaxone, and ceftazidime) all have enhanced potency against many enteric Gram-negative bacilli. As with all cephalosporins, they are less active against enterococci and *Listeria*; only ceftazidime has significant activity against *Pseudomonas*. Cefotaxime and ceftriaxone have been used very successfully to treat meningitis caused by pneumococcus (mostly penicillin-susceptible strains), *H influenzae* type b, meningococcus, and susceptible strains of *E coli* meningitis. These drugs have the greatest usefulness for treating Gram-negative bacillary infections due to their safety, compared with other classes of antibiotics. Because ceftriaxone is excreted, to a large extent, via the liver, it can be used with little dosage adjustment in patients with renal failure. With a serum half-life of 4 to 7 hours, it can be given once a day for all infections, including meningitis, that are caused by susceptible organisms.

Cefepime, a fourth-generation cephalosporin approved for use in children in 1999, exhibits (1) enhanced antipseudomonal activity over ceftazidime; (2) the Gram-positive activity of second-generation cephalosporins; (3) better activity against Gram-negative enteric bacilli; and (4) stability against the inducible ampC beta-lactamases of *Enterobacter* and *Serratia* (and some strains of *Proteus* and *Citrobacter*) that can hydrolyze third-generation cephalosporins. It can be used as single-drug antibiotic therapy against these pathogens, rather than paired with an aminoglycoside to prevent the emergence of ampC resistance.

Ceftaroline is a fifth-generation cephalosporin, the first of the cephalosporins with activity against MRSA. Ceftaroline was approved by the US Food and Drug Administration (FDA) in December 2010 for adults and approved for children in June 2016 for treatment of complicated skin infections (including MRSA) and community-acquired pneumonia. The pharmacokinetics of ceftaroline have been evaluated in all pediatric age groups, including neonates; clinical studies for pediatric community-acquired pneumonia and complicated skin infection have now been published.[1] Global studies in neonatal sepsis are in progress. Based on these published data and review by the FDA, for infants and children 2 months and older, ceftaroline should be as effective and safer than vancomycin for treatment of MRSA infections. Just as beta-lactams are preferred over vancomycin for methicillin-susceptible *S aureus* infections, ceftaroline should be considered preferred treatment over vancomycin for MRSA infection. Neither renal function nor drug levels need to be followed with ceftaroline therapy.

Penicillinase-Resistant Penicillins (dicloxacillin [capsules only]; nafcillin and oxacillin [parenteral only]). "Penicillinase" refers specifically to the beta-lactamase produced by *S aureus* in this case and not those produced by Gram-negative bacteria. These antibiotics are active against penicillin-resistant *S aureus* but not against MRSA. Nafcillin differs pharmacologically from the others in being excreted primarily by the liver rather than by the kidneys, which may explain the relative lack of nephrotoxicity compared with methicillin, which is no longer available in the United States. Nafcillin pharmacokinetics are erratic in persons with liver disease and often painful with IV infusion.

Antipseudomonal Beta-lactams (ticarcillin/clavulanate, piperacillin, piperacillin/tazobactam, aztreonam, ceftazidime, cefepime, meropenem, and imipenem). Timentin (ticarcillin/clavulanate), Zosyn (piperacillin/tazobactam), and Zerbaxa (ceftolozane/tazobactam) represent combinations of 2 beta-lactam drugs. One beta-lactam drug in the combination, known as a "beta-lactamase inhibitor" (clavulanic acid or tazobactam in these combinations), binds irreversibly to and neutralizes specific beta-lactamase enzymes produced by the organism, allowing the second beta-lactam drug (ticarcillin, piperacillin, or ceftolozane) to act as the active antibiotic to bind effectively to the intracellular target site (transpeptidase), resulting in death of the organism. Thus, the combination only adds to the spectrum of the original antibiotic when the mechanism of resistance is a beta-lactamase enzyme and only when the beta-lactamase inhibitor is capable of binding to and inhibiting that particular organism's beta-lactamase enzyme(s). The combinations extend the spectrum of activity of the primary antibiotic to include many beta-lactamase–positive bacteria, including some strains of enteric Gram-negative bacilli (*E coli, Klebsiella,* and *Enterobacter*), *S aureus,* and *B fragilis.* Ticarcillin/clavulanate, piperacillin/tazobactam, and ceftolozane/tazobactam have no significant activity against *Pseudomonas* beyond that of ticarcillin, piperacillin, or ceftolozane because their beta-lactamase inhibitors do not effectively inhibit all the many relevant beta-lactamases of *Pseudomonas.*

Pseudomonas has an intrinsic capacity to develop resistance following exposure to any beta-lactam, based on the activity of several inducible chromosomal beta-lactamases, upregulated efflux pumps, and changes in the permeability of the cell wall. Because development of resistance during therapy is not uncommon (particularly beta-lactamase–mediated resistance against ticarcillin, piperacillin, or ceftazidime), an aminoglycoside such as tobramycin is often used in combination, in hopes that the tobramycin will kill strains developing resistance to the beta-lactams. Cefepime, meropenem, and imipenem are relatively stable to the beta-lactamases induced while on therapy and can be used as single-agent therapy for most *Pseudomonas* infections, but resistance may still develop to these agents based on other mechanisms of resistance. For *Pseudomonas* infections in compromised hosts or in life-threatening infections, these drugs, too, should be used in combination with an aminoglycoside or a second active agent. The benefits of the additional antibiotic should be weighed against the potential for additional toxicity and alteration of host flora.

Aminopenicillins (amoxicillin and amoxicillin/clavulanate [oral formulations only, in the United States], ampicillin [oral and parenteral], and ampicillin/sulbactam [parenteral only]). Amoxicillin is very well absorbed, good tasting, and associated with very few side effects. Augmentin is a combination of amoxicillin and clavulanate (see Antipseudomonal Beta-lactams for more information on beta-lactam/beta-lactamase inhibitor combinations) that is available in several fixed proportions that permit amoxicillin to remain active against many beta-lactamase–producing bacteria, including *H influenzae* and *S aureus* (but not MRSA). Amoxicillin/clavulanate has undergone many changes in formulation since its introduction. The ratio of amoxicillin to clavulanate was originally 4:1, based on susceptibility data of pneumococcus and *Haemophilus* during the 1970s. With the emergence of penicillin-resistant pneumococcus, recommendations for increasing the dosage of amoxicillin, particularly for upper respiratory tract infections, were made. However, if one increases the dosage of clavulanate even slightly, the incidence of diarrhea increases dramatically. If one keeps the dosage of clavulanate constant while increasing the dosage of amoxicillin, one can treat the relatively resistant pneumococci while not increasing gastrointestinal side effects of the combination. The original 4:1 ratio is present in suspensions containing 125-mg and 250-mg amoxicillin/5 mL and the 125-mg and 250-mg chewable tablets. A higher 7:1 ratio is present in the suspensions containing 200-mg and 400-mg amoxicillin/5 mL and in the 200-mg and 400-mg chewable tablets. A still higher ratio of 14:1 is present in the suspension formulation Augmentin ES-600 that contains 600-mg amoxicillin/5 mL; this preparation is designed to deliver 90 mg/kg/day of amoxicillin, divided twice daily, for the treatment of ear (and sinus) infections. The high serum and middle ear fluid concentrations achieved with 45 mg/kg/dose, combined with the long middle ear fluid half-life (4–6 hours) of amoxicillin, allow for a therapeutic antibiotic exposure to pathogens in the middle ear with a twice-daily regimen. However, the prolonged half-life in the middle ear fluid is not necessarily found in other infection sites (eg, skin, lung tissue, joint tissue), for which dosing of amoxicillin and Augmentin should continue to be 3 times daily for most susceptible pathogens.

For older children who can swallow tablets, the amoxicillin to clavulanate ratios are as follows: 500-mg tablet (4:1); 875-mg tablet (7:1); 1,000-mg tablet (16:1).

Sulbactam, another beta-lactamase inhibitor like clavulanate, is combined with ampicillin in the parenteral formulation Unasyn. The cautions regarding spectrum of activity for piperacillin/tazobactam with respect to the limitations of the beta-lactamase inhibitor in increasing the spectrum of activity (see Antipseudomonal Beta-lactams) also apply to ampicillin/sulbactam that does not even have the extended activity against the enteric bacilli seen with piperacillin/tazobactam.

Carbapenems. Meropenem, imipenem, doripenem, and ertapenem are carbapenems with a broader spectrum of activity than any other class of beta-lactam currently available. Meropenem, imipenem, and ertapenem are approved by the FDA for use in children. At present, we recommend them for treatment of infections caused by bacteria resistant to standard therapy or for mixed infections involving aerobes and anaerobes. Imipenem has greater central nervous system irritability compared with other carbapenems, leading to an increased risk of seizures in children with meningitis. Meropenem was not associated with an increased rate of seizures, compared with cefotaxime in children with meningitis. Imipenem and meropenem are active against virtually all coliform bacilli, including cefotaxime-resistant (extended spectrum beta-lactamase–producing or ampC-producing) strains, against *Pseudomonas aeruginosa* (including most ceftazidime-resistant strains), and against anaerobes, including *B fragilis*. While ertapenem lacks the excellent activity against *P aeruginosa* of the other carbapenems, it has the advantage of a prolonged serum half-life, which allows for once-daily dosing in adults and children aged 13 years and older and twice-daily dosing in younger children. Newly emergent strains of *Klebsiella pneumoniae* contain *K pneumoniae* carbapenemases that degrade and inactivate all the carbapenems. These strains, as well as strains carrying the less common New Delhi metallo-beta-lactamase, which is also active against carbapenems, have begun to spread to many parts of the world, reinforcing the need to keep track of your local antibiotic susceptibility patterns.

Macrolides

Erythromycin is the prototype of macrolide antibiotics. Almost 30 macrolides have been produced, but only 3 are FDA approved for children in the United States: erythromycin, azithromycin (also called an azalide), and clarithromycin, while a fourth, telithromycin (also called a ketolide), is approved for adults and only available in tablet form. As a class, these drugs achieve greater concentrations intracellularly than in serum, particularly with azithromycin and clarithromycin. As a result, measuring serum concentrations is usually not clinically useful. Gastrointestinal intolerance to erythromycin is caused by the breakdown products of the macrolide ring structure. This is much less of a problem with azithromycin and clarithromycin. Azithromycin, clarithromycin, and telithromycin extend the activity of erythromycin to include *Haemophilus;* azithromycin and clarithromycin also have substantial activity against certain mycobacteria. Azithromycin is also active in vitro and effective against many enteric Gram-negative pathogens, including *Salmonella* and *Shigella*. Solithromycin, a fluoroketolide with enhanced activity against Gram-positive organisms, including MRSA, is currently in pediatric clinical trials.

Aminoglycosides

Although 5 aminoglycoside antibiotics are available in the United States, only 3 are widely used for systemic therapy of aerobic Gram-negative infections and for synergy in the treatment of certain Gram-positive and Gram-negative infections: gentamicin, tobramycin, and amikacin. Streptomycin and kanamycin have more limited utility due to increased toxicity compared with the other agents. Resistance in Gram-negative bacilli to aminoglycosides is caused by bacterial enzymes that adenylate, acetylate, or phosphorylate the aminoglycoside, resulting in inactivity. The specific activities of each enzyme against each agent in each pathogen are highly variable. As a result, antibiotic susceptibility tests must be done for each aminoglycoside drug separately. There are small differences in toxicities to the kidneys and eighth cranial nerve hearing/vestibular function, although it is uncertain whether these small differences are clinically significant. For all children receiving a full treatment course, it is advisable to monitor peak and trough serum concentrations early in the course of therapy, as the degree of drug exposure correlates with toxicity and elevated trough concentrations may predict impending drug accumulation. With amikacin, desired peak concentrations are 20 to 35 µg/mL and trough drug concentrations are less than 10 µg/mL; for gentamicin and tobramycin, depending on the frequency of dosing, peak concentrations should be

5 to 10 µg/mL and trough concentrations less than 2 µg/mL. Children with cystic fibrosis require greater dosages to achieve equivalent therapeutic serum concentrations due to enhanced clearance. Inhaled tobramycin has been very successful in children with cystic fibrosis as an adjunctive therapy of Gram-negative bacillary infections. The role of inhaled aminoglycosides in other Gram-negative pneumonias (eg, ventilator-associated pneumonia) has not yet been defined.

Once-Daily Dosing of Aminoglycosides. Once-daily dosing of 5 to 7.5 mg/kg gentamicin or tobramycin has been studied in adults and in some neonates and children; peak serum concentrations are greater than those achieved with dosing 3 times daily. Aminoglycosides demonstrate concentration-dependent killing of pathogens, suggesting a potential benefit to higher serum concentrations achieved with once-daily dosing. Regimens giving the daily dosage as a single infusion, rather than as traditionally split doses every 8 hours, are effective and safe for normal adult hosts and immune-compromised hosts with fever and neutropenia and may be less toxic. Experience with once-daily dosing in children is increasing, with similar results, as noted, for adults. A recent Cochrane review for children (and adults) with cystic fibrosis comparing once-daily with 3-times–daily administration found equal efficacy but decreased toxicity in children.[2] Once-daily dosing should be considered as effective as multiple, smaller doses per day and may be safer for children.

Fluoroquinolones

More than 40 years ago, fluoroquinolone (FQ) toxicity to cartilage in weight-bearing joints in experimental juvenile animals was documented to be dose and duration of therapy dependent. Pediatric studies were, therefore, not initially undertaken with ciprofloxacin or other FQs. However, with increasing antibiotic resistance in pediatric pathogens and an accumulating database in pediatrics suggesting that joint toxicity may be uncommon, the FDA allowed prospective studies to proceed in 1998. As of July 2017, no cases of documented FQ-attributable joint toxicity have occurred in children with FQs that are approved for use in the United States. Limited published data are available from prospective, blinded studies to accurately assess this risk. A prospective, randomized, double-blind study of moxifloxacin for intra-abdominal infection, with 1-year follow-up specifically designed to assess tendon/joint toxicity, demonstrated no concern for toxicity. Unblinded studies with levofloxacin for respiratory tract infections and unpublished randomized studies comparing ciprofloxacin versus other agents for complicated urinary tract infection suggest the possibility of an uncommon, reversible, FQ-attributable arthralgia, but these data should be interpreted with caution. The use of FQs in situations of antibiotic resistance where no other active agent is available is reasonable, weighing the benefits of treatment against the low risk of toxicity of this class of antibiotics. The use of an oral FQ in situations in which the only alternative is parenteral therapy is also justified.[3]

Ciprofloxacin usually has very good Gram-negative activity (with great regional variation in susceptibility) against enteric bacilli (*E coli*, *Klebsiella*, *Enterobacter*, *Salmonella*, and *Shigella*) and against *P aeruginosa*. However, it lacks substantial Gram-positive coverage and should not be used to treat streptococcal, staphylococcal, or pneumococcal infections. Newer-generation FQs are more active against these pathogens; levofloxacin has documented efficacy and safety in pediatric clinical trials for respiratory tract infections, acute otitis media, and community-acquired pneumonia. Children with any question of joint/tendon/bone toxicity in the levofloxacin studies were followed up to 5 years after treatment, with no difference in outcomes in these randomized studies, compared with the standard FDA-approved antibiotics used as comparators in these studies.[4] None of the newer-generation FQs are more active against Gram-negative pathogens than ciprofloxacin. Quinolone antibiotics are bitter tasting. Ciprofloxacin and levofloxacin are currently available in a suspension form; ciprofloxacin is FDA approved in pediatrics for complicated urinary tract infections and inhalation anthrax, while levofloxacin is approved for inhalation anthrax only, as the sponsor chose not to apply for approval for pediatric respiratory tract infections. For reasons of safety and to prevent the emergence of widespread resistance, FQs should still not be used for primary therapy of pediatric infections and should be limited to situations in which safe and effective oral therapy with other classes of antibiotics does not exist.

2. Choosing Among Antifungal Agents: Polyenes, Azoles, and Echinocandins

Separating antifungal agents by class, much like navigating the myriad of antibacterial agents, allows one to best understand the underlying mechanisms of action and then appropriately choose which agent would be optimal for empirical therapy or a targeted approach. There are certain helpful generalizations that should be considered; for example, echinocandins are fungicidal against yeast and fungistatic against molds, while azoles are the opposite. Coupled with these concepts is the need for continued surveillance for fungal resistance patterns. While some fungal species are inherently or very often resistant to specific agents or even classes, there are also an increasing number of fungal isolates that are developing resistance due to environmental pressure or chronic use in individual patients. Additionally, new (often resistant) fungal species emerge that deserve special attention, such as *Candida auris*. In 2018, there are 14 individual antifungal agents approved by the US Food and Drug Administration (FDA) for systemic use, and several more in development. For each agent, there are sometimes several formulations, each with unique pharmacokinetics that one has to understand to optimize the agent, particularly in patients who are critically ill. Therefore, it is more important than ever to establish a firm foundation in understanding how these antifungal agents work to optimize pharmacokinetics and where they work best to target fungal pathogens most appropriately.

Polyenes

Amphotericin B (AmB) is a polyene antifungal antibiotic that has been available since 1958. A *Streptomyces* species, isolated from the soil in Venezuela, produced 2 antifungals whose names originated from the drug's amphoteric property of reacting as an acid as well as a base. Amphotericin A was not as active as AmB, so only AmB is used clinically. Nystatin is another polyene antifungal, but, due to systemic toxicity, it is only used in topical preparations. It was named after the research laboratory where it was discovered, the New York State Health Department Laboratory. AmB remains the most broad-spectrum antifungal available for clinical use. This lipophilic drug binds to ergosterol, the major sterol in the fungal cell membrane, and creates transmembrane pores that compromise the integrity of the cell membrane and create a rapid fungicidal effect through osmotic lysis. Toxicity is likely due to the cross-reactivity with the human cholesterol bi-lipid membrane, which resembles ergosterol. The toxicity of the conventional formulation, AmB deoxycholate (AmB-D)—the parent molecule coupled with an ionic detergent for clinical use—can be substantial from the standpoints of systemic reactions (fever, rigors) and acute and chronic renal toxicity. Premedication with acetaminophen, diphenhydramine, and meperidine is often required to prevent systemic reactions during infusion. Renal dysfunction manifests primarily as decreased glomerular filtration with a rising serum creatinine concentration, but substantial tubular nephropathy is associated with potassium and magnesium wasting, requiring supplemental potassium for many neonates and children, regardless of clinical symptoms associated with infusion. Fluid loading with saline pre– and post–AmB-D infusion seems to mitigate renal toxicity.

Three lipid preparations approved in the mid-1990s decrease toxicity with no apparent decrease in clinical efficacy. Decisions on which lipid AmB preparation to use should, therefore, largely focus on side effects and costs. Two clinically useful lipid formulations exist: one in which ribbonlike lipid complexes of AmB are created (amphotericin B lipid complex [ABLC]), Abelcet, and one in which AmB is incorporated into true liposomes (liposomal amphotericin B [L-AmB]), AmBisome. The classic clinical dosage used of these preparations is 5 mg/kg/day, in contrast to the 1 mg/kg/day of AmB-D. In most studies, the side effects of L-AmB were somewhat less than those of ABLC, but both have significantly fewer side effects than AmB-D. The advantage of the lipid preparations is the ability to safely deliver a greater overall dose of the parent AmB drug. The cost of conventional AmB-D is substantially less than either lipid formulation. A colloidal dispersion of AmB in cholesteryl sulfate, Amphotec, which is no longer available in the United States, with decreased nephrotoxicity but infusion-related side effects, is closer to AmB-D than to the lipid formulations and precludes recommendation for its use. The decreased nephrotoxicity of the 3 lipid preparations is thought to be due to the preferential binding of its AmB to high-density lipoproteins, compared with AmB-D binding to low-density lipoproteins. Despite in vitro concentration-dependent killing, a clinical trial comparing L-AmB at doses of 3 mg/kg/day versus 10 mg/kg/day found no efficacy benefit for the higher dose and only greater toxicity.[1] Recent pharmacokinetic analyses of L-AmB found that while children receiving L-AmB at lower doses exhibit linear pharmacokinetics, a significant proportion of children receiving L-AmB at daily doses greater than 5 mg/kg/day exhibit nonlinear pharmacokinetics with significantly higher peak concentrations and some toxicity.[2,3] Therefore, it is generally not recommended to use any lipid AmB preparations at very high dosages (>5 mg/kg/day), as it will likely only incur greater toxicity with no real therapeutic advantage. There are reports of using higher dosing in very difficult infections where a lipid AmB formulation is the first-line therapy (eg, mucormycosis), and while experts remain divided on this practice, it is clear that at least 5 mg/kg/day of a lipid AmB formulation should be used. AmB has a long terminal half-life and, coupled with the concentration-dependent killing, the agent is best used as single daily doses. These pharmacokinetics explain the use in some studies of once-weekly, or even once every 2 weeks,[4] AmB for antifungal prophylaxis or preemptive therapy. If the overall AmB exposure needs to be decreased due to toxicity, it is best to increase the dosing interval (eg, 3 times weekly) but retain the full mg/kg dose for optimal pharmacokinetics.

AmB-D has been used for nonsystemic purposes, such as in bladder washes, intraventricular instillation, intrapleural instillation, and other modalities, but there are no firm data supporting those clinical indications, and it is likely that the local toxicities outweigh the theoretic benefits. One exception is aerosolized AmB for antifungal prophylaxis (not treatment) in lung transplant recipients due to the different pathophysiology of invasive aspergillosis (often originating at the bronchial anastomotic site, more so than parenchymal disease) in that specific patient population. Due to the lipid chemistry, the L-AmB does not interact well with renal tubules and L-AmB is recovered from the urine at lower levels than AmB-D, so there is a theoretic concern with using a lipid formulation, as opposed to AmB-D, when treating isolated urinary fungal disease. This theoretic concern is likely outweighed by the real concern of toxicity with AmB-D. Most experts believe AmB-D should be reserved for use in resource-limited settings in which no alternative agents (eg, lipid formulations) are available. An exception is in neonates, where limited retrospective data suggest that the AmB-D formulation had better efficacy.[5] Importantly, there are several pathogens that are inherently or functionally resistant to AmB, including *Candida lusitaniae, Trichosporon* spp, *Aspergillus terreus, Fusarium* spp, and *Pseudallescheria boydii (Scedosporium apiospermum)* or *Scedosporium prolificans.*

Azoles

This class of systemic agents was first approved in 1981 and is divided into imidazoles (ketoconazole), triazoles (fluconazole, itraconazole), and second-generation triazoles (voriconazole, posaconazole, and isavuconazole) based on the number of nitrogen atoms in the azole ring. All the azoles work by inhibition of ergosterol synthesis (fungal cytochrome P450 [CYP] sterol 14-demethylation) that is required for fungal cell membrane integrity. While the polyenes are rapidly fungicidal, the azoles are fungistatic against yeasts and fungicidal against molds. However, it is important to note that ketoconazole and fluconazole have no mold activity. The only systemic imidazole is ketoconazole, which is primarily active against *Candida* spp and is available in an oral formulation. Three azoles (itraconazole, voriconazole, posaconazole) need therapeutic drug monitoring with trough levels within the first 4 to 7 days (when patient is at pharmacokinetic steady state); it is unclear at present if isavuconazole will require drug-level monitoring. It is less clear if therapeutic drug monitoring is required during primary azole prophylaxis, although low levels have been associated with a higher probability of breakthrough infection.

Fluconazole is active against a broader range of fungi than ketoconazole and includes clinically relevant activity against *Cryptococcus, Coccidioides,* and *Histoplasma.* The pediatric treatment dose is 12 mg/kg/day, which targets exposures that are observed in critically ill adults who receive 800 mg of fluconazole per day. Like most other azoles, fluconazole requires a loading dose on the first day, and this approach is routinely used in adult patients. A loading dose of 25 mg/kg on the first day has been nicely studied in infants[6] and is likely also beneficial, but it has not been definitively studied yet in all children. The exception is children on extracorporeal membrane oxygenation, for whom, because of the higher volume of distribution, a higher loading dose (35 mg/kg) is required to achieve comparable exposure.[7] Fluconazole achieves relatively high concentrations in urine and cerebrospinal fluid (CSF) compared with AmB due to its low lipophilicity, with urinary concentrations often so high that treatment against even "resistant" pathogens that are isolated only in the urine is possible. Fluconazole remains one of the most active and, so far, one of the safest systemic antifungal agents for the treatment of most *Candida* infections. *Candida albicans* remains generally sensitive to fluconazole, although some resistance is present in many non-*albicans Candida* spp as well as in *C albicans* in children repeatedly exposed to fluconazole. For instance, *Candida krusei* is considered inherently resistant to fluconazole, *Candida glabrata* demonstrates dose-dependent resistance to fluconazole (and usually voriconazole), *Candida tropicalis* is developing more resistant strains, and the newly identified *Candida auris* is often fluconazole resistant. Fluconazole is available in parenteral and oral (with >90% bioavailability) formulations and toxicity is unusual and primarily hepatic.

Itraconazole is active against an even broader range of fungi and, unlike fluconazole, includes molds such as *Aspergillus*. It is currently available as a capsule or oral solution (the intravenous [IV] form was discontinued); the oral solution provides higher, more consistent serum concentrations than capsules and should be used preferentially. Absorption using itraconazole oral solution is improved on an empty stomach (unlike the capsule form, which is best administered under fed conditions and with a cola beverage to increase absorption), and monitoring itraconazole serum concentrations, like most azole antifungals, is a key principal in management (generally, itraconazole serum trough levels should be 1–2 µg/mL; trough levels >5 µg/mL may be associated with increased toxicity). Concentrations should be checked after 1 to 2 weeks of therapy to ensure adequate drug exposure. When measured by high-pressure liquid chromatography, itraconazole and its bioactive hydroxy-itraconazole metabolite are reported, the sum of which should be considered in assessing drug levels. In adult patients, itraconazole is recommended to be loaded at 200 mg twice daily for 2 days, followed by 200 mg daily starting on the third day. Loading dose studies have not been performed in children. Dosing itraconazole in children requires twice-daily dosing throughout treatment. Limited pharmacokinetic data are available in children; itraconazole has not been approved by the FDA for pediatric indications. Itraconazole is indicated in adults for therapy of mild/moderate disease with blastomycosis, histoplasmosis, and others. Although it possesses antifungal activity, itraconazole is not indicated as primary therapy against invasive aspergillosis, as voriconazole is a far superior option. Itraconazole is not active against *Zygomycetes* (eg, mucormycosis). Toxicity in adults is primarily hepatic.

Voriconazole was approved in 2002 and is only FDA approved for children 12 years and older, although there are now substantial pharmacokinetic data and experience for children aged 2 to 12 years.[8] Voriconazole is a fluconazole derivative, so think of it as having the greater tissue and CSF penetration of fluconazole but the added antifungal spectrum to include molds. While the bioavailability of voriconazole in adults is approximately 96%, multiple studies have shown that it is only approximately 50% to 60% in children, requiring clinicians to carefully monitor voriconazole trough concentrations in patients taking the oral formulation, further complicated by great inter-patient variability in clearance. Voriconazole serum concentrations are tricky to interpret, but monitoring concentrations is essential to using this drug, like all azole antifungals, and especially important in circumstances of suspected treatment failure or possible toxicity. Most experts suggest voriconazole trough concentrations of 2 µg/mL (at a minimum, 1 µg/mL) or greater, which would generally exceed the pathogen's minimum inhibitory concentration, but, generally, toxicity will not be seen until concentrations of approximately 6 µg/mL or greater. One important point is the acquisition of an accurate trough concentration, one obtained just before the next dose is due and not obtained through a catheter infusing the drug. These simple trough parameters will make interpretation possible. The fundamental voriconazole pharmacokinetics are different in adults versus children; in adults, voriconazole is metabolized in a nonlinear fashion, whereas in children, the drug is metabolized in a linear fashion. This explains the increased pediatric starting dosing for voriconazole at 9 mg/kg/dose versus loading with 6 mg/kg/dose in adult patients. Younger children, especially those younger than 3 years, require even higher dosages of voriconazole and also have a larger therapeutic window for dosing. However, many studies have shown an inconsistent relationship, on a population level, between dosing and levels, highlighting the need for close monitoring after the initial dosing scheme and then dose adjustment as needed in the individual patient. For children younger than 2 years, some have proposed 3-times–daily dosing to achieve sufficient serum levels.[9] Given the poor clinical and microbiological response of *Aspergillus* infections to AmB, voriconazole is now the treatment of choice for invasive aspergillosis and many other mold infections (eg, pseudallescheriasis, fusariosis). Importantly, infections with *Zygomycetes* (eg, mucormycosis) are resistant to voriconazole. Voriconazole retains activity against most *Candida* spp, including some that are fluconazole resistant, but it is unlikely to replace fluconazole for treatment of fluconazole-susceptible *Candida* infections. Importantly, there are increasing reports of *C glabrata* resistance to voriconazole. Voriconazole produces some unique transient visual field abnormalities in about 10% of adults and children. There are an increasing number of reports, seen in as high as 20% of patients, of a photosensitive sunburn-like erythema that is not aided by sunscreen (only sun avoidance). In some rare long-term (mean of 3 years of therapy) cases, this voriconazole phototoxicity has developed into cutaneous squamous cell carcinoma. Discontinuing voriconazole is recommended in patients experiencing chronic phototoxicity. The rash is the most common indication for switching from voriconazole to posaconazole/isavuconazole if a triazole antifungal is required. Hepatotoxicity is uncommon, occurring only in 2% to 5% of patients. Voriconazole is CYP metabolized (CYP2C19), and allelic polymorphisms in the population could lead to personalized dosing.[10] Results have shown that some Asian patients will achieve higher toxic serum concentrations than other patients. Voriconazole also interacts with many similarly P450 metabolized drugs to produce some profound changes in serum concentrations of many concurrently administered drugs.

Posaconazole, an itraconazole derivative, was FDA approved in 2006 as an oral suspension for adolescents 13 years and older. An extended-release tablet formulation was approved in November 2013, also for 13 years and older, and an IV formulation was approved in March 2014 for patients 18 years and older. Effective absorption of the oral suspension strongly requires taking the medication with food, ideally a high-fat meal; taking posaconazole on an empty stomach will result in approximately one-fourth of the absorption as in the fed state. The tablet formulation has significantly better absorption due to its delayed release in the small intestine, but absorption will still be slightly increased with food. If the patient can take the (relatively large) tablets, the extended-release tablet is the preferred form due to the ability to easily obtain higher and more consistent drug levels. Due to the low pH (<5) of IV posaconazole, a central venous catheter is required for administration. The IV formulation contains only slightly lower amounts of the cyclodextrin vehicle than voriconazole, so similar theoretic renal accumulation concerns exist. The exact pediatric dosing for posaconazole has not been completely determined and requires consultation with a pediatric infectious diseases expert. The pediatric oral suspension dose recommended by some experts for treating invasive disease is 18 mg/kg/day divided 3 times daily, but the true answer is likely higher and serum trough level monitoring is recommended. A study with a new pediatric formulation for suspension, essentially the tablet form that is able to be suspended, is underway. Importantly, the current tablet cannot be broken for use due to its chemical coating. Pediatric dosing with the current IV or extended-release tablet dosing is completely unknown, but adolescents can likely follow the adult dosing schemes. In adult patients, IV posaconazole is loaded at 300 mg twice daily on the first day, and then 300 mg once daily starting on the second day. Similarly, in adult patients, the extended-release tablet is dosed as 300 mg twice daily on the first day, and then 300 mg once daily starting on the second day. In adult patients, the maximum amount of posaconazole oral suspension given is 800 mg per day due to its excretion, and that has been given as 400 mg twice daily or 200 mg 4 times a day in severely ill patients due to findings of a marginal increase in exposure with more frequent dosing. Greater than 800 mg per day is not indicated in any patient. Like voriconazole and itraconazole, trough levels should be monitored, and most experts feel that posaconazole levels for treatment should be greater than or equal to 1 µg/mL. The in vitro activity of posaconazole against *Candida* spp is better than that of fluconazole and similar to voriconazole. Overall in vitro antifungal activity against *Aspergillus* is also equivalent to voriconazole, but, notably, it is the first triazole with substantial activity against some *Zygomycetes,* including *Rhizopus* spp and *Mucor* spp, as well as activity against *Coccidioides, Histoplasma,* and *Blastomyces* and the pathogens of phaeohyphomycosis. Posaconazole treatment of invasive aspergillosis in patients with chronic granulomatous disease appears to be superior to voriconazole in this specific patient population for an unknown reason. Posaconazole is eliminated by hepatic glucuronidation but does demonstrate inhibition of the CYP3A4 enzyme system, leading to many drug interactions with other P450 metabolized drugs. It is currently approved for prophylaxis of *Candida* and *Aspergillus* infections in high-risk adults and for treatment of *Candida* oropharyngeal disease or esophagitis in adults. Posaconazole, like itraconazole, has generally poor CSF penetration.

Isavuconazole is a new triazole that was FDA approved in March 2015 for treatment of invasive aspergillosis and invasive mucormycosis with oral (capsules only) and IV formulations. Isavuconazole has a similar antifungal spectrum as voriconazole and some activity against *Zygomycetes* (yet, potentially, not as potent against *Zygomycetes* as posaconazole). A phase 3 clinical trial in adult patients demonstrated non-inferiority versus voriconazole against invasive aspergillosis and other mold infections,[11] and an open-label study showed activity against mucormycosis.[12] Isavuconazole is actually dispensed as the prodrug isavuconazonium sulfate. Dosing in adult patients is loading with isavuconazole 200 mg (equivalent to 372-mg isavuconazonium sulfate) every 8 hours for 2 days (6 doses), followed by 200 mg once daily for maintenance dosing. The half-life is long (>5 days), there is 98% bioavailability in adults, and there is no reported food effect with oral isavuconazole. The IV formulation does not contain the vehicle cyclodextrin, unlike voriconazole, which could make it more attractive in patients with renal failure. Early experience suggests a much lower rate of photosensitivity and skin disorders as well as visual disturbances compared with voriconazole. No specific pediatric dosing data exist for isavuconazole yet, but studies are set to begin soon.

Echinocandins

This class of systemic antifungal agents was first approved in 2001. The echinocandins inhibit cell wall formation (in contrast to acting on the cell membrane by the polyenes and azoles) by noncompetitively inhibiting beta-1,3-glucan synthase, an enzyme present in fungi but absent in mammalian cells. These agents are generally very safe, as there is no beta-1,3-glucan in humans. The echinocandins are not metabolized through the CYP system, so fewer drug interactions are problematic, compared with the azoles. There is no need to dose-adjust in renal failure, but one needs a lower dosage in the setting of very severe hepatic dysfunction. As a class, these antifungals generally have poor CSF penetration, although animal studies have shown adequate brain parenchyma levels, and do not penetrate the urine well. While the 3 clinically available echinocandins each individually have some unique and important dosing and pharmacokinetic parameters, especially in children, efficacy is generally equivalent. Opposite the azole class, the echinocandins are fungicidal against yeasts but fungistatic against molds. The fungicidal activity against yeasts has elevated the echinocandins to the preferred therapy against invasive candidiasis. Echinocandins are thought to be best utilized against invasive aspergillosis only as salvage therapy if a triazole fails or in a patient with suspected triazole resistance, but never as primary monotherapy against invasive aspergillosis or any other mold infection. Improved efficacy with combination therapy with the echinocandins and triazoles against *Aspergillus* infections is unclear, with disparate results in multiple smaller studies and a definitive clinical trial demonstrating minimal benefit over voriconazole monotherapy in only certain patient populations. Some experts have used combination therapy in invasive aspergillosis with a triazole plus echinocandin only during the initial phase of waiting for triazole drug levels to be appropriately high. There are reports of echinocandin resistance in *Candida* spp, as high as 12% in *C glabrata* in some studies, and the echinocandins as a class have previously been shown to be somewhat less active against *Candida parapsilosis* isolates (approximately 10%–15% respond poorly, but most are still susceptible, and guidelines still recommend echinocandin empiric therapy for invasive candidiasis).

Caspofungin received FDA approval for children aged 3 months to 17 years in 2008 for empiric therapy of presumed fungal infections in febrile, neutropenic children; treatment of candidemia as well as *Candida* esophagitis, peritonitis, and empyema; and salvage therapy of invasive aspergillosis. Due to its earlier approval, there are generally more reports with caspofungin than the other echinocandins. Caspofungin dosing in children is calculated according to body surface area, with a loading dose on the first day of 70 mg/m², followed by daily maintenance dosing of 50 mg/m², and not to exceed 70 mg regardless of the calculated dose. Significantly higher doses of caspofungin have been studied in adult patients without any clear added benefit in efficacy, but if the 50 mg/m^2 dose is tolerated and does not provide adequate clinical response, the daily dose can be increased to 70 mg/m^2. Dosing for caspofungin in neonates is 25 mg/m^2/day.

Micafungin was approved in adults in 2005 for treatment of candidemia, *Candida* esophagitis and peritonitis, and prophylaxis of *Candida* infections in stem cell transplant recipients, and in 2013 for pediatric patients aged 4 months and older. Micafungin has the most pediatric and neonatal data available of all 3 echinocandins, including more extensive pharmacokinetic studies surrounding dosing and several efficacy studies.[13-15] Micafungin dosing in children is age dependent, as clearance increases dramatically in the younger age groups (especially neonates), necessitating higher doses for younger children. Doses in children are generally thought to be 2 mg/kg/day, with higher doses likely needed for younger patients, and preterm neonates dosed at 10 mg/kg/day. Adult micafungin dosing (100 or 150 mg once daily) is to be used in patients who weigh more than 40 kg. Unlike the other echinocandins, a loading dose is not required for micafungin.

Anidulafungin was approved for adults for candidemia and *Candida* esophagitis in 2006 and is not officially approved for pediatric patients. Like the other echinocandins, anidulafungin is not P450 metabolized and has not demonstrated significant drug interactions. Limited clinical efficacy data are available in children, with only some pediatric pharmacokinetic data suggesting weight-based dosing (3 mg/kg/day loading dose, followed by 1.5 mg/kg/day maintenance dosing).[16] The adult dose for invasive candidiasis is a loading dose of 200 mg on the first day, followed by 100 mg daily.

3. How Antibiotic Dosages Are Determined Using Susceptibility Data, Pharmacodynamics, and Treatment Outcomes

Factors Involved in Dosing Recommendations

Our view of the optimal use of antimicrobials is continually changing. As the published literature and our experience with each drug increases, our recommendations evolve as we compare the efficacy, safety, and cost of each drug in the context of current and previous data from adults and children. Every new antibiotic must demonstrate some degree of efficacy and safety in adults before we attempt to treat children. Occasionally, due to unanticipated toxicities and unanticipated clinical failures at a specific dosage, we will modify our initial recommendations for an antibiotic.

Important considerations in any recommendations we make include (1) the susceptibilities of pathogens to antibiotics, which are constantly changing, are different from region to region, and are often hospital- and unit-specific; (2) the antibiotic concentrations achieved at the site of infection over a 24-hour dosing interval; (3) the mechanism of how antibiotics kill bacteria; (4) how often the dose we select produces a clinical and microbiological cure; (5) how often we encounter toxicity; (6) how likely the antibiotic exposure will lead to antibiotic resistance in the treated child and in the population in general; and (7) the effect on the child's microbiome.

Susceptibility

Susceptibility data for each bacterial pathogen against a wide range of antibiotics are available from the microbiology laboratory of virtually every hospital. This antibiogram can help guide you in antibiotic selection for empiric therapy while you wait for specific susceptibilities to come back from your cultures. Many hospitals can separate the inpatient culture results from outpatient results, and many can give you the data by hospital ward (eg, pediatric ward vs neonatal intensive care unit vs adult intensive care unit). Susceptibility data are also available by region and by country from reference laboratories or public health laboratories. The recommendations made in *Nelson's Pediatric Antimicrobial Therapy* reflect overall susceptibility patterns present in the United States. Tables A and B in Chapter 7 provide some overall guidance on susceptibility of Gram-positive and Gram-negative pathogens, respectively. Wide variations may exist for certain pathogens in different regions of the United States and the world. New techniques for rapid molecular diagnosis of a bacterial, mycobacterial, fungal, or viral pathogen based on polymerase chain reaction or next-generation sequencing may quickly give you the name of the pathogen, but with current molecular technology, susceptibility data are not available.

Drug Concentrations at the Site of Infection

With every antibiotic, we can measure the concentration of antibiotic present in the serum. We can also directly measure the concentrations in specific tissue sites, such as spinal fluid or middle ear fluid. Because free, nonprotein-bound antibiotic is required to inhibit and kill pathogens, it is also important to calculate the amount of free drug available at the site of infection. While traditional methods of measuring antibiotics focused on the peak concentrations in serum and how rapidly the drugs were excreted, complex models of drug distribution in plasma and tissue sites (eg, cerebrospinal fluid, urine, peritoneal fluid) and elimination from plasma and tissue compartments now exist. Antibiotic exposure to pathogens at the site of infection can be described mathematically in many ways: (1) the percentage of time in a 24-hour dosing interval that the antibiotic concentrations are above the minimum inhibitory concentration (MIC; the antibiotic concentration required for inhibition of growth of an organism) at the site of infection (%T>MIC); (2) the mathematically calculated area below the serum concentration-versus-time curve (area under the curve [AUC]); and (3) the maximal concentration of drug achieved at the tissue site (Cmax). For each of these 3 values, a ratio of that value to the MIC of the pathogen in question can be calculated and provides more useful information on specific drug activity against a specific pathogen than simply looking at the MIC. It allows us to compare the exposure of different antibiotics (that achieve quite different concentrations in tissues) to a pathogen (where the MIC for each drug may be different) and to assess the activity of a single antibiotic that may be used for empiric therapy against the many different pathogens (potentially with many different MICs) that may be causing an infection at that tissue site.

Pharmacodynamics

Pharmacodynamic descriptions provide the clinician with information on *how* the bacterial pathogens are killed (see Suggested Reading). Beta-lactam antibiotics tend to eradicate bacteria following prolonged exposure of the antibiotic to the pathogen at the site of infection, usually expressed as the percent of time over a dosing interval that the antibiotic is present at the site of infection in concentrations greater than the MIC (%T>MIC). For example, amoxicillin needs to be present at the site of pneumococcal infection (eg, middle ear) at a concentration above the MIC for only 40% of a 24-hour dosing interval. Remarkably, neither higher concentrations of amoxicillin nor a more prolonged exposure will substantially increase the cure rate. On the other hand, gentamicin's activity against *Escherichia coli* is based primarily on the absolute concentration of free antibiotic at the site of infection, in the context of the MIC of the pathogen (Cmax:MIC). The more antibiotic you can deliver to the site of infection, the more rapidly you can sterilize the tissue; we are only limited by the toxicities of gentamicin. For fluoroquinolones like ciprofloxacin, the antibiotic exposure best linked to clinical and microbiologic success is, like aminoglycosides, concentration-dependent. However, the best mathematical correlate to microbiologic (and clinical) outcomes for fluoroquinolones is the AUC:MIC, rather than Cmax:MIC. All 3 metrics of antibiotic exposure are linked to the MIC of the pathogen.

Assessment of Clinical and Microbiological Outcomes

In clinical trials of anti-infective agents, most adults and children will hopefully be cured, but a few will fail therapy. For those few, we may note unanticipated inadequate drug exposure (eg, more rapid drug elimination in a particular patient; the inability of a particular antibiotic to penetrate to the site of infection in its active form, not bound to salts or proteins) or infection caused by a pathogen with a particularly high MIC. By analyzing the successes and the failures based on the appropriate exposure parameters outlined previously (%T>MIC, AUC:MIC, or Cmax:MIC), we can often observe a particular value of exposure, above which we observe a higher rate of cure and below which the cure rate drops quickly. Knowing this target value in adults (the "antibiotic exposure break point") allows us to calculate the dosage that will create treatment success in most children. We do not evaluate antibiotics in children with study designs that have failure rates sufficient to calculate a pediatric exposure break point. It is the adult *exposure value* that leads to success that we all (including the US Food and Drug Administration [FDA] and pharmaceutical companies) subsequently share with you, a pediatric health care practitioner, as one likely to cure your patient. US FDA-approved break points that are reported by microbiology laboratories (S, I, and R) are now determined by outcomes linked to drug pharmacokinetics and exposure, the MIC, and the pharmacodynamic parameter for that agent. Recommendations to the FDA for break points for the United States often come from "break point organizations," such as the US Committee on Antimicrobial Susceptibility Testing (www.uscast.org) or the Clinical Laboratory Standards Institute Subcommittee on Antimicrobial Susceptibility Testing.

Suggested Reading

Bradley JS, et al. *Pediatr Infect Dis J.* 2010;29(11):1043–1046 PMID: 20975453

Drusano GL. *Clin Infect Dis.* 2007;45(Suppl 1):S89–S95 PMID: 17582578

Onufrak NJ, et al. *Clin Ther.* 2016;38(9):1930–1947 PMID: 27449411

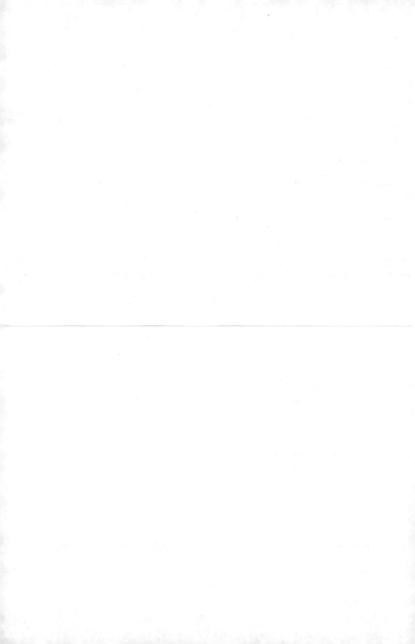

4. Approach to Antibiotic Therapy of Drug-Resistant Gram-negative Bacilli and Methicillin-Resistant *Staphylococcus aureus*

Multidrug-Resistant Gram-negative Bacilli

Increasing antibiotic resistance in Gram-negative bacilli, primarily the enteric bacilli *Pseudomonas aeruginosa* and *Acinetobacter* spp, has caused profound difficulties in management of patients around the world; some of the pathogens are now resistant to all available agents. At this time, a limited number of pediatric tertiary care centers in North America have reported isolated outbreaks, but sustained transmission of completely resistant organisms has not yet been reported, likely due to the critical infection control strategies in place to prevent spread within pediatric health care institutions. However, for complicated hospitalized neonates, infants, and children, multiple treatment courses of antibiotics for documented or suspected infections can create substantial resistance to many classes of agents, particularly in *P aeruginosa*. These pathogens have the genetic capability to express resistance to virtually any antibiotic used, as a result of more than one hundred million years of exposure to antibiotics elaborated by other organisms in their environment. Inducible enzymes to cleave antibiotics and modify binding sites, efflux pumps, and Gram-negative cell wall alterations to prevent antibiotic penetration (and combinations of mechanisms) all may be present. Some mechanisms of resistance, if not intrinsic, can be acquired from other bacilli. By using antibiotics, we "awaken" resistance; therefore, only using antibiotics when appropriate limits the selection, or induction, of resistance for all children. Community prevalence, as well as health care institution prevalence, of resistant organisms, such as extended-spectrum beta-lactamase (ESBL)-containing *Escherichia coli,* is increasing.

In Figure 4-1, we assume that the clinician has the antibiotic susceptibility report in hand. Each tier provides increasingly broader spectrum activity, from the narrowest of the Gram-negative agents to the broadest (and most toxic), colistin. Tier 1 is ampicillin, safe and widely available but not active against *Klebsiella, Enterobacter,* or *Pseudomonas* and only active against about half of *E coli* in the community setting. Tier 2 contains antibiotics that have a broader spectrum but are also very safe and effective (trimethoprim/sulfamethoxazole [TMP/SMX] and cephalosporins), with decades of experience. In general, use an antibiotic from tier 2 before going to broader spectrum agents. Please be aware that many enteric bacilli (the SPICE bacteria, *Enterobacter, Citrobacter, Serratia,* and indole-positive *Proteus*) have inducible beta-lactam resistance (including third-generation cephalosporins cefotaxime, ceftriaxone, and ceftazidime), which may manifest only after exposure of the pathogen to the antibiotic. Tier 3 is made up of very broad-spectrum antibiotics (aminoglycosides, carbapenems, piperacillin/tazobactam) and aminoglycosides with significantly more toxicity than beta-lactam antibacterial agents, although we have used them safely for decades. As with tier 2, use any antibiotic from tier 3 before going to broader spectrum agents. Tier 4 is fluoroquinolones, to be used only when lower-tier antibiotics cannot be used due to potential (and not yet verified in children) toxicities. Tier 5 is represented by a new set of beta-lactam/beta-lactamase inhibitor combinations, represented by ceftazidime/

Figure 4-1. Enteric Bacilli: Bacilli and *Pseudomonas* With Known Susceptibilities (See Text for Interpretation)

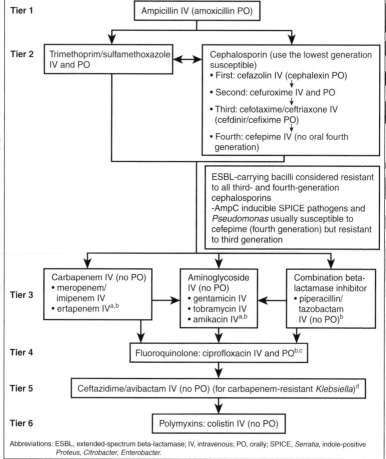

Abbreviations: ESBL, extended-spectrum beta-lactamase; IV, intravenous; PO, orally; SPICE, *Serratia*, indole-positive *Proteus*, *Citrobacter*, *Enterobacter*.

[a] Ertapenem is the only carbapenem *not* active against *Pseudomonas*. Ertapenem and amikacin can be given once daily as outpatient IV/intramuscular (IM) therapy for infections where these drugs achieve therapeutic concentrations (eg, urinary tract). Some use once-daily gentamicin or tobramycin.

[b] For ESBL infections caused by organisms susceptible only to IV/IM therapy, except for fluoroquinolones, oral fluoroquinolone therapy is preferred over IV/IM therapy for infections amenable to treatment by oral therapy.

[c] If you have susceptibility to only a few remaining agents, consider combination therapy to prevent the emergence of resistance to your last-resort antibiotics (no prospective, controlled data in these situations).

[d] Active against carbapenem-resistant *Klebsiella pneumoniae* strains; US Food and Drug Administration approved for adults; pharmacokinetic data published for children.

Approach to Antibiotic Therapy of Drug-Resistant Gram-negative Bacilli and Methicillin-Resistant *Staphylococcus aureus*

4

avibactam, which is active against certain carbapenem-resistant *Klebsiella* spp and *E coli;* it is approved for adults, with clinical trials almost completed in children. Tier 6 is colistin, one of the broadest-spectrum agents available. Colistin was US Food and Drug Administration (FDA) approved in 1962 with significant toxicity and limited clinical experience in children. Many new drugs for multidrug-resistant Gram-negative organisms are currently investigational.

Community-Associated Methicillin-Resistant *Staphylococcus aureus*

Community-associated methicillin-resistant *Staphylococcus aureus* (CA-MRSA) is a community pathogen for children (that can also spread from child to child in hospitals) that first appeared in the United States in the mid-1990s and currently represents 30% to 80% of all community isolates in various regions of the United States (check your hospital microbiology laboratory for your local rate); it is increasingly present in many areas of the world, with some strain variation documented. CA-MRSA is resistant to beta-lactam antibiotics, except for ceftaroline, a fifth-generation cephalosporin antibiotic FDA approved for pediatrics in June 2016 (see Chapter 2).

There are an undetermined number of pathogenicity factors that make CA-MRSA more aggressive than methicillin-susceptible *S aureus* (MSSA) strains. CA-MRSA seems to cause greater tissue necrosis, an increased host inflammatory response, an increased rate of complications, and an increased rate of recurrent infections compared with MSSA. Response to therapy with non–beta-lactam antibiotics (eg, vancomycin, clindamycin) seems to be inferior compared with the response of MSSA to oxacillin/nafcillin or cefazolin, but it is unknown whether poorer outcomes are due to a hardier, better-adapted, more aggressive CA-MRSA or whether these alternative agents are just not as effective against MRSA as beta-lactam agents are against MSSA. Studies in children using ceftaroline to treat skin infections (many caused by MRSA) were conducted using a non-inferiority clinical trial design, compared with vancomycin, with the finding that ceftaroline was equivalent to vancomycin. Guidelines for management of MRSA infections (2011) and management of skin and soft tissue infections (2014) have been published by the Infectious Diseases Society of America[1] and are available at www.idsociety.org.

Antimicrobials for CA-MRSA

Vancomycin (intravenous [IV]) has been the mainstay of parenteral therapy of MRSA infections for the past 4 decades and continues to have activity against more than 98% of strains isolated from children. A few cases of intermediate resistance and "heteroresistance" (transient moderately increased resistance based on thickened staphylococcal cell walls) have been reported, most commonly in adults who are receiving long-term therapy or who have received multiple exposures to vancomycin. Unfortunately, the response to therapy using standard vancomycin dosing of 40 mg/kg/day in the treatment of many CA-MRSA strains has not been as predictably successful as in the past with MSSA. Increasingly, data in adults suggest that serum trough concentrations of vancomycin in treating serious CA-MRSA infections should be kept in the range of 15 to 20 µg/mL, which frequently causes toxicity in adults. For

4

Approach to Antibiotic Therapy of Drug-Resistant Gram-negative Bacilli and Methicillin-Resistant *Staphylococcus aureus* children, serum trough concentrations of 15 to 20 µg/mL can usually be achieved using the old pediatric "meningitis dosage" of vancomycin of 60 mg/kg/day but have also been associated with renal toxicity. Although no prospectively collected data are available, it appears that this dosage in children is reasonably effective and not associated with the degree of nephrotoxicity observed in adults. For vancomycin, the ratio of the area under the serum concentration curve to minimum inhibitory concentration (AUC:MIC) that appears to be the exposure that best predicts a successful outcome is about 400 or greater (see Chapter 3 for more on the AIC:MIC). This ratio is achievable for CA-MRSA strains with in vitro MIC values of 1 µg/mL or less but difficult to achieve for strains with 2 µg/mL or greater.[2] Recent data suggest that vancomycin MICs may actually be decreasing in children for MRSA, causing bloodstream infections as they increase for MSSA.[3] Strains with MIC values of 4 µg/mL or greater should generally be considered resistant to vancomycin. When using these higher "meningitis" treatment dosages, one needs to follow renal function carefully for the development of toxicity.

Clindamycin (oral [PO] or IV) is active against approximately 70% to 90% of strains of either MRSA or MSSA, with great geographic variability (again, check with your hospital laboratory).[4] The dosage for moderate to severe infections is 30 to 40 mg/kg/day, in 3 divided doses, using the same mg/kg dose PO or IV. Clindamycin is not as bactericidal as vancomycin but achieves higher concentrations in abscesses (based on high intracellular concentrations in neutrophils). Some CA-MRSA strains are susceptible to clindamycin on initial testing but have inducible clindamycin resistance (methylase-mediated) that is usually assessed by the "D-test" and, more recently, in automated multi-well microtiter plates. Within each population of these CA-MRSA organisms, a rare organism (between 1 in 10^9 and 10^{11} organisms) will have a mutation that allows for constant (rather than induced) resistance.[5] Although still somewhat controversial, clindamycin should be effective therapy for infections that have a relatively low organism load (cellulitis, small or drained abscesses) and are unlikely to contain a significant population of these constitutive methylase-producing mutants that are truly resistant (in contrast to the strains that are not already producing methylase and, in fact, are actually poorly induced by clindamycin). Infections with a high organism load (empyema) may have a greater risk of failure (as a large population is more likely to have a significant number of truly resistant organisms), and clindamycin should not be used as the preferred agent for these strains. Many laboratories no longer report D-test results but simply call the organism "resistant." This forces the clinician to use alternative therapy that may not be needed.

Clindamycin is used to treat most CA-MRSA infections that are not life-threatening, and, if the child responds, therapy can be switched from IV to PO (although the oral solution is not very well tolerated). *Clostridium difficile* enterocolitis is a concern; however, despite a great increase in the use of clindamycin in children during the past decade, recent published data do not document a clinically significant increase in the rate of this complication in children.

Trimethoprim/sulfamethoxazole (TMP/SMX) (PO, IV), Bactrim/Septra, is active against CA-MRSA in vitro. Prospective comparative data on treatment of skin or skin structure infections in adults and children document efficacy equivalent to clindamycin.[6] Given our current lack of prospective, comparative information in MRSA bacteremia, pneumonia, and osteomyelitis (in contrast to skin infections), TMP/SMX should not be used routinely to treat these more serious infections at this time.

Linezolid (PO, IV), Zyvox, active against virtually 100% of CA-MRSA strains, is another reasonable alternative but is considered bacteriostatic and has relatively frequent hematologic toxicity in adults (neutropenia, thrombocytopenia) and some infrequent neurologic toxicity (peripheral neuropathy, optic neuritis), particularly when used for courses of 2 weeks or longer (a complete blood cell count should be checked every week or 2 in children receiving prolonged linezolid therapy). The cost of linezolid is substantially more than clindamycin or vancomycin.

Daptomycin (IV), FDA approved for adults for skin infections in 2003 and, subsequently, for bacteremia/endocarditis, was approved for use for children with skin infections in April 2017. It is a unique class of antibiotic, a lipopeptide, and is highly bactericidal. Daptomycin should be considered for treatment of skin infection and bacteremia in failures with other, better studied antibiotics. **Daptomycin should not be used to treat pneumonia,** as it is inactivated by pulmonary surfactant. Pediatric studies for skin infections have been completed and published,[7] and those for bacteremia and osteomyelitis have concluded, but data from the trials have not yet been analyzed or presented. Some newborn animal neurologic toxicity data suggest additional **caution for the use of daptomycin in infants younger than 1 year,** prompting a warning in the package label. Pediatric clinical trial investigations in young infants are not proceeding at this time.

Tigecycline and fluoroquinolones, both of which may show in vitro activity, are not generally recommended for children if other agents are available and are tolerated due to potential toxicity issues for children with tetracyclines and fluoroquinolones and rapid emergence of resistance with fluoroquinolones.

Ceftaroline, a fifth-generation cephalosporin antibiotic, the first FDA-approved beta-lactam antibiotic to be active against MRSA, was approved for children in June 2016. The Gram-negative coverage is similar to cefotaxime, with no activity against *Pseudomonas*. Published data are available for pediatric pharmacokinetics, as well as for prospective, randomized comparative treatment trials of skin and skin structure infections[8] and community-acquired pneumonia.[9,10] The efficacy and toxicity profile in adults is what one would expect from most cephalosporins. Based on these published data and review by the FDA, for infants and children 2 months and older, ceftaroline should be effective and safer than vancomycin for treatment of MRSA infections. Just as beta-lactams are preferred over vancomycin for MSSA infections, ceftaroline should be considered preferred treatment over vancomycin for MRSA infections. Neither renal function nor drug levels need to be followed with ceftaroline therapy. We will be closely following post-marketing experience in children, and recommendations may change if unexpected clinical data on lack of efficacy or unexpected toxicity (beyond what may be expected with beta-lactams) should be presented.

Combination therapy for serious infections, with vancomycin and rifampin (for deep abscesses) or vancomycin and gentamicin (for bacteremia), is often used, but no prospective, controlled human clinical data exist on improved efficacy over single antibiotic therapy. Some experts use vancomycin and clindamycin in combination, particularly for children with a toxic-shock clinical presentation. Ceftaroline has also been used in combination therapy with other agents in adults, but no prospective, controlled clinical data exist to assess benefits.

Investigational Agents Recently Approved for Adults That Are Being Studied in Children

Dalbavancin and Oritavancin. Both antibiotics are IV glycopeptides, structurally very similar to vancomycin but with enhanced in vitro activity against MRSA and a much longer serum half-life, allowing once-weekly dosing or even just a single dose to treat skin infections.

Telavancin. A glyco-lipopeptide with mechanisms of activity that include cell wall inhibition and cell membrane depolarization, telavancin is administered once daily.

Tedizolid. A second-generation oxazolidinone like linezolid, tedizolid is more potent in vitro against MRSA than linezolid, with somewhat decreased toxicity to bone marrow in adult clinical studies.

Recommendations for Empiric Therapy of Suspected MRSA Infections

Life-threatening and Serious Infections. If any CA-MRSA is present in your community, empiric therapy for presumed staphylococcal infections that are life-threatening or infections for which any risk of failure is unacceptable (eg, meningitis) should follow the recommendations for CA-MRSA and include *high-dose* vancomycin, clindamycin, or linezolid, in addition to nafcillin or oxacillin (beta-lactam antibiotics are considered better than vancomycin or clindamycin for MSSA). Ceftaroline is now another option, particularly for children with some degree of renal injury.

Moderate Infections. If you live in a location with greater than 10% methicillin resistance, consider using the CA-MRSA recommendations for hospitalized children with presumed staphylococcal infections of any severity, and start empiric therapy with clindamycin (usually active against >80% of CA-MRSA), ceftaroline, vancomycin, or linezolid IV.

In skin and skin structure abscesses, drainage of the abscess may be completely curative in some children, and antibiotics may not be necessary following incision and drainage.

Mild Infections. For nonserious, presumed staphylococcal infections in regions with significant CA-MRSA, empiric topical therapy with mupirocin (Bactroban) or retapamulin (Altabax) ointment, or oral therapy with TMP/SMX or clindamycin, are preferred. For older children, doxycycline and minocycline are also options based on data in adults.

Prevention of Recurrent Infections

For children with problematic, recurrent infections, no well-studied, prospectively collected data provide a solution. Bleach baths (one-half cup of bleach in a full bathtub)[11] seems to be able to transiently decrease the numbers of colonizing organisms but was not shown to decrease the number of infections in a prospective, controlled study in children with eczema. Similarly, a regimen to decolonize with twice-weekly bleach baths in an attempt to prevent recurrent infection did not lead to a statistically significant decrease.[12] Bathing with chlorhexidine (Hibiclens, a preoperative antibacterial skin disinfectant) daily or 2 to 3 times each week should provide topical anti-MRSA activity for several hours following a bath. Treating the entire family with decolonization regimens will provide an additional decrease in risk of recurrence for the index child.[13] Nasal mupirocin ointment (Bactroban) designed to eradicate colonization may also be used. All these measures have advantages and disadvantages and need to be used together with environmental measures (eg, washing towels frequently, using hand sanitizers, not sharing items of clothing). Helpful advice can be found on the Centers for Disease Control and Prevention Web site at www.cdc.gov/mrsa (accessed September 28, 2017).

Vaccines are being investigated but are not likely to be available for several years.

5. Antimicrobial Therapy for Newborns

NOTES

- Prospectively collected data in newborns continue to become available, thanks in large part to federal legislation (including the US Food and Drug Administration [FDA] Safety and Innovation Act of 2012 that mandates neonatal studies). In situations of inadequate data, suggested doses are based on efficacy, safety, and pharmacological data from older children or adults. These may not account for the effect of developmental changes (effect of ontogeny) on drug metabolism that occur during early infancy and among preterm and full-term newborns.[1] These values may vary widely, particularly for the unstable preterm newborn. Oral convalescent therapy for neonatal infections has not been well studied but may be used cautiously in non–life-threatening infections in adherent families with ready access to medical care.[2]

- The recommended antibiotic dosages and intervals of administration are given in the tables at the end of this chapter.

- **Adverse drug reaction:** Neonates should not receive intravenous (IV) ceftriaxone while receiving IV calcium-containing products, including parenteral nutrition, by the same or different infusion lines, as fatal reactions with ceftriaxone-calcium precipitates in lungs and kidneys in neonates have occurred. There are no data on interactions between IV ceftriaxone and oral calcium-containing products or between intramuscular ceftriaxone and IV or oral calcium-containing products. Current information is available on the FDA Web site.[3] Cefotaxime is preferred over ceftriaxone for neonates.[4]

- **Abbreviations:** 3TC, lamivudine; ABLC, lipid complex amphotericin; ABR, auditory brainstem response; ALT, alanine transaminase; AmB, amphotericin B; AmB-D, AmB deoxycholate; amox/clav, amoxicillin/clavulanate; AOM, acute otitis media; AST, aspartate transaminase; AUC, area under the curve; bid, twice daily; CBC, complete blood cell count; CDC, Centers for Disease Control and Prevention; CLD, chronic lung disease; CMV, cytomegalovirus; CNS, central nervous system; CSF, cerebrospinal fluid; CT, computed tomography; div, divided; echo, echocardiogram; ECMO, extracorporeal membrane oxygenation; ESBL, extended spectrum beta-lactamase; FDA, US Food and Drug Administration; GA, gestational age; GBS, group B streptococcus; G-CSF, granulocyte colony stimulating factor; HIV, human immunodeficiency virus; HSV, herpes simplex virus; IAI, intra-abdominal infection; ID, infectious diseases; IM, intramuscular; IUGR, intrauterine growth restriction; IV, intravenous; IVIG, intravenous immune globulin; L-AmB, liposomal AmB; MIC, minimal inhibitory concentration; MRSA, methicillin-resistant *Staphylococcus aureus;* MSSA, methicillin-susceptible *S aureus;* NEC, necrotizing enterocolitis; NICU, neonatal intensive care unit; NVP, nevirapine; PCR, polymerase chain reaction; pip/tazo, piperacillin/tazobactam; PMA, postmenstrual age; PO, orally; RSV, respiratory syncytial virus; spp, species; tid, 3 times daily; TIG, tetanus immune globulin; TMP/SMX, trimethoprim/sulfamethoxazole; UCSF, University of California, San Francisco; UTI, urinary tract infection; VCUG, voiding cystourethrogram; VDRL, Venereal Disease Research Laboratories; ZDV, zidovudine.

A. RECOMMENDED THERAPY FOR SELECTED NEWBORN CONDITIONS

Condition	Therapy (evidence grade) *See Tables 5B–D for neonatal dosages.*	Comments
Conjunctivitis		
– Chlamydial[5-8]	Azithromycin 10 mg/kg/day PO for 1 day, then 5 mg/kg/day PO for 4 days (AII), or erythromycin ethylsuccinate PO for 10–14 days (AII)	Macrolides PO preferred to topical eye drops to prevent development of pneumonia; association of erythromycin and pyloric stenosis in young neonates.[9] Alternative: 3-day course of higher-dose azithromycin at 10 mg/kg/dose once daily, although safety not well defined in neonates (CIII). Oral sulfonamides may be used after the immediate neonatal period for infants who do not tolerate erythromycin.
– Gonococcal[10-14]	Ceftriaxone 25–50 mg/kg (max 125 mg) IV, IM once, AND azithromycin 10 mg/kg PO q24h for 5 days (AIII)	Ceftriaxone no longer recommended as single agent therapy due to increasing cephalosporin resistance; therefore, addition of azithromycin recommended (no data in neonates; azithromycin dose given is that recommended for pertussis). Cefotaxime is preferred for neonates with hyperbilirubinemia and those at risk for calcium drug interactions (see Table 5B). Saline irrigation of eyes. Evaluate for chlamydial infection. All neonates born to mothers with untreated gonococcal infection (regardless of symptoms) require therapy. Cefixime and ciprofloxacin no longer recommended for empiric maternal therapy.
– *Staphylococcus aureus*[15-17]	Topical therapy sufficient for mild *S aureus* cases (AII), but oral or IV therapy may be considered for moderate to severe conjunctivitis. MSSA: oxacillin/nafcillin IV or cefazolin (for non-CNS infections) IM, IV for 7 days. MRSA: vancomycin IV or clindamycin IV, PO.	Neomycin or erythromycin PO ophthalmic drops or ointment No prospective data for MRSA conjunctivitis (BIII) Cephalexin PO for mild–moderate disease caused by MSSA Increased *S aureus* resistance with ciprofloxacin/levofloxacin ophthalmic formulations (AII)

Pseudomonas aeruginosa[18-20]	Ceftazidime IM, IV AND tobramycin IM, IV for 7–10 days (alternatives: meropenem, cefepime, pip/tazo) (BIII)	Aminoglycoside or polymyxin B–containing ophthalmic drops or ointment as adjunctive therapy
– Other Gram-negative	Aminoglycoside or polymyxin B–containing ophthalmic drops or ointment if mild (AII) Systemic therapy if moderate to severe or unresponsive to topical therapy (AIII)	Duration of therapy is dependent on clinical course and may be as short as 5 days if clinically resolved.
Cytomegalovirus		
– Congenital[21-25]	For moderately to severely symptomatic neonates with congenital infection syndrome and multisystem disease: oral valganciclovir at 16 mg/kg/dose PO bid for 6 mo[24] (AI); IV ganciclovir 6 mg/kg/dose IV q12h can be used for some of or all the first 6 wk of therapy if oral therapy not advised, but provides no added benefit over oral valganciclovir (AII).	Benefit for hearing loss and neurodevelopmental outcomes (AI). Treatment recommended for neonates with moderate or severe symptomatic congenital CMV disease, with or without CNS involvement. Treatment is not routinely recommended for "mildly symptomatic" neonates congenitally infected with CMV (eg, only 1 or perhaps 2 manifestations of congenital CMV infection, which are mild in scope [eg, slight IUGR, mild hepatomegaly] or transient and mild in nature [eg, a single platelet count of 80,000 or an ALT of 130]), as the risks of treatment may not be balanced by benefits in mild disease that is often reversible without long-term sequelae.[25] This includes neonates who are asymptomatic except for sensorineural hearing loss. Treatment for asymptomatic neonates congenitally infected with CMV is not recommended. Neutropenia in 20% (oral valganciclovir) to 68% (IV ganciclovir) of neonates on long-term therapy (responds to G-CSF or temporary discontinuation of therapy). Treatment for congenital CMV should start within the first month after birth. CMV-IVIG not recommended for infants.

Antimicrobial Therapy for Newborns

A. RECOMMENDED THERAPY FOR SELECTED NEWBORN CONDITIONS (continued)

Condition	Therapy (evidence grade) See Tables 5B–D for neonatal dosages.	Comments
– Perinatally or postnatally acquired[23]	Ganciclovir 12 mg/kg/day IV div q12h for 14–21 days (AIII)	Antiviral treatment has not been studied in this population but can be considered in patients with acute, severe, visceral (end-organ) disease, such as pneumonia, hepatitis, encephalitis, necrotizing enterocolitis, or persistent thrombocytopenia. If such patients are treated with parenteral ganciclovir, a reasonable approach is to treat for 2 wk and then reassess responsiveness to therapy. If clinical data suggest benefit of treatment, an additional 1 wk of parenteral ganciclovir can be considered if symptoms and signs have not fully resolved. Observe for possible relapse after completion of therapy (AIII).

Fungal infections (See also Chapter 8.)

– Candidiasis[26-34]	**Treatment** AmB-D (1 mg/kg/day) is recommended therapy (AII). Fluconazole (12 mg/kg/day q24h, after a load of 25 mg/kg/day) is an alternative if patient has not been on fluconazole prophylaxis (AII).[26] For treatment of neonates and young infants (<120 days) on ECMO, fluconazole loading dose is 35 mg/kg on day 1, then 12 mg/kg q24h (BII). Lipid formulation AmB is an alternative but carries a theoretical risk of less urinary tract penetration compared with AmB-D (CIII). Duration of therapy for candidemia without obvious metastatic complications is for 2 wk after documented clearance and resolution of symptoms.	Neonates are at high risk of urinary tract and CNS infection, problematic for echinocandins with poor penetration at those sites; therefore, AmB-D is preferred, followed by fluconazole, and echinocandins discouraged, despite their fungicidal activity. Evaluate for other sites of infection: CSF analysis, echo, abdominal ultrasound to include bladder; retinal eye examination. Length of therapy dependent on disease (BIII), usually 2 wk after all clearance. Antifungal susceptibility testing is suggested with persistent disease. Candida krusei inherently resistant to fluconazole; Candida parapsilosis may be less susceptible to echinocandins; increasing resistance of Candida glabrata to fluconazole and echinocandins. No proven benefit for combination antifungal therapy in candidiasis. Change from AmB or fluconazole to echinocandin if cultures persistently positive (BIII). Although fluconazole prophylaxis has been shown to reduce colonization, it has not reduced mortality.[29] Lumbar puncture and dilated retinal examination recommended in neonates with cultures positive for Candida spp from blood (AIII).

Prophylaxis

In nurseries with high rates of candidiasis (>10%),[35] IV or oral fluconazole prophylaxis (AI) (3–6 mg/kg twice weekly for 6 wk) in high-risk neonates (birth weight <1,000 g) is recommended. Oral nystatin, 100,000 units 3 times daily for 6 wk, is an alternative to fluconazole in neonates with birth weights <1,500 g if availability or resistance preclude fluconazole use (CII).

Neonates and children on ECMO: fluconazole 12 mg/kg on day 1, followed by 6 mg/kg/day (BII).

Same recommended for all infants with birth weight <1,500 g with candiduria with or without candidemia (AIII).

CT or ultrasound imaging of genitourinary tract, liver, and spleen should be performed if blood culture results are persistently positive (AIII).

Meningoencephalitis in the neonate occurs at a higher rate than in older children/adults.

Central venous catheter removal strongly recommended.

Infected CNS devices, including ventriculostomy drains and shunts, should be removed, if possible.

See Skin and soft tissues later in this Table for management of congenital cutaneous candidiasis.

Echinocandins should be used with caution and generally limited to salvage therapy or situations in which resistance or toxicity preclude use of AmB-D or fluconazole (CIII).

Role of flucytosine in neonates with meningitis is questionable and not routinely recommended due to toxicity concerns. The addition of flucytosine (100 mg/kg/day div q6h) may be considered as salvage therapy in patients who have not had a clinical response to initial AmB therapy, but adverse effects are frequent (CIII).

5

A. RECOMMENDED THERAPY FOR SELECTED NEWBORN CONDITIONS (continued)

Condition	Therapy (evidence grade) See Tables 5B–D for neonatal dosages.	Comments
– Aspergillosis (usually cutaneous infection with systemic dissemination)[24,36-38]	Voriconazole initial dosing same as pediatric ≥2 y: 18 mg/kg/day IV div q12h for a loading dose on the first day, then 16 mg/kg/day IV div q12h as a maintenance dose. Continued dosing is guided by monitoring of trough serum concentrations (AII). When stable, may switch from voriconazole IV to voriconazole PO 18 mg/kg/day div bid (AII). Unlike in adults, PO bioavailability in children is only approximately 60%. Trough monitoring is crucial after switch.[23] Alternatives for primary therapy when voriconazole cannot be administered: L-AmB 5 mg/kg/day (AII). ABLC is another possible alternative. Echinocandin primary monotherapy should not be used for treating invasive aspergillosis (CII). AmB-D should be used only in resource-limited settings in which no alternative agent is available (AII).	Aggressive antifungal therapy, early debridement of skin lesions (AIII). Voriconazole is preferred primary antifungal therapy for all clinical forms of aspergillosis (AI). Early initiation of therapy in patients with strong suspicion of disease is important while a diagnostic evaluation is conducted. Therapeutic voriconazole trough serum concentrations of 2–5 mg/L are important for success. It is critical to monitor trough concentrations to guide therapy due to high inter-patient variability.[25] Low voriconazole concentrations are a leading cause of clinical failure. Neonatal and infant voriconazole dosing is not well defined, but doses required to achieve therapeutic troughs are generally higher than in children >2 y (AIII). No experience with posaconazole or isavuconazole in neonates. Total treatment course is for a minimum of 6–12 wk, largely dependent on the degree and duration of immunosuppression and evidence of disease improvement. Salvage antifungal therapy options after failed primary therapy include a change of antifungal class (using L-AmB or an echinocandin), switching to posaconazole (trough concentrations >0.7 μg/mL), or using combination antifungal therapy. Combination therapy with voriconazole + an echinocandin may be considered in select patients. In vitro data suggest some synergy with 2 (but not 3) drug combinations: an azole + an echinocandin is the most well studied. If combination therapy is employed, this is likely best done initially when voriconazole trough concentrations may not yet be therapeutic.[26] Routine susceptibility testing is not recommended but is suggested for patients suspected of having an azole-resistant isolate or who are unresponsive to therapy.

Azole-resistant *Aspergillus fumigatus* is increasing. If local epidemiology suggests >10% azole resistance, empiric initial therapy should be voriconazole + echinocandin OR + L-AmB, and subsequent therapy guided based on antifungal susceptibilities.[39] Micafungin likely has equal efficacy to caspofungin against aspergillosis.[27]

Gastrointestinal infections

Condition	Therapy	Comments
– NEC or peritonitis secondary to bowel rupture[40-45]	Ampicillin IV AND gentamicin IM, IV for ≥10 days (AII). Alternatives: pip/tazo AND gentamicin (AII); ceftazidime/cefotaxime AND gentamicin ± metronidazole (BIII); OR meropenem (B). ADD fluconazole if known to have gastrointestinal colonization with *Candida* (BIII).	Surgical drainage (AII). Definitive antibiotic therapy based on culture results (aerobic, anaerobic, and fungal); meropenem or cefepime if ceftazidime-resistant Gram-negative bacilli isolated. Vancomycin rather than ampicillin if MRSA prevalent. *Bacteroides* colonization may occur as early as the first week after birth (AIII).[45] Duration of therapy dependent on clinical response and risk of persisting intra-abdominal abscess (AIII). Probiotics may prevent NEC in neonates born <1,500 g, but agent, dose, and safety not fully known.[42,45]
– *Salmonella*[46]	Ampicillin IM, IV (if susceptible) OR cefotaxime IM, IV for 7–10 days (AII)	Observe for focal complications (eg, meningitis, arthritis) (AIII).

Herpes simplex infection

Condition	Therapy	Comments
– CNS and disseminated disease[47-49]	Acyclovir 60 mg/kg/day div q8h IV for 21 days (AII) (if eye disease present, ADD topical 1% trifluridine or 0.15% ganciclovir ophthalmic gel) (AII).	For babies with CNS involvement, perform CSF HSV PCR near end of 21 days of therapy and continue acyclovir until PCR negative. Serum AST/ALT may help identify early disseminated infection. Foscarnet for acyclovir-resistant disease. Acyclovir PO (300 mg/m²/dose tid) suppression for 6 mo recommended following parenteral therapy (AI).[50] Monitor for neutropenia during suppressive therapy. Different dosages than those listed in Table 5B have been modeled, but there are no safety or efficacy data in humans to support them.[50]

5

A. RECOMMENDED THERAPY FOR SELECTED NEWBORN CONDITIONS (continued)

Condition	Therapy (evidence grade) See Tables 5B–D for neonatal dosages.	Comments
– Skin, eye, or mouth disease[47–49]	Acyclovir 60 mg/kg/day div q8h IV for 14 days (AII) (if eye disease present, ADD topical 1% trifluridine or 0.15% ganciclovir ophthalmic gel) (AII). Obtain CSF PCR for HSV to assess for CNS infection.	Acyclovir PO (300 mg/m²/dose tid) suppression for 6 mo recommended following parenteral therapy (AI).[51] Monitor for neutropenia during suppressive therapy. Different dosages than those listed in Table 5B have been modeled, but there are no safety or efficacy data in humans to support them.[50]
Human immunodeficiency virus infection[52,53]	There has been recent interest in using "treatment" antiretroviral regimens for high-risk, exposed neonates in an attempt to achieve a remission or possibly even a cure. This was initially stimulated by the experience of a baby from Mississippi: high-risk neonate treated within the first 2 days after birth with subsequent infection documentation; off therapy at 18 mo of age without evidence of circulating virus until 4 y of age, at which point virus became detectable.[54] While a clinical trial is ongoing to study issues further, full treatment dosing of high-risk neonates is not currently recommended due to lack of safety and dosing data and lack of defined efficacy. Peripartum presumptive preventive therapy for HIV-exposed newborns: ZDV for the first 6 wk of age (AI). Note: if the mother was treated with combination antiretroviral therapy during pregnancy with complete viral suppression, newborn prevention therapy for 4 wk is recommended (BIII). GA ≥35 wk: ZDV 8 mg/kg/day PO div bid OR 6 mg/kg/day IV div q8h for 6 wk. GA 30–34 wk: ZDV 4 mg/kg/day PO (OR 3 mg/kg/day IV) div q12h. Increase at 2 wk of age to 6 mg/kg/day PO div 4.5 mg/kg/day IV) div q12h. GA ≤29 wk: ZDV 4 mg/kg/day PO (OR 3 mg/kg/day IV) div q12h. Increase at 4 wk of age to 6 mg/kg/day PO (OR	For detailed information: https://aidsinfo.nih.gov/guidelines/html/3/perinatal-guidelines/0/# (accessed October 2, 2017). UCSF Clinician Consultation Center (888/448-8765) provides free clinical consultation. Start prevention therapy as soon after delivery as possible but by 6–8 h of age for best effectiveness (AII). Monitor CBC at birth and 4 wk (AII). Some experts consider the use of ZDV in combination with other antiretroviral drugs in certain situations (eg, mothers with minimal intervention before delivery, with high viral load, and/or with known resistant virus). Consultation with a pediatric HIV specialist is recommended (BIII). Perform HIV-1 PCR or RNA assays at 14–21 days, 1–2 mo, and 4–6 mo (AI). Initiate prophylaxis for pneumocystis pneumonia at 6 wk of age if HIV infection not yet excluded (AI). NVP dosing and safety not established for infants whose birth weight

	For newborns whose mothers received NO antenatal antiretroviral therapy, add 3 doses of NVP (first dose at 0–48 h; second dose 48 h later; third dose 96 h after second dose) to the 6 wk of ZDV treatment (AI). NVP dose (not per kg): birth weight 1.5–2 kg: 8 mg/dose PO; birth weight >2 kg: 12 mg/dose PO (AI).[55] The preventive ZDV doses listed herein for neonates are also treatment doses for infants with diagnosed HIV infection. Note that antiretroviral treatment doses for neonates are established only for ZDV and 3TC (4 mg/kg/day div q12h). Treatment of HIV-infected neonates should be considered only with expert consultation.	
Influenza A and B viruses[56-59]	Preterm, <38 wk PMA: 1 mg/kg/dose PO bid Preterm, 38–40 wk PMA: 1.5 mg/kg/dose PO bid Preterm, >40 wk PMA: 3 mg/kg/dose PO bid[57] Term, birth–8 mo: 3 mg/kg/dose PO bid[57,60]	Oseltamivir chemoprophylaxis not recommended for infants <3 mo unless the situation is judged critical because of limited safety and efficacy data in this age group.[61] Studies of parenteral zanamivir have been completed in children.[61] However, this formulation of the drug is not yet approved in the United States.
Omphalitis and funisitis		
– Empiric therapy for omphalitis and necrotizing funisitis direct therapy against coliform bacilli, *S aureus* (consider MRSA), and anaerobes[62-64]	Cefotaxime OR gentamicin, AND clindamycin for ≥10 days (AII)	Need to culture to direct therapy. Alternatives for coliform coverage if resistance likely: cefepime, meropenem. For suspect MRSA: ADD vancomycin. Alternative for combined MSSA and anaerobic coverage: pip/tazo. Appropriate wound management for infected cord and necrotic tissue (AIII).

A. RECOMMENDED THERAPY FOR SELECTED NEWBORN CONDITIONS (continued)

Condition	Therapy (evidence grade) See Tables 5B–D for neonatal dosages.	Comments
– Group A or B streptococci[65]	Penicillin G IV for ≥7–14 days (shorter course for superficial funisitis without invasive infection) (AII)	Group A streptococcus usually causes "wet cord" without pus and with minimal erythema; single dose of benzathine penicillin IM adequate. Consultation with pediatric ID specialist is recommended for necrotizing fasciitis (AII).
– S aureus[64]	MSSA: oxacillin/nafcillin IV, IM for ≥5–7 days (shorter course for superficial funisitis without invasive infection) (AIII) MRSA: vancomycin (AIII)	Assess for bacteremia and other focus of infection. Alternatives for MRSA: linezolid, clindamycin (if susceptible).
– Clostridium spp[66]	Clindamycin OR penicillin G IV for ≥10 days, with additional agents based on culture results (AII)	Crepitation and rapidly spreading cellulitis around umbilicus Mixed infection with other Gram-positive and Gram-negative bacteria common

Osteomyelitis, suppurative arthritis[67–69]
Obtain cultures (aerobic; fungal if NICU) of bone or joint fluid before antibiotic therapy.
Duration of therapy dependent on causative organism and normalization of erythrocyte sedimentation rate and C-reactive protein; minimum for osteomyelitis 3 wk and arthritis therapy 2–3 wk if no organism identified (AIII).
Surgical drainage of pus (AIII); physical therapy may be needed (BIII).

– Empiric therapy	Nafcillin/oxacillin IV (or vancomycin if MRSA is a concern) AND cefotaxime or gentamicin IV, IM (AIII)	
– Coliform bacteria (eg, Escherichia coli, Klebsiella spp, Enterobacter spp)	For E coli and Klebsiella: cefotaxime OR gentamicin OR ampicillin (if susceptible) (AIII). For Enterobacter, Serratia, or Citrobacter: ADD gentamicin IV, IM to cefotaxime or ceftriaxone, OR use cefepime or meropenem alone (AIII).	Meropenem for ESBL-producing coliforms (AIII). Pip/tazo or cefepime are alternatives for susceptible bacilli (BIII).

– Gonococcal arthritis and tenosynovitis[11-14]	Ceftriaxone IV, IM OR cefotaxime IV AND azithromycin 10 mg/kg PO q24h for 5 days (AIII)	Ceftriaxone no longer recommended as single agent therapy due to increasing cephalosporin resistance; therefore, addition of azithromycin recommended (no data in neonates; azithromycin dose is that recommended for pertussis). Cefotaxime is preferred for neonates with hyperbilirubinemia and those at risk for calcium drug interactions (see Table 5B).
– S aureus	MSSA: oxacillin/nafcillin IV (AII) MRSA: vancomycin IV (AIII)	Alternative for MSSA: cefazolin (AIII) Alternatives for MRSA: linezolid, clindamycin (if susceptible) (BIII) Addition of rifampin if persistently positive cultures
– Group B streptococcus	Ampicillin or penicillin G IV (AII)	
– Haemophilus influenzae	Ampicillin IV OR cefotaxime IV, IM if ampicillin resistant	Start with IV therapy and switch to oral therapy when clinically stable. Amox/clav PO OR amoxicillin PO if susceptible (AIII).
Otitis media[70]	No controlled treatment trials in newborns; if no response, obtain middle ear fluid for culture.	In addition to Pneumococcus and Haemophilus, coliforms and S aureus may also cause AOM in neonates (AIII).
– Empiric therapy[71]	Oxacillin/nafcillin AND cefotaxime or gentamicin	Start with IV therapy and switch to oral therapy when clinically stable. Amox/clav (AIII).
– E coli (therapy of other coliforms based on susceptibility testing)	Cefotaxime OR gentamicin	Start with IV therapy and switch to oral therapy when clinically stable. For ESBL-producing strains, use meropenem (AII). Amox/clav if susceptible (AIII).
– S aureus	MSSA: oxacillin/nafcillin IV MRSA: vancomycin or clindamycin IV (if susceptible)	Start with IV therapy and switch to oral therapy when clinically stable. MSSA: cephalexin PO for 10 days or cloxacillin PO (AIII). MRSA: linezolid PO or clindamycin PO (BII).
– Group A or B streptococci	Penicillin G or ampicillin IV, IM	Start with IV therapy and switch to oral therapy when clinically stable. Amoxicillin 30–40 mg/kg/day PO div q8h for 10 days.
Parotitis, suppurative[72]	Oxacillin/nafcillin IV AND gentamicin IV, IM for 10 days; consider vancomycin if MRSA suspected (AIII).	Usually staphylococcal but occasionally coliform. Antimicrobial regimen without incision/drainage is adequate in >75% of cases.

Antimicrobial Therapy for Newborns

Antimicrobial Therapy for Newborns

5

A. RECOMMENDED THERAPY FOR SELECTED NEWBORN CONDITIONS (continued)

Condition	Therapy (evidence grade) See Tables 5B–D for neonatal dosages.	Comments
Pulmonary infections		
– Empiric therapy of the neonate with early onset of pulmonary infiltrates (within the first 48–72 h after birth)	Ampicillin IV, IM AND gentamicin or cefotaxime IV, IM for 10 days; many neonatologists treat low-risk neonates for ≤7 days (see Comments).	For newborns with no additional risk factors for bacterial infection (eg, maternal chorioamnionitis) who (1) have negative blood cultures, (2) have little need for > 8 h of oxygen, and (3) are asymptomatic at 48 h into therapy, 4 days may be sufficient therapy, based on limited data.[73]
– Aspiration pneumonia[74]	Ampicillin IV, IM AND gentamicin IV, IM for 7–10 days (AIII)	Early onset neonatal pneumonia may represent aspiration of amniotic fluid, particularly if fluid is not sterile. Mild aspiration episodes may not require antibiotic therapy.
– Chlamydia trachomatis[75]	Azithromycin PO, IV q24h for 5 days OR erythromycin ethylsuccinate PO for 14 days (AII)	Association of erythromycin and azithromycin with pyloric stenosis in infants treated <6 wk of age[76]
– Mycoplasma hominis[77,78]	Clindamycin PO, IV for 10 days (Organisms are resistant to macrolides.)	Pathogenic role in pneumonia not well defined and clinical efficacy unknown; no association with bronchopulmonary dysplasia (BIII)
– Pertussis[79]	Azithromycin 10 mg/kg PO, IV q24h for 5 days OR erythromycin ethylsuccinate PO for 14 days (AII)	Association of erythromycin and azithromycin with pyloric stenosis in infants treated <6 wk of age Alternatives: for >1 mo of age, clarithromycin for 7 days; for >2 mo of age, TMP/SMX for 14 days
– P aeruginosa[80]	Ceftazidime IV, IM AND tobramycin IV, IM for 10–14 days (AIII)	Alternatives: cefepime or meropenem, OR pip/tazo AND tobramycin
– Respiratory syncytial virus[81]	Treatment: see Comments. Prophylaxis: palivizumab (Synagis, a monoclonal antibody) 15 mg/kg IM monthly (maximum: 5 doses) for these high-risk infants (AI).	Aerosol ribavirin (6-g vial to make 20-mg/mL solution in sterile water), aerosolized over 18–20 h daily for 3–5 days (BII), provides little benefit and should only be used for life-threatening infection with RSV. Difficulties in administration, complications with airway reactivity, and concern for potential toxicities to health care workers preclude routine use.

In first y after birth, palivizumab prophylaxis is recommended for infants born before 29 wk 0 days' gestation.

Palivizumab prophylaxis is not recommended for otherwise healthy infants born at ≥29 wk 0 days' gestation.

In first y after birth, palivizumab prophylaxis is recommended for preterm infants with CLD of prematurity, defined as birth at <32 wk 0 days' gestation and a requirement for >21% oxygen for at least 28 days after birth.

Clinicians may administer palivizumab prophylaxis in the first y after birth to certain infants with hemodynamically significant heart disease.

Palivizumab does not provide benefit in the treatment of an active RSV infection.

Palivizumab prophylaxis may be considered for children <24 mo who will be profoundly immunocompromised during the RSV season.

Palivizumab prophylaxis is not recommended in the second y after birth except for children who required at least 28 days of supplemental oxygen after birth and who continue to require medical support (supplemental oxygen, chronic corticosteroid therapy, or diuretic therapy) during the 6-mo period before the start of the second RSV season.

Monthly prophylaxis should be discontinued in any child who experiences a breakthrough RSV hospitalization.

Children with pulmonary abnormality or neuromuscular disease that impairs the ability to clear secretions from the upper airways may be considered for prophylaxis in the first y after birth.

Insufficient data are available to recommend palivizumab prophylaxis for children with cystic fibrosis or Down syndrome.

The burden of RSV disease and costs associated with transport from remote locations may result in a broader use of palivizumab for RSV prevention in Alaska Native populations and possibly in selected other American Indian populations.[82,83]

Palivizumab prophylaxis is not recommended for prevention of health care–associated RSV disease.

— S aureus[17,84-86]

MSSA: oxacillin/nafcillin IV (AIII).

MRSA: vancomycin IV OR clindamycin IV if susceptible (AIII).

Duration of therapy depends on extent of disease (pneumonia vs pulmonary abscesses vs empyema) and should be individualized with therapy up to 21 days or longer.

Alternative for MSSA: cefazolin IV

Addition of rifampin or linezolid if persistently positive cultures (AIII)

Thoracostomy drainage of empyema

A. RECOMMENDED THERAPY FOR SELECTED NEWBORN CONDITIONS (continued)

Condition	Therapy (evidence grade) See Tables 5B–D for neonatal dosages.	Comments
– Group B streptococcus[87,88]	Penicillin G IV OR ampicillin IV, IM for 10 days (AIII)	For serious infections, ADD gentamicin for synergy until clinically improved. No prospective, randomized data on the efficacy of a 7-day treatment course.
– Ureaplasma spp (urealyticum or parvum)[89]	Azithromycin[90] PO, IV 20 mg/kg once daily for 3 days (BII)	Pathogenic role of Ureaplasma not well defined and no prophylaxis recommended for CLD Many Ureaplasma spp resistant to erythromycin Association of erythromycin and pyloric stenosis in young infants
Sepsis and meningitis[86,91,92]	NOTE: Duration of therapy: 10 days for sepsis without a focus (AIII); minimum of 21 days for Gram-negative meningitis (or at least 14 days after CSF is sterile) and 14–21 days for GBS meningitis and other Gram-positive bacteria (AIII)	There are no prospective, controlled studies on 5- or 7-day courses for mild or presumed sepsis.
– Initial therapy, organism unknown	Ampicillin IV AND a second agent, either cefotaxime IV or gentamicin IV, IM (AII)	Cefotaxime preferred if meningitis suspected or cannot be excluded clinically or by lumbar puncture (AIII). For locations with a high rate (≥10%) of ESBL-producing E coli, and empiric therapy with meropenem (or cefepime) is preferred over cefotaxime. For empiric therapy of sepsis without meningitis, in areas with a high rate of ESBL E coli, gentamicin is preferred. Initial empiric therapy of nosocomial infection should be based on each hospital's pathogens and susceptibilities. Always narrow antibiotic coverage once susceptibility data are available.
– Bacteroides fragilis	Metronidazole or meropenem IV, IM (AIII)	Alternative: clindamycin, but increasing resistance reported
– Enterococcus spp	Ampicillin IV, IM AND gentamicin IV, IM (AIII); for ampicillin-resistant organisms: vancomycin AND gentamicin (AIII)	Gentamicin needed with ampicillin or vancomycin for bactericidal activity; continue until clinical and microbiological response documented (AIII)

Organism	Therapy	Comments
		For vancomycin-resistant enterococci that are also ampicillin resistant: linezolid (AIII).
– Enterovirus	Supportive therapy; no antivirals currently FDA approved	Pocapavir PO is currently under investigation for enterovirus (poliovirus). Pleconaril PO is currently under consideration for approval at FDA for treatment of neonatal enteroviral sepsis syndrome.[93]
– E coli[91,92]	Cefotaxime IV or gentamicin IV, IM (AII)	Cefotaxime preferred if meningitis suspected or cannot be excluded clinically or by lumbar puncture (AII). For locations with a high rate (≥10%) of ESBL-producing E coli, and meningitis is suspected, empiric therapy with meropenem (or cefepime) is preferred over cefotaxime.
– Gonococcal[11–14]	Ceftriaxone IV, IM OR cefotaxime IV, IM, AND azithromycin 10 mg/kg PO q24h for 5 days (AIII)	Ceftriaxone no longer recommended as single agent therapy due to increasing cephalosporin resistance; therefore, addition of azithromycin recommended (no data in neonates; azithromycin dose is that recommended for pertussis). Cefotaxime is preferred for neonates with hyperbilirubinemia and those at risk for calcium drug interactions (see Table 5B).
– Listeria monocytogenes[94]	Ampicillin IV, IM AND gentamicin IV, IM (AIII)	Gentamicin is synergistic in vitro with ampicillin. Continue until clinical and microbiological response documented (AIII).
– P aeruginosa	Ceftazidime IV, IM AND tobramycin IV, IM (AIII)	Meropenem, cefepime, and tobramycin are suitable alternatives (AIII). Pip/tazo should not be used for CNS infection.
– S aureus[17,84–86,95,96]	MSSA: oxacillin/nafcillin IV, IM or cefazolin IV, IM (AII) MRSA: vancomycin IV (AIII)	Alternatives for MRSA: clindamycin, linezolid
– Staphylococcus epidermidis (or any coagulase-negative staphylococci)	Vancomycin IV (AIII)	If organism susceptible and infection not severe, oxacillin/nafcillin or cefazolin are alternatives for methicillin-susceptible strains. Cefazolin does not enter CNS. Add rifampin if cultures persistently positive.[97] Alternative: linezolid.
– Group A streptococcus	Penicillin G or ampicillin IV (AII)	

Antimicrobial Therapy for Newborns

5

A. RECOMMENDED THERAPY FOR SELECTED NEWBORN CONDITIONS (continued)

Condition	Therapy (evidence grade) See Tables 5B–D for neonatal dosages.	Comments
– Group B streptococcus[87]	Ampicillin or penicillin G IV AND gentamicin IV, IM (AI)	Continue gentamicin until clinical and microbiological response documented (AIII). Duration of therapy: 10 days for bacteremia/sepsis (AII); minimum of 14 days for meningitis (AII).
Skin and soft tissues		
– Breast abscess[98]	Oxacillin/nafcillin IV, IM (for MSSA) or vancomycin IV (for MRSA). ADD cefotaxime OR gentamicin if Gram-negative rods seen on Gram stain (AIII).	Gram stain of expressed pus guides empiric therapy; vancomycin if MRSA prevalent in community; alternative to vancomycin: clindamycin, linezolid, may need surgical drainage to minimize damage to breast tissue. Treatment duration individualized until clinical findings have completely resolved (AIII).
– Congenital cutaneous candidiasis[99]	Amphotericin B for 14 days, or 10 days if CSF culture negative (AII). Fluconazole alternative if Candida albicans or known sensitive Candida.	Treat promptly when rash presents with full IV dose, not prophylactic dosing or topical therapy. Diagnostic workup includes aerobic cultures of rash surface, blood, and CSF. Pathology examination of placenta and umbilical cord if possible.
– Erysipelas (and other group A streptococcal infections)	Penicillin G IV for 5–7 days, followed by oral therapy (if bacteremia not present) to complete a 10-day course (AIII)	Alternative: ampicillin. GBS may produce similar cellulitis or nodular lesions.
– Impetigo neonatorum	MSSA: oxacillin/nafcillin IV, IM OR cephalexin (AIII) MRSA: vancomycin IV for 5 days (AIII)	Systemic antibiotic therapy usually not required for superficial impetigo; local chlorhexidine cleansing may help with or without topical mupirocin (MRSA) or bacitracin (MSSA). Alternatives for MRSA: clindamycin IV, PO or linezolid IV, PO.
– S aureus[17,84,86,100]	MSSA: oxacillin/nafcillin IV, IM (AII) MRSA: vancomycin IV (AIII)	Surgical drainage may be required. MRSA may cause necrotizing fasciitis. Alternatives for MRSA: clindamycin IV or linezolid IV. Convalescent oral therapy if infection responds quickly to IV therapy.

– Group B streptococcus[87]	Penicillin G IV OR ampicillin IV, IM	Usually no pus formed Treatment course dependent on extent of infection, 7–14 days
Syphilis, congenital (<1 mo of age)[101]	During periods when availability of penicillin is compromised, contact CDC.	Evaluation and treatment do not depend on mother's HIV status. Obtain follow-up serology every 2–3 mo until nontreponemal test nonreactive or decreased 4-fold. If CSF positive, repeat spinal tap with CSF VDRL at 6 mo and, if abnormal, re-treat.
– Proven or highly probable disease: (1) abnormal physical examination; (2) serum quantitative nontreponemal serologic titer 4-fold higher than mother's titer; or (3) positive dark field or fluorescent antibody test of body fluid(s)	Aqueous penicillin G 50,000 U/kg/dose q12h (day of life 1–7), q8h (>7 days) IV OR procaine penicillin G 50,000 U/kg IM q24h for 10 days (AII)	Evaluation to determine type and duration of therapy: CSF analysis (VDRL, cell count, protein), CBC, and platelet count. Other tests, as clinically indicated, including long-bone radiographs, chest radiograph, liver function tests, cranial ultrasound, ophthalmologic examination, and hearing test (ABR). If >1 day of therapy is missed, entire course is restarted.
– Normal physical examination, serum quantitative nontreponemal serologic titer ≤maternal titer, and maternal treatment was (1) none, inadequate, or undocumented; (2) erythromycin, azithromycin, or other non-penicillin regimen; or (3) <4 wk before delivery.	Evaluation abnormal or not done completely: aqueous penicillin G 50,000 U/kg/dose q12h (day of life 1–7), q8h (>7 days) IV OR procaine penicillin G 50,000 U/kg IM q24h for 10 days (AII) Evaluation normal: aqueous penicillin G 50,000 U/kg/dose q12h (day of life 1–7), q8h (>7 days) IV OR procaine penicillin G 50,000 U/kg IM q24h for 10 days; OR benzathine penicillin G 50,000 units/kg/dose IM in a single dose (AII)	Evaluation: CSF analysis, CBC with platelets, long-bone radiographs. If >1 day of therapy is missed, entire course is restarted. Reliable follow-up important if only a single dose of benzathine penicillin given.

A. RECOMMENDED THERAPY FOR SELECTED NEWBORN CONDITIONS (continued)

Condition	Therapy (evidence grade) See Tables 5B–D for neonatal dosages.	Comments
– Normal physical examination, serum quantitative nontreponemal serologic titer ≤maternal titer, mother treated adequately during pregnancy and >4 wk before delivery; no evidence of reinfection or relapse in mother	Benzathine penicillin G 50,000 units/kg/dose IM in a single dose (AIII)	No evaluation required. Some experts would not treat but provide close serologic follow-up.
– Normal physical examination, serum quantitative nontreponemal serologic titer ≤maternal titer, mother's treatment adequate before pregnancy	No treatment	No evaluation required. Some experts would treat with benzathine penicillin G 50,000 U/kg as a single IM injection, particularly if follow-up is uncertain.
Syphilis, congenital (>1 mo of age)[101]	Aqueous crystalline penicillin G 200,000–300,000 U/kg/day IV div q4–6h for 10 days (AII)	Evaluation to determine type and duration of therapy: CSF analysis (VDRL, cell count, protein), CBC and platelet count. Other tests as clinically indicated, including long-bone radiographs, chest radiograph, liver function tests, neuroimaging, ophthalmologic examination, and hearing evaluation. If no clinical manifestations of disease, CSF examination is normal, and CSF VDRL test result is nonreactive, some specialists would treat with up to 3 weekly doses of benzathine penicillin G 50,000 U/kg IM.

Tetanus neonatorum[102]	Metronidazole IV, PO (alternative: penicillin G IV) for 10–14 days (AIII) Human TIG 3,000–6,000 U IM for 1 dose (AIII)	Some experts would provide a single dose of benzathine penicillin G 50,000 U/kg IM after 10 days of parenteral treatment, but value of this additional therapy is not well documented. Wound cleaning and debridement vital; IVIG (200–400 mg/kg) is an alternative if TIG not available; equine tetanus antitoxin not available in the United States but is alternative to TIG.
Toxoplasmosis, congenital[103,104]	Sulfadiazine 100 mg/kg/day PO div q12h AND pyrimethamine 2 mg/kg PO daily for 2 days (loading dose), then 1 mg/kg PO q24h for 2–6 mo, then 3 times weekly (M-W-F) up to 1 y (AII) Folinic acid (leucovorin) 10 mg 3 times weekly (AII)	Corticosteroids (1 mg/kg/day div q12h) if active chorioretinitis or CSF protein >1 g/dL (AIII). Start sulfa after neonatal jaundice has resolved. Therapy is only effective against active trophozoites, not cysts.
Urinary tract infection[105]	Initial empiric therapy with ampicillin AND gentamicin; OR ampicillin AND cefotaxime pending culture and susceptibility test results for 7–10 days	Investigate for kidney disease and abnormalities of urinary tract: VCUG indicated after first UTI. Oral therapy acceptable once neonate asymptomatic and culture sterile. No prophylaxis for grades 1–3 reflux.[106] In neonates with reflux, prophylaxis reduces recurrences but increases likelihood of recurrences being due to resistant organisms. Prophylaxis does not affect renal scarring.[101]
– Coliform bacteria (eg, *E coli, Klebsiella, Enterobacter, Serratia*)	Cefotaxime IV, IM OR, in absence of renal or perinephric abscess, gentamicin IV, IM for 7–10 days (AII)	Ampicillin used for susceptible organisms.
– *Enterococcus*	Ampicillin IV, IM for 7 days for cystitis, may need 10–14 days for pyelonephritis; add gentamicin until cultures are sterile (AIII); for ampicillin resistance, use vancomycin, add gentamicin until cultures are sterile.	Aminoglycoside needed with ampicillin or vancomycin for synergistic bactericidal activity (assuming organisms susceptible to an aminoglycoside).
– *P aeruginosa*	Ceftazidime IV, IM OR, in absence of renal or perinephric abscess, tobramycin IV, IM for 7–10 days (AIII)	Meropenem or cefepime are alternatives.

5

Antimicrobial Therapy for Newborns

A. RECOMMENDED THERAPY FOR SELECTED NEWBORN CONDITIONS (continued)

Condition	Therapy (evidence grade) See Tables 5B–D for neonatal dosages.	Comments
– *Candida* spp[31–33]	AmB-D (1 mg/kg/day) is recommended therapy (AII). Lipid formulation AmB is an alternative but carries a theoretical risk of less urinary tract penetration compared with AmB-D (CIII). Fluconazole (12 mg/kg/day q24h, after a load of 25 mg/kg/day) is an alternative if patient has not been on fluconazole prophylaxis (AII).[45] Duration of therapy for candidemia without obvious metastatic complications is for 2 wk after documented clearance and resolution of symptoms. Echinocandins should be used with caution and generally limited to salvage therapy or to situations in which resistance or toxicity preclude the use of AmB-D or fluconazole (CIII). Role of flucytosine in neonates with meningitis is questionable and not routinely recommended due to toxicity concerns. The addition of flucytosine (100 mg/kg/day div q6h) may be considered as salvage therapy in patients who have not had a clinical response to initial AmB therapy, but adverse effects are frequent (CIII).	Neonatal *Candida* disease is usually systemic; isolated UTI is uncommon. Treat *Candida* identified in the urine as systemic infection until proven otherwise. See Fungal infections earlier in Table. Echinocandins are not renally eliminated and should not be used to treat isolated neonatal UTI. Central venous catheter removal strongly recommended. Length of therapy dependent on disease (BIII), usually 2 wk after all clearance. Antifungal susceptibility testing is suggested with persistent disease. (*C krusei* inherently resistant to fluconazole; *C parapsilosis* may be less susceptible to echinocandins; *C glabrata* demonstrates increasing resistance to fluconazole and echinocandins.) No proven benefit for combination antifungal therapy in candidiasis. Change from AmB or fluconazole to micafungin/caspofungin if cultures persistently positive (BII). Although fluconazole prophylaxis has been shown to reduce colonization, it has not reduced mortality.[29] Lumbar puncture and dilated retinal examination recommended in neonates with cultures positive for *Candida* spp from blood (AIII). Same recommended for all infants with birth weight <1,500 g with candiduria with or without candidemia (AIII). CT or ultrasound imaging of genitourinary tract, liver, and spleen should be performed if blood cultures are persistently positive (AIII). Meningoencephalitis in the neonate occurs at a higher rate than in older children/adults. Infected CNS devices, including ventriculostomy drains and shunts, should be removed, if possible.

B. ANTIMICROBIAL DOSAGES FOR NEONATES—Lead author Jason Sauberan, assisted by the editors and John Van Den Anker

NOTE: This table contains empiric dosage recommendations for each agent listed. See Table 5A (Recommended Therapy for Selected Newborn Conditions) for more details of dosages for specific pathogens in specific tissue sites and for information on anti-influenza and antiretroviral drug dosages.

Antibiotic	Route	Chronologic Age ≤28 days				Chronologic Age 29–60 days
		Body Weight ≤2,000 g		Body Weight >2,000 g		
		0–7 days old	8–28 days old	0–7 days old	8–28 days old	
Acyclovir	IV	40 div q12h	60 div q8h	60 div q8h	60 div q8h	60 div q8h
	PO	—	$900/m^2$/day div q8h	—	$900/m^2$/day div q8h	$900/m^2$/day div q8h
Amoxicillin–clavulanate[a]	PO	—	—	30 div q12h	30 div q12h	30 div q12h
Amphotericin B						
– deoxycholate	IV	1 q24h	1 q24h	1 q24h	1 q24h	1 q24h
– lipid complex	IV	5 q24h	5 q24h	5 q24h	5 q24h	5 q24h
– liposomal	IV	5 q24h	5 q24h	5 q24h	5 q24h	5 q24h
Ampicillin[b]	IV, IM	100 div q12h	150 div q12h	150 div q8h	150 div q8h	200 div q6h
Anidulafungin[c]	IV	1.5 q24h	1.5 q24h	1.5 q24h	1.5 q24h	1.5 q24h
Azithromycin[d]	PO	10 q24h	10 q24h	10 q24h	10 q24h	10 q24h
	IV	10 q24h	10 q24h	10 q24h	10 q24h	10 q24h
Aztreonam	IV, IM	60 div q12h	90 div q8h[e]	90 div q8h	120 div q6h	120 div q6h

Only parenteral acyclovir should be used for the treatment of acute neonatal HSV disease. Oral suppression therapy for 6 mo duration after completion of initial neonatal HSV treatment. See text in Table 5A, Herpes simplex infection.

5

Antimicrobial Therapy for Newborns

Antimicrobial Therapy for Newborns

B. ANTIMICROBIAL DOSAGES FOR NEONATES (continued)—Lead author Jason Sauberan, assisted by the editors and John van den Anker

Antibiotic	Route	Dosages (mg/kg/day) and Intervals of Administration				Chronologic Age 29–60 days
		Chronological Age ≤28 days				
		Body Weight ≤2,000 g		Body Weight >2,000 g		
		0–7 days old	8–28 days old	0–7 days old	8–28 days old	
Caspofungin[f]	IV	25/m² q24h	25/m² q24h	25/m² q24h	25/m² q24h	25/m² q24h
Cefazolin	IV, IM	50 div q12h	75 div q8h[e]	50 div q12h	75 div q8h	75 div q8h
Cefepime	IV, IM	60 div q12h	60 div q12h	100 div q12h	100 div q12h	150 div q8h[g]
Cefotaxime	IV, IM	100 div q12h	150 div q8h[e]	100 div q12h	150 div q8h	200 div q6h
Cefoxitin	IV, IM	70 div q12h	100 div q8h[e]	100 div q8h	100 div q8h	120 div q6h
Ceftazidime	IV, IM	100 div q12h	150 div q8h[e]	100 div q12h	150 div q8h	150 div q8h
Ceftriaxone[h]	IV, IM	—	—	50 q24h	50 q24h	50 q24h
Cefuroxime	IV, IM	100 div q12h	150 div q8h[e]	100 div q12h	150 div q8h	150 div q8h
Chloramphenicol[i]	IV, IM	25 q24h	50 div q12h[e]	25 q24h	50 div q12h	50–100 div q6h
Clindamycin	IV, IM, PO	15 div q8h	15 div q8h	21 div q8h	27 div q8h	30 div q8h
Daptomycin (Potential neurotoxicity; use cautiously if no other options.)	IV	12 div q12h	12 div q12h	12 div q12h	12 div q12h	12 div q12h
Erythromycin	PO	40 div q6h	40 div q6h	40 div q6h	40 div q6h	40 div q6h
Fluconazole						
– treatment[j]	IV, PO	12 q24h	12 q24h	12 q24h	12 q24h	12 q24h
– prophylaxis	IV, PO	6 mg/kg/dose twice weekly	6 mg/kg/dose twice weekly	6 mg/kg/dose twice weekly	6 mg/kg/dose twice weekly	6 mg/kg/dose twice weekly

Drug	Route						
Flucytosine[k]	PO	100 div q6h[e]	100 div q6h	100 div q6h	100 div q6h[e]	100 div q6h	75 div q8h
Ganciclovir	IV	Insufficient data	12 div q12h	12 div q12h	Insufficient data	12 div q12h	Insufficient data
Linezolid	IV, PO	30 div q8h	30 div q8h	30 div q8h	30 div q8h	30 div q8h	20 div q12h
Meropenem							
– sepsis, IAI[l]	IV	90 div q8h	90 div q8h	60 div q8h	60 div q8h[l]	60 div q8h	40 div q12h
– meningitis	IV	120 div q8h	120 div q8h	120 div q8h	120 div q8h[l]	120 div q8h	80 div q12h
Metronidazole[m]	IV, PO	30 div q8h	30 div q8h	22.5 div q8h	15 div q12h	15 div q12h	15 div q12h
Micafungin	IV	10 q24h	10 q24h	10 q24h	10 q24h	10 q24h	10 q24h
Nafcillin,[n] oxacillin[n]	IV, IM	150 div q6h	100 div q6h	75 div q8h	75 div q8h[e]	75 div q8h	50 div q12h
Penicillin G benzathine	IM	50,000 U	50,000 U	50,000 U	50,000 U	50,000 U	50,000 U
Penicillin G crystalline (GBS sepsis, congenital syphilis)	IV	200,000 U div q6h	150,000 U div q8h	100,000 U div q12h	150,000 U div q8h	100,000 U div q12h	100,000 U div q12h
Penicillin G crystalline (GBS meningitis)	IV	400,000 U div q6h	400,000 U div q6h	400,000 U div q6h	400,000 U div q6h	400,000 U div q6h	400,000 U div q6h
Penicillin G procaine	IM	50,000 U q24h	50,000 U q24h	50,000 U q24h	50,000 U q24h	50,000 U q24h	50,000 U q24h
Piperacillin/tazobactam	IV	320 div q6h	320 div q6h	320 div q6h	320 div q6h[o]	320 div q6h	300 div q8h
Rifampin	IV, PO	10 q24h	10 q24h	10 q24h	10 q24h	10 q24h	10 q24h
Valganciclovir	PO	32 div q12h	32 div q12h	32 div q12h	Insufficient data	32 div q12h	Insufficient data
Voriconazole[p]	IV	16 div q12h	16 div q12h	16 div q12h	16 div q12h	16 div q12h	16 div q12h

5

Antimicrobial Therapy for Newborns

B. ANTIMICROBIAL DOSAGES FOR NEONATES (continued)—Lead author Jason Sauberan, assisted by the editors and John van den Anker

Antibiotic	Route	Dosages (mg/kg/day) and Intervals of Administration				Chronologic Age 29–60 days
		Chronologic Age ≤28 days				
		Body Weight ≤2,000 g		Body Weight >2,000 g		
		0–7 days old	8–28 days old	0–7 days old	8–28 days old	
Zidovudine	IV	3 div q12h[q]	3 div q12h[q]	6 div q12h	6 div q12h	See Table 5A, Human immunodeficiency virus infection.
	PO	4 div q12h[q]	4 div q12h[q]	8 div q12h	8 div q12h	See Table 5A, Human immunodeficiency virus infection.

[a] 25- or 50-mg/mL concentration.

[b] 300 mg/kg/day for GBS meningitis div q8h for all neonates ≤7 days of age and q6h >7 days of age.

[c] Loading dose 3 mg/kg followed 24 h later by maintenance dose listed.

[d] See Table 5A for pathogen-specific dosing.

[e] Use 0–7 days old dosing until 14 days old if birth weight <1,000 g.

[f] Higher dosage of 50 mg/m² may be needed for Aspergillus.

[g] May require infusion over 3 h, or 200 mg/kg/day div q6h, to treat organisms with MIC ≥8 mg/L.

[h] Usually avoided in neonates. Can be considered for transitioning to outpatient treatment of GBS bacteremia in well-appearing neonates at low risk for hyperbilirubinemia. Contraindicated if concomitant intravenous calcium; see Pediatrics. 2009;123(4):e609–e613.

[i] Desired serum concentration 15–25 mg/L.

[j] Loading dose 25 mg/kg followed 24 h later by maintenance dose listed.

[k] Desired serum concentrations peak 50–100 mg/L, trough 25–50 mg/L. Dose range 50–100 mg/kg/day.

[l] Adjust dosage after 14 days of age instead of after 7 days of age.

[m] Loading dose 15 mg/kg.

[n] Double the dose for meningitis.

[o] When PMA reaches >30 weeks.

[p] Initial loading dose of 18 mg/kg div q12h on day 1. Desired serum concentrations, trough 2–5 mg/L. See Table 5A, Aspergillosis.

[q] Starting dose if gestational age <35+0 wk and postnatal ≤14 days. See Table 5A, Human immunodeficiency virus infection, for ZDV dosage after 2 wk of age and for NVP

Empiric Dosage (mg/kg/dose) by Gestational and Postnatal Age

Medication	Route	<30 wk		30–34 wk		≥35 wk	
		0–14 days	>14 days	0–10 days	>10 days	0–7 days	>7 days[a]
Amikacin[b]	IV, IM	15 q48h	15 q24h	15 q24h	15 q24h	15 q24h	17.5 q24h
Gentamicin[c]	IV, IM	5 q48h	5 q36h	5 q36h	5 q36h	4 q24h	5 q24h
Tobramycin[c]	IV, IM	5 q48h	5 q36h	5 q36h	5 q36h	4 q24h	5 q24h

[a] If >60 days of age, see Chapter 11.
[b] Desired serum concentrations: 20–35 mg/L or 10 × MIC (peak), <7 mg/L (trough).
[c] Desired serum concentrations: 6–12 mg/L or 10 × MIC (peak), <2 mg/L (trough).

D. VANCOMYCIN[a,b,c]

Empiric Dosage (mg/kg/dose) by Gestational Age and Serum Creatinine (Begin with a 20 mg/kg loading dose.)

≤28 wk			>28 wk		
Serum Creatinine	Dose	Frequency	Serum Creatinine	Dose	Frequency
<0.5	15	q12h	<0.7	15	q12h
0.5–0.7	20	q24h	0.7–0.9	20	q24h
0.8–1.0	15	q24h	1.0–1.2	15	q24h
1.1–1.4	10	q24h	1.3–1.6	10	q24h
>1.4	15	q48h	>1.6	15	q48h

[a] Serum creatinine concentrations normally fluctuate and are partly influenced by transplacental maternal creatinine in the first wk after birth. Cautious use of creatinine-based dosing strategy with frequent reassessment of renal function and vancomycin serum concentrations are recommended in neonates ≤7 days old.
[b] Desired serum concentrations; a 24-h AUC:MIC of 400 mg·h/L is recommended based on adult studies of invasive MRSA infections. The AUC is best calculated from 2 concentrations (ie, peak and trough) rather than 1 trough serum concentration measurement. In situations in which AUC calculation is not feasible, a trough concentration 10–12 mg/L is very highly likely (>90%) to achieve the goal AUC target in neonates when the MIC is 1 mg/L.
[c] If >60 days of age, see Chapter 11.

5

Antimicrobial Therapy for Newborns

E. Use of Antimicrobials During Pregnancy or Breastfeeding

The use of antimicrobials during pregnancy and lactation should balance benefit to the mother with the risk of fetal and infant toxicity (including anatomic anomalies with fetal exposure). A number of factors determine the degree of transfer of antibiotics across the placenta: lipid solubility, degree of ionization, molecular weight, protein binding, placental maturation, and placental and fetal blood flow. The FDA traditionally provided 5 categories to indicate the level of risk to the fetus: (1) Category A: fetal harm seems remote, as controlled studies have not demonstrated a risk to the fetus; (2) Category B: animal reproduction studies have not shown a fetal risk, but no controlled studies in pregnant women have been done, or animal studies have shown an adverse effect that has not been confirmed in human studies (penicillin, amoxicillin, ampicillin, cephalexin/cefazolin, azithromycin, clindamycin, vancomycin, zanamivir); (3) Category C: studies in animals have shown an adverse effect on the fetus, but there are no studies in women; the potential benefit of the drug may justify the possible risk to the fetus (chloramphenicol, ciprofloxacin, gentamicin, levofloxacin, oseltamivir, rifampin); (4) Category D: evidence exists of human fetal risk, but the benefits may outweigh such risk (doxycycline); (5) Category X: the drug is contraindicated because animal or human studies have shown fetal abnormalities or fetal risk (ribavirin). Prescription drugs approved after June 30, 2015, are required to conform to a new pregnancy risk labeling format.[107]

Fetal serum antibiotic concentrations (or cord blood concentrations) following maternal administration have not been systematically studied.[108] The following commonly used drugs appear to achieve fetal concentrations that are equal to or only slightly less than those in the mother: penicillin G, amoxicillin, ampicillin, sulfonamides, trimethoprim, and tetracyclines, as well as oseltamivir.[109] The aminoglycoside concentrations in fetal serum are 20% to 50% of those in maternal serum. Cephalosporins, carbapenems, nafcillin, oxacillin, clindamycin, and vancomycin[110] penetrate poorly (10%–30%), and fetal concentrations of erythromycin and azithromycin are less than 10% of those in the mother.

The most current, updated information on the pharmacokinetics and safety of antimicrobials and other agents in human milk can be found at the National Library of Medicine LactMed Web site (http://toxnet.nlm.nih.gov/newtoxnet/lactmed.htm; accessed October 2, 2017).[111]

In general, neonatal exposure to antimicrobials in human milk is minimal or insignificant. Aminoglycosides, beta-lactams, ciprofloxacin, clindamycin, macrolides, fluconazole, and agents for tuberculosis are considered safe for the mother to take during breastfeeding.[112] The most common reported neonatal side effect of maternal antimicrobial use during breastfeeding is increased stool output. Clinicians should recommend mothers alert their pediatric health care professional if stool output changes occur. Maternal treatment with sulfa-containing antibiotics should be approached with caution in the breastfed infant who is jaundiced or ill.

6. Antimicrobial Therapy According to Clinical Syndromes

NOTES

- This chapter should be considered a rough guidance for a typical patient. Dosage recommendations are for patients with relatively normal hydration, renal function, and hepatic function. Because the dose required is based on the exposure of the antibiotic to the pathogen at the site of infection, higher dosages may be necessary if the antibiotic does not penetrate well into the infected tissue (eg, meningitis) or if the child eliminates the antibiotic from the body more quickly than average. Higher dosages/longer courses may also be needed if the child is immunocompromised and the immune system cannot help clear the infection, as it is becoming clearer that the host contributes significantly to microbiologic and clinical cure above and beyond the antimicrobial-attributable effect.

- Duration of treatment should be individualized. Those recommended are based on the literature, common practice, and general experience. Critical evaluations of duration of therapy have been carried out in very few infectious diseases. In general, a longer duration of therapy should be used (1) for tissues in which antibiotic concentrations may be relatively low (eg, undrained abscess, central nervous system [CNS] infection); (2) for tissues in which repair following infection-mediated damage is slow (eg, bone); (3) when the organisms are less susceptible; (4) when a relapse of infection is unacceptable (eg, CNS infections); or (5) when the host is immunocompromised in some way. An assessment after therapy will ensure that your selection of antibiotic, dose, and duration of therapy were appropriate. Until prospective, comparative studies are performed for different durations, we cannot assign a specific increased risk of failure for shorter courses. We support the need for these studies in a controlled clinical research setting, either outpatient or inpatient.

- Diseases in this chapter are arranged by body systems. Please consult the index for the alphabetized listing of diseases and chapters 7 through 10 for the alphabetized listing of pathogens and for uncommon organisms not included in this chapter.

- A more detailed description of treatment options for methicillin-resistant *Staphylococcus aureus* infections and multidrug resistant Gram-negative bacilli infections is provided in Chapter 4.

- Therapy of *Pseudomonas aeruginosa* systemic infections has evolved from intravenous (IV) ceftazidime plus tobramycin to single-drug IV therapy with cefepime for most infections in immune-competent children, due to the relative stability of cefepime to beta-lactamases, compared with ceftazidime. Oral therapy with ciprofloxacin has replaced IV therapy in otherwise normal children who are compliant and able to take oral therapy, particularly for "step-down" therapy of invasive infections.

- **Abbreviations:** AAP, American Academy of Pediatrics; ADH, antidiuretic hormone; AFB, acid-fast bacilli; AHA, American Heart Association; ALT, alanine transaminase; AmB, amphotericin B; amox/clav, amoxicillin/clavulanate; AOM, acute otitis media;

ARF, acute rheumatic fever; AST, aspartate transaminase; AUC:MIC, area under the serum concentration vs time curve: minimum inhibitory concentration; bid, twice daily; CA-MRSA, community-associated methicillin-resistant *Staphylococcus aureus;* cap, capsule; CDC, Centers for Disease Control and Prevention; CMV, cytomegalo-virus; CNS, central nervous system; CRP, C-reactive protein; CSD, cat-scratch disease; CSF, cerebrospinal fluid; CT, computed tomography; DAT, diphtheria antitoxin; div, divided; DOT, directly observed therapy; EBV, Epstein-Barr virus; ESBL, extended spectrum beta-lactamase; ESR, erythrocyte sedimentation rate; ETEC, enterotoxin-producing *Escherichia coli;* FDA, US Food and Drug Administration; GI, gastrointes-tinal; HACEK, *Haemophilus aphrophilus, Aggregatibacter* (formerly *Actinobacillus) actinomycetemcomitans, Cardiobacterium hominis, Eikenella corrodens, Kingella* spp; HIV, human immunodeficiency virus; HSV, herpes simplex virus; HUS, hemolytic uremic syndrome; I&D, incision and drainage; IDSA, Infectious Diseases Society of America; IM, intramuscular; INH, isoniazid; IV, intravenous; IVIG, intravenous immune globulin; KPC, *Klebsiella pneumoniae* carbapenemase; L-AmB, liposomal amphotericin B; LFT, liver function test; LP, lumbar puncture; MDR, multidrug resis-tant; MRI, magnetic resonance imaging; MRSA, methicillin-resistant *S aureus;* MRSE, methicillin-resistant *Staphylococcus epidermidis;* MSSA, methicillin-susceptible *S aureus;* MSSE, methicillin-sensitive *S epidermidis;* ophth, ophthalmic; PCR, poly-merase chain reaction; PCV13, Prevnar 13-valent pneumococcal conjugate vaccine; pen-R, penicillin-resistant; pen-S, penicillin-susceptible; PIDS, Pediatric Infectious Diseases Society; pip/tazo, piperacillin/tazobactam; PMA, post-menstrual age; PO, oral; PPD, purified protein derivative; PZA, pyrazinamide; qd, once daily; qid, 4 times daily; qod, every other day; RIVUR, Randomized Intervention for Children with Vesicoureteral Reflux; RSV, respiratory syncytial virus; soln, solution; SPAG-2, small particle aerosol generator-2; spp, species; STEC, Shiga toxin-producing *E coli;* STI, sex-ually transmitted infection; tab, tablet; TB, tuberculosis; Td, tetanus, diphtheria; Tdap, tetanus, diphtheria, acellular pertussis; ticar/clav, ticarcillin/clavulanate; tid, 3 times daily; TIG, tetanus immune globulin; TMP/SMX, trimethoprim/sulfamethoxazole; ULN, upper limit of normal; UTI, urinary tract infection; VDRL, Venereal Disease Research Laboratories; WBC, white blood cell.

A. SKIN AND SOFT TISSUE INFECTIONS

Clinical Diagnosis	Therapy (evidence grade)	Comments
NOTE: CA-MRSA (see Chapter 4) is prevalent in most areas of the world. Recommendations for staphylococcal infections are given for 2 scenarios: standard and CA-MRSA. Antibiotic recommendations "for CA-MRSA" should be used for empiric therapy in regions with greater than 5% to 10% of invasive staphylococcal infections caused by MRSA, in situations where CA-MRSA is suspected, and for documented CA-MRSA infections, while "standard recommendations" refer to treatment of MSSA. During the past few years, clindamycin resistance in MRSA has increased to 40% in some areas but remained stable at 5% in others, although this increase may be an artifact of changes in reporting, with many laboratories now reporting all clindamycin-susceptible but D-test-positive strains as resistant. Please check your local susceptibility data for *Staphylococcus aureus* before using clindamycin for empiric therapy. For MSSA, oxacillin/nafcillin are considered equivalent agents.		
Adenitis, acute bacterial[1–7] (*S aureus*, including CA-MRSA, and group A streptococcus; consider *Bartonella* [CSD] for subacute adenitis.)[8]	Empiric therapy Standard: oxacillin/nafcillin 150 mg/kg/day IV div q6h OR cefazolin 100 mg/kg/day IV div q8h (AI); OR cephalexin 50–75 mg/kg/day PO div qid CA-MRSA: clindamycin 30 mg/kg/day IV or PO (AI) div q8h OR ceftaroline: 2 mo—<2 y, 24 mg/kg/ day IV div q8h; ≥2 y, 36 mg/kg/day IV div q8h (max single dose 400 mg); >33 kg, either 400 mg/dose IV q8h or 600 mg/dose IV q12h (BI), OR vancomycin 40 mg/kg/day IV q8h (BII), OR daptomycin: 1–<2 y, 10 mg/kg IV qd; 2–6 y, 9 mg/kg IV qd; 7–11 y, 7 mg/kg qd; 12–17 y, 5 mg/kg qd (BI) CSD: azithromycin 12 mg/kg qd (max 500 mg) for 5 days (BIII)	Avoid daptomycin in infants until 1 y due to potential toxicity. May need surgical drainage for staph/strep infection; not usually needed for CSD. Following drainage of mild to moderate suppurative adenitis caused by staph or strep, additional antibiotics may not be required. For oral therapy for MSSA: cephalexin or amox/clav; for CA-MRSA: clindamycin, TMP/SMX, or linezolid. For oral therapy of group A strep: amoxicillin or penicillin V. Total IV plus PO therapy for 7–10 days. For CSD: this is the same high dose of azithromycin that is recommended routinely for strep pharyngitis.
Adenitis, nontuberculous (atypical) mycobacterial[9–12]	Excision usually curative (BII); azithromycin PO OR clarithromycin PO for 6–12 wk (with or without rifampin) if susceptible (BII)	Antibiotic susceptibility patterns are quite variable; cultures should guide therapy: excision >97% effective; medical therapy 60%–70% effective. Newer data suggest toxicity of antimicrobials may not be worth the small clinical benefit of medical therapy over surgery.

6

Antimicrobial Therapy According to Clinical Syndromes

Antimicrobial Therapy According to Clinical Syndromes

A. SKIN AND SOFT TISSUE INFECTIONS (continued)

Clinical Diagnosis	Therapy (evidence grade)	Comments
Adenitis, tuberculous[13,14] (*Mycobacterium tuberculosis* and *Mycobacterium bovis*)	INH 10–15 mg/kg/day (max 300 mg) PO, IV qd, for 6 mo AND rifampin 10–20 mg/kg/day (max 600 mg) PO, IV qd, for 6 mo AND PZA 20–40 mg/kg/day PO qd for first 2 mo therapy (BI); if suspected multidrug resistance, add ethambutol 20 mg/kg/day PO qd.	Surgical excision usually not indicated because organisms are treatable. Adenitis caused by *M bovis* (unpasteurized dairy product ingestion) is uniformly resistant to PZA. Treat 9–12 mo with INH and rifampin, if susceptible (BII). No contraindication to fine needle aspirate of node for diagnosis.
Anthrax, cutaneous[15]	Empiric therapy: ciprofloxacin 20–30 mg/kg/day PO div bid OR doxycycline 4 mg/kg/day (max 200 mg) PO div bid (regardless of age) (AIII)	If susceptible, amoxicillin or clindamycin (BIII). Ciprofloxacin and levofloxacin are FDA approved for inhalational anthrax and should be effective for skin infection (BIII).
Bites, dog and cat[1,16-20] (*Pasteurella multocida*; *S aureus*, including CA-MRSA; — *Streptococcus* spp, anaerobes; *Capnocytophaga canimorsus*, particularly in asplenic hosts)	Amox/clav 45 mg/kg/day PO div tid (amox/clav 7:1; see Chapter 1, Aminopenicillins) for 5–10 days (AII); for hospitalized children, use ampicillin AND clindamycin (BII) OR ceftriaxone AND clindamycin (BII) OR cefaroline: 2 mo–<2 y, 24 mg/kg/day IV div q8h; ≥2 y, 36 mg/kg/day IV div q8h (max single dose 400 mg); >33 kg, either 400 mg/dose IV q8h or 600 mg/dose IV q12h (BII).	Amox/clav has good *Pasteurella*, MSSA, and anaerobic coverage but lacks MRSA coverage. Ampicillin/amox plus clindamycin has good *Pasteurella*, MSSA, MRSA, and anaerobic coverage. Ceftaroline has good *Pasteurella*, MSSA, and MRSA coverage but lacks *Bacteroides fragilis* anaerobic coverage.[21] Ampicillin/sulbactam also lacks MRSA coverage. Consider rabies prophylaxis[22] for bites from at-risk animals (observe animal for 10 days, if possible) (AI); consider tetanus prophylaxis. For penicillin allergy, ciprofloxacin (for *Pasteurella*) plus clindamycin (BIII). Doxycycline may be considered for *Pasteurella* coverage.
Bites, human[1,19,23] (*Eikenella corrodens*; *S aureus*, including CA-MRSA; — *Streptococcus* spp, anaerobes)	Amox/clav 45 mg/kg/day PO div tid (amox/clav 7:1; see Chapter 1, Aminopenicillins) for 5–10 days (AII); for hospitalized children, use ampicillin and clindamycin (BII) OR ceftriaxone and clindamycin (BII).	Human bites have a very high rate of infection (do not routinely close open wounds). Amox/clav has good *Eikenella*, MSSA, and anaerobic coverage but lacks MRSA coverage. Ampicillin/sulbactam also lacks MRSA coverage.

6

	For penicillin allergy, ciprofloxacin (for *Pasteurella*) plus clindamycin (BIII). Doxycycline and TMP-SMX may be considered for *Pasteurella* coverage.
Bullous impetigo [1,2,5,6] (usually *S aureus*, including CA-MRSA)	Standard: cephalexin 50–75 mg/kg/day PO div tid OR amox/clav 45 mg/kg/day PO div tid (CII) CA-MRSA: clindamycin 30 mg/kg/day PO div tid OR TMP/SMX 8 mg/kg/day of TMP PO div bid; for 5–7 days (CI)	For topical therapy if mild infection: mupirocin or retapamulin ointment
Cellulitis of unknown etiology (usually *S aureus*, including CA-MRSA, or group A streptococcus) [1–3,5–7,24–26]	Empiric IV therapy Standard: oxacillin/nafcillin 150 mg/kg/day IV div q6h OR cefazolin 100 mg/kg/day IV div q8h (BII) CA-MRSA: clindamycin 30 mg/kg/day IV div q8h OR ceftaroline: 2 mo—<2 y, 36 mg/kg/day IV div q8h (max single dose 400 mg); ≥2 y, either 400 mg/dose IV q8h or 600 mg/dose IV q12h (BII) OR vancomycin 40 mg/kg/day IV q8h (BII) OR daptomycin: 1—<2 y, 10 mg/kg IV qd; 2–6 y, 9 mg/kg IV qd; 7–11 y, 7 mg/kg qd; 12–17 y, 5 mg/kg qd (BI) For oral therapy for MSSA: cephalexin (AII) OR amox/clav 45 mg/kg/day PO div tid (BII); for CA-MRSA: clindamycin (BII), TMP/SMX (AII), or linezolid (BII)	For periorbital or buccal cellulitis, also consider *Streptococcus pneumoniae* or *Haemophilus influenzae* type b in unimmunized infants. Total IV plus PO therapy for 7–10 days. Since nonsuppurative cellulitis is most often caused by group A streptococcus, cephalexin alone is usually effective.
Cellulitis, buccal (for unimmunized infants and preschool-aged children, *H influenzae* type b) [27]	Cefotaxime 100–150 mg/kg/day IV div q8h OR ceftriaxone 50 mg/kg/day (AI) IV, IM q24h; for 2–7 days parenteral therapy before switch to oral (BII)	Rule out meningitis (larger dosages may be needed). For penicillin allergy, levofloxacin IV/PO covers pathogens, but no clinical data available. Oral therapy: amoxicillin if beta-lactamase negative; amox/clav or oral 2nd- or 3rd-generation cephalosporin if beta-lactamase positive.

6

Antimicrobial Therapy According to Clinical Syndromes

Antimicrobial Therapy According to Clinical Syndromes

A. SKIN AND SOFT TISSUE INFECTIONS (continued)

Clinical Diagnosis	Therapy (evidence grade)	Comments
Cellulitis, erysipelas (streptococcal)[1,2,7,28]	Penicillin G 100,000–200,000 U/kg/day IV div q4–6h (BII) initially, then penicillin V 100 mg/kg/day PO div qid (BIII) or tid OR amoxicillin 50 mg/kg/day PO tid (BIII) for 10 days	Clindamycin and macrolides are also effective.
Gas gangrene (See Necrotizing fasciitis.)		
Impetigo (S aureus, including CA-MRSA; occasionally group A streptococcus)[1,2,6,7,29,30]	Mupirocin OR retapamulin topically (BII) to lesions tid; OR for more extensive lesions, oral therapy Standard: cephalexin 50–75 mg/kg/day PO div tid OR amox/clav 45 mg/kg/day PO div tid (AII) CA-MRSA: clindamycin 30 mg/kg/day PO div tid OR TMP/SMX 8 mg/kg/day TMP PO div bid (AII); for 5–7 days	
Ludwig angina[31]	Penicillin G 200,000–250,000 U/kg/day IV div q6h AND clindamycin 40 mg/kg/day IV div q8h (CIII)	Alternatives: ceftriaxone/clindamycin, meropenem, imipenem, pip/tazo if Gram-negative aerobic bacilli also suspected (CIII); high risk of respiratory tract obstruction from inflammatory edema
Lymphadenitis (See Adenitis, acute bacterial.)		
Lymphangitis (usually group A streptococcus)[1,2,7]	Penicillin G 200,000 U/kg/day IV div q6h (BII) initially, then penicillin V 100 mg/kg/day PO div qid OR amoxicillin 50 mg/kg/day PO div tid for 10 days	Cefazolin IV (for group A strep or MSSA) or clindamycin IV (for group A strep, most MSSA and MRSA) For mild disease, penicillin V 50 mg/kg/day PO div qid for 10 days Some recent reports of S aureus as a cause
Myositis, suppurative[32] (S aureus, including CA-MRSA; synonyms: tropical myositis, pyomyositis)	Standard: oxacillin/nafcillin 150 mg/kg/day IV div q6h OR cefazolin 100 mg/kg/day IV div q8h (CII)	Surgical debridement is usually necessary.

	CA-MRSA: clindamycin 40 mg/kg/day IV div q8h OR ceftaroline: 2 mo–<2 y, 24 mg/kg/day IV div q8h; ≥2 y, 36 mg/kg/day IV div q8h (max single dose 400 mg); >33 kg, either 400 mg/dose IV q8h or 600 mg/dose IV q12h (BI) OR vancomycin 40 mg/kg/day IV q8h (CIII) OR daptomycin: 1–<2 y, 10 mg/kg IV qd; 2–6 y, 9 mg/kg IV qd; 7–11 y, 7 mg/kg qd; 12–17 y, 5 mg/kg qd (BIII)	Aggressive, emergent debridement; use clindamycin to help decrease toxin production (BIII); consider IVIG to bind bacterial toxins for life-threatening disease (CIII); abscesses may develop with CA-MRSA while on therapy.
Necrotizing fasciitis (Pathogens vary depending on the age of the child and location of infection. Single pathogen: group A streptococcus; *Clostridia* spp, *S aureus* [including CA-MRSA], *Pseudomonas aeruginosa, Vibrio* spp, *Aeromonas.* Multiple pathogen, mixed aerobic/anaerobic synergistic fasciitis: any organism[s] above, plus Gram-negative bacilli, plus *Bacteroides* spp, and other anaerobes.)[1,33–36]	Empiric therapy: ceftazidime 150 mg/kg/day IV div q8h, or cefepime 150 mg/kg/day IV div q8h or cefotaxime 200 mg/kg/day IV div q6h AND clindamycin 40 mg/kg/day IV div q8h (BIII); OR meropenem 60 mg/kg/day IV div q8h; OR pip/tazo 400 mg/kg/day pip component IV div q6h (AIII). ADD vancomycin OR ceftaroline for suspect CA-MRSA, pending culture results (AIII). Group A streptococcal: penicillin G 200,000–250,000 U/kg/day div q6h AND clindamycin 40 mg/kg/day div q8h (AIII). Mixed aerobic/anaerobic/Gram-negative: meropenem or pip/tazo AND clindamycin (AIII).	Aggressive emergent wound debridement (AII). ADD clindamycin to inhibit synthesis of toxins during the first few days of therapy (AIII). If CA-MRSA identified and susceptible to clindamycin, additional vancomycin is not required. Consider IVIG to bind bacterial toxins for life-threatening disease (BIII). Value of hyperbaric oxygen is not established (CIII).[37] Focus definitive antimicrobial therapy based on culture results.
Pyoderma, cutaneous abscesses (*S aureus,* including CA-MRSA; group A streptococcus)[2,3,5–7,24,25,38–40]	Standard: cephalexin 50–75 mg/kg/day PO div tid OR amox/clav 45 mg/kg/day PO div tid (BII) CA-MRSA: clindamycin 30 mg/kg/day PO div tid (BII) OR TMP/SMX 8 mg/kg/day of TMP PO div bid (AI)	I&D when indicated; IV for serious infections. For prevention of recurrent CA-MRSA infection, use bleach baths twice weekly (½ cup of bleach per full bathtub) (BII), OR bathe with chlorhexidine soap daily or qod (BIII). Decolonization with nasal mupirocin may also be helpful, as is decolonization of the entire family.[41]
Rat-bite fever (*Streptobacillus moniliformis, Spirillum minus*)[42]	Penicillin G 100,000–200,000 U/kg/day IV div q6h (BII) for 7–10 days; for endocarditis, ADD gentamicin for 4–6 wk (CIII). For mild disease, oral therapy with amox/clav (CIII).	Organisms are normal oral flora for rodents. High rate of associated endocarditis. Alternatives: doxycycline; 2nd- and 3rd-generation cephalosporins (CIII).

Antimicrobial Therapy According to Clinical Syndromes

A. SKIN AND SOFT TISSUE INFECTIONS (continued)

Clinical Diagnosis	Therapy (evidence grade)	Comments
Staphylococcal scalded skin syndrome[6,43,44]	Standard: oxacillin 150 mg/kg/day IV div q6h OR cefazolin 100 mg/kg/day IV div q8h (CII) CA-MRSA: clindamycin 30 mg/kg/day IV div q8h (CIII) OR ceftaroline: 2 mo—<2 y, 24 mg/kg/day IV div q8h; ≥2 y, 36 mg/kg/day IV div q8h (max single dose 400 mg); >33 kg, either 400 mg/dose IV q8h or 600 mg/dose IV q12h (BI), OR vancomycin 40 mg/kg/day IV q8h (CIII) OR daptomycin: 1–<2 y, 10 mg/kg IV qd; 2–6 y, 9 mg/kg IV qd; 7–11 y, 7 mg/kg qd; 12–17 y, 5 mg/kg qd (BI)	Burow or Zephiran compresses for oozing skin and intertriginous areas. Corticosteroids are contraindicated.

B. SKELETAL INFECTIONS

Clinical Diagnosis	Therapy (evidence grade)	Comments

NOTE: CA-MRSA (see Chapter 4) is prevalent in most areas of the world. Recommendations are given for CA-MRSA and MSSA. Antibiotic recommendations for empiric therapy should include CA-MRSA when it is suspected or documented, while treatment for MSSA with beta-lactam antibiotics (eg, cephalexin) is preferred over clindamycin. During the past few years, clindamycin resistance in MRSA has increased to 40% in some areas but remained stable at 5% in others, although this increase may be an artifact of changes in reporting, with many laboratories now reporting all clindamycin-susceptible but D-test–positive strains as resistant. Please check your local susceptibility data for *Staphylococcus aureus* before using clindamycin for empiric therapy. For MSSA, oxacillin/nafcillin are considered equivalent agents. The first pediatric-specific PIDS/IDSA guidelines for bacterial osteomyelitis and bacterial arthritis are currently being written.

Arthritis, bacterial[45–50]	Switch to appropriate high-dose oral therapy when clinically improved, CRP decreasing (see Chapter 13).[47,51,52]	
– Newborns	See Chapter 5.	

	Empiric therapy	Comments
– Infants (S aureus, including CA-MRSA; group A streptococcus; Kingella kingae; in unimmunized or immunocompromised children: pneumococcus, Haemophilus influenzae type b) — Children (S aureus, including CA-MRSA; group A streptococcus; K kingae) For Lyme disease and brucellosis, see page 115 in Table 6L, Miscellaneous Systemic Infections.	Empiric therapy: clindamycin (to cover CA-MRSA unless clindamycin resistance locally is >10%, then use vancomycin). For serious infections, ADD cefazolin to provide better MSSA coverage and add Kingella coverage. See Comments for discussion of dexamethasone adjunctive therapy. For CA-MRSA: clindamycin 30 mg/kg/day IV div q8h (AI) OR ceftaroline: 2 mo–<2 y, 24 mg/kg/day IV div q8h; ≥2 y, 36 mg/kg/day IV div q8h (max single dose 400 mg); >33 kg, either 400 mg/dose IV q8h or 600 mg/dose IV q12h (BI) OR vancomycin 40 mg/kg/day IV div q8h (BI). For MSSA: oxacillin/nafcillin 150 mg/kg/day IV div q6h OR cefazolin 100 mg/kg/day IV div q8h (AI). For Kingella: cefazolin 100 mg/kg/day IV div q8h OR ampicillin 150 mg/kg/day IV div q6h, OR ceftriaxone 50 mg/kg/day IV, IM q24h (AII). For pen-S pneumococci or group A streptococcus: penicillin G 200,000 U/kg/day IV div q6h (BII). For pen-R pneumococci or Haemophilus: ceftriaxone 50–75 mg/kg/day IV, IM q24h, OR cefotaxime (BII). Total therapy (IV plus PO) for up to 21 days with normal ESR; low-risk, non-hip MSSA arthritis may respond to a 10-day course (AII).[49]	Dexamethasone adjunctive therapy (0.15 mg/kg/dose every 6 h for 4 days in one study) demonstrated significant benefit in decreasing symptoms and earlier hospital discharge (but with some "rebound" symptoms).[53,54] NOTE: children with rheumatologic, postinfectious fungal/mycobacterial infections or malignant conditions are also likely to improve with steroid therapy. Oral step-down therapy options For CA-MRSA: clindamycin OR linezolid.[49] For MSSA: cephalexin OR dicloxacillin caps for older children. For Kingella, most penicillins or cephalosporins (but not clindamycin).
– Gonococcal arthritis or tenosynovitis[55,56]	Ceftriaxone 50 mg/kg IV, IM q24h (BII) for 7 days AND azithromycin 20 mg/kg PO as a single dose	Combination therapy with azithromycin to decrease risk of development of resistance. Cefixime 8 mg/kg/day PO as a single daily dose may not be effective due to increasing resistance. Ceftriaxone IV, IM is preferred over cefixime PO.
– Other bacteria	See Chapter 7 for preferred antibiotics.	
Osteomyelitis[45,47–49,57–62]	Step down to appropriate high-dose oral therapy when clinically improved (see Chapter 13).[47,49,51,60]	

6

Antimicrobial Therapy According to Clinical Syndromes

6

B. SKELETAL INFECTIONS (continued)

Clinical Diagnosis	Therapy (evidence grade)	Comments
– Newborns	See Chapter 5.	
– Infants and children, acute infection (usually S aureus, including CA-MRSA; group A streptococcus; K kingae)	Empiric therapy: clindamycin (for coverage of MSSA and MRSA in most locations). For serious infections, ADD cefazolin to provide better MSSA coverage and add Kingella coverage (CIII). For CA-MRSA: clindamycin 30 mg/kg/day IV div q8h OR vancomycin 40 mg/kg/day IV q8h (BII). For MSSA: oxacillin/nafcillin 150 mg/kg/day IV div q6h OR cefazolin 100 mg/kg/day IV div q8h (AII). For Kingella: cefazolin 100 mg/kg/day IV div q8h OR ampicillin 150 mg/kg/day IV div q6h, OR ceftriaxone 50 mg/kg/day IV, IM q24h (BIII). Total therapy (IV plus PO) usually 4–6 wk for MSSA (with end-of-therapy normal ESR, radiograph to document healing) but may be as short as 3 wk for mild infection. May need longer than 4–6 wk for CA-MRSA (BII). Follow closely for clinical response to empiric therapy.	In children with open fractures secondary to trauma, add ceftazidime for extended aerobic Gram-negative bacilli activity. Kingella is often resistant to clindamycin and vancomycin. For MSSA (BI) and Kingella (BIII), step-down oral therapy with cephalexin 100 mg/kg/day PO div tid. Kingella is usually susceptible to amoxicillin. Oral step-down therapy options for CA-MRSA include clindamycin and linezolid,[63] with insufficient data to recommend TMP/SMX.[59] For prosthetic devices, biofilms may impair microbial eradication, requiring the addition of rifampin or other agents.[61]
– Acute, other organisms	See Chapter 7 for preferred antibiotics.	
– Chronic (staphylococcal)	For MSSA: cephalexin 100 mg/kg/day PO div tid OR dicloxacillin caps 75–100 mg/kg/day PO div qid for 3–6 mo or longer (CIII) For CA-MRSA: clindamycin or linezolid (CIII)	Surgery to debride sequestrum is usually required for cure. For prosthetic joint infection caused by staphylococci, add rifampin (CIII).[61] Watch for beta-lactam–associated neutropenia with high-dose, long-term therapy and linezolid-associated neutropenia/thrombocytopenia with long-term (>2 wk) therapy.[63]

Osteomyelitis of the foot[64,65]

(osteochondritis after a puncture wound)

Pseudomonas aeruginosa

(occasionally *S aureus*, including CA-MRSA)

Cefepime 150 mg/kg/day IV div q8h (BIII); OR meropenem 60 mg/kg/day IV div q8h (BIII); OR ceftazidime 150 mg/kg/day IM, IV div q8h (BIII); AND tobramycin 6–7.5 mg/kg/day IM, IV div q8h (BIII); ADD vancomycin 40 mg/kg/day IV div q8h OR clindamycin 30 mg/kg/day IV div q8h for serious infection (for CA-MRSA), pending culture results.

Cefepime and meropenem will provide coverage for MSSA in addition to *Pseudomonas*. Thorough surgical debridement required for *Pseudomonas* (second drainage procedure needed in at least 20% of children); oral convalescent therapy with ciprofloxacin (BIII).[66]

Treatment course 7–10 days after surgery.

C. EYE INFECTIONS

Clinical Diagnosis	Therapy (evidence grade)	Comments
Cellulitis, orbital[67-69] (also called post-septal cellulitis; cellulitis of the contents of the orbit; may be associated with orbital abscess; usually secondary to sinus infection; caused by respiratory tract flora and *Staphylococcus aureus*, including CA-MRSA)	Cefotaxime 150 mg/kg/day div q8h or ceftriaxone 50 mg/kg/day q24h; ADD clindamycin 30 mg/kg/day IV div q8h (for *S aureus*, including CA-MRSA) OR ceftaroline: 2 mo–<2 y, 24 mg/kg/day IV div q8h; ≥2 y, 36 mg/kg/day IV div q8h (max single dose 400 mg); >33 kg, either 400 mg/dose IV q8h or 600 mg/dose IV q12h (BIII) OR vancomycin 40 mg/kg/day IV q8h (AIII). If MSSA isolated, use oxacillin/nafcillin IV OR cefazolin IV.	Surgical drainage of significant orbital or subperiosteal abscess if present by CT scan or MRI. Try medical therapy alone for small abscess (BIII).[70] Treatment course for 10–14 days after surgical drainage, up to 21 days. CT scan or MRI can confirm cure (BIII).
Cellulitis, periorbital[71] (preseptal infection)	Periorbital tissues are TENDER with cellulitis. Periorbital edema with sinusitis can look identical but is NOT tender.	
– Associated with entry site lesion on skin (*S aureus*, including CA-MRSA, group A streptococcus) in the fully immunized child	Standard: oxacillin/nafcillin 150 mg/kg/day IV div q6h OR cefazolin 100 mg/kg/day IV div q8h (BII) CA-MRSA: clindamycin 30 mg/kg/day IV div q8h or ceftaroline: 2 mo–<2 y, 24 mg/kg/day IV div q8h; ≥2 y, 36 mg/kg/day IV div q8h (max single dose 400 mg); >33 kg, either 400 mg/dose IV q8h or 600 mg/dose IV q12h (BII)	Oral antistaphylococcal antibiotic (eg, clindamycin) for empiric therapy of less severe infection; treatment course for 7–10 days

6

Antimicrobial Therapy According to Clinical Syndromes

Antimicrobial Therapy According to Clinical Syndromes

C. EYE INFECTIONS (continued)

Clinical Diagnosis	Therapy (evidence grade)	Comments
– No associated entry site (in febrile, unimmunized infants); pneumococcal or *Haemophilus influenzae* type b	Ceftriaxone 50 mg/kg/day q24h OR cefotaxime 100–150 mg/kg/day IV, IM div q8h OR cefuroxime 150 mg/kg/day IV div q8h (AII)	Treatment course for 7–10 days; rule out meningitis if bacteremic with *H influenzae*. Alternative agents: other 2nd-, 3rd-, or 4th-generation cephalosporins or amoxicillin/clavulanate.
– Periorbital, non-tender erythematous swelling (not true cellulitis, usually associated with sinusitis); sinus pathogens *rarely* may erode anteriorly, causing cellulitis.	Ceftriaxone 50 mg/kg/day q24h OR cefotaxime 100–150 mg/kg/day IV, IM div q8h OR cefuroxime 150 mg/kg/day IV div q8h (BII). ADD clindamycin 30 mg/kg/day IV div q8h for more severe infection with suspect *S aureus* including CA-MRSA or for chronic sinusitis (covers anaerobes) (AIII).	For oral convalescent antibiotic therapy, see Sinusitis, acute; total treatment course of 14–21 days or 7 days after resolution of symptoms.
Conjunctivitis, acute (*Haemophilus* and pneumococcus predominantly)[72–74]	Polymyxin/trimethoprim ophth solution OR polymyxin/bacitracin ophth ointment OR ciprofloxacin ophth solution (BII), for 7–10 days. For neonatal infection, see Chapter 5. Steroid-containing therapy only if HSV ruled out.	Other topical antibiotics (gentamicin, tobramycin ophth solution erythromycin, besifloxacin, moxifloxacin, norfloxacin, ofloxacin, levofloxacin) may offer advantages for particular pathogens (CII). High rates of resistance to sulfacetamide.
Conjunctivitis, herpetic[75–78]	1% trifluridine or 0.15% ganciclovir ophth gel (AII) AND acyclovir PO (80 mg/kg/day div qid; max daily dose: 3,200 mg/day) has been effective in limited studies (BIII). Oral valacyclovir (60 mg/kg/day div tid) has superior pharmacokinetics to oral acyclovir and can be considered for systemic treatment, as can parenteral (IV) acyclovir if extent of disease is severe (CIII).	Refer to ophthalmologist. Recurrences common; corneal scars may form. Topical steroids for keratitis concurrent with topical antiviral solution. Long-term prophylaxis (≥1 y, and oftentimes for several years) for suppression of recurrent infection with oral acyclovir 300 mg/m²/dose PO tid (max 400 mg/dose). Potential risks must balance potential benefits to vision (BII).

6

Dacryocystitis	Warm compresses; may require surgical probing of nasolacrimal duct.
	No antibiotic usually needed; oral therapy for more symptomatic infection, based on Gram stain and culture of pus; topical therapy as for conjunctivitis may be helpful.

Endophthalmitis[79,80]

NOTE: Subconjunctival/sub-tenon antibiotics are likely to be required (vancomycin/ceftazidime or clindamycin/gentamicin); steroids commonly used; requires anterior chamber or vitreous tap for microbiological diagnosis. Listed systemic antibiotics to be used in addition to ocular injections.

– Empiric therapy following open globe injury	Vancomycin 40 mg/kg/day IV div q8h AND cefepime 150 mg/kg/day IV div q8h (AIII)	Refer to ophthalmologist; vitrectomy may be necessary for advanced endophthalmitis. No prospective, controlled studies.
– Staphylococcal	Vancomycin 40 mg/kg/day IV div q8h pending susceptibility testing; oxacillin/nafcillin 150 mg/kg/day IV div q6h if susceptible (AIII)	Consider ceftaroline for MRSA treatment as it may penetrate the vitreous better than vancomycin.
– Pneumococcal, meningococcal, *Haemophilus*	Ceftriaxone 100 mg/kg/day IV q24h; penicillin G 250,000 U/kg/day IV div q4h if susceptible (AIII)	Rule out meningitis; treatment course for 10–14 days.
– Gonococcal	Ceftriaxone 50 mg/kg q24h IV, IM (AIII)	ADD azithromycin. Treatment course 7 days or longer.
– *Pseudomonas*	Cefepime 150 mg/kg/day IV div q8h for 10–14 days (AIII)	Cefepime is preferred over ceftazidime for *Pseudomonas* based on decreased risk of development of resistance on therapy; meropenem IV or imipenem IV are alternatives (no clinical data). Very poor outcomes.

6

Antimicrobial Therapy According to Clinical Syndromes

Antimicrobial Therapy According to Clinical Syndromes

C. EYE INFECTIONS (continued)

Clinical Diagnosis	Therapy (evidence grade)	Comments
– *Candida*[81]	Fluconazole (25 mg/kg loading, then 12 mg/kg/day IV), OR voriconazole (9 mg/kg loading, then 8 mg/kg/day IV); for resistant strains, L-AmB (5 mg/kg/day IV). For chorioretinitis, systemic antifungals PLUS intravitreal amphotericin 5–10 µg/0.1-mL sterile water OR voriconazole 100 µg/0.1-mL sterile water or physiologic (normal) saline soln (AIII). Duration of therapy is at least 4–6 wk (AIII).	Echinocandins given IV may not be able to achieve adequate antifungal activity in the eye.
Hordeolum (sty) or chalazion	None (topical antibiotic not necessary)	Warm compresses; I&D when necessary
Retinitis		
– CMV[82–84] For neonatal, see Chapter 5. For HIV-infected children, https://aidsinfo.nih.gov/guidelines/html/5/pediatric-opportunistic-infection/401/cytomegalovirus (accessed November 8, 2017).	Ganciclovir 10 mg/kg/day IV div q12h for 2 wk (BIII); if needed, continue at 5 mg/kg/day q24h to complete 6 wk total (BIII).	Neutropenia risk increases with duration of therapy. Foscarnet IV and cidofovir IV are alternatives but demonstrate significant toxicities. Oral valganciclovir has not been evaluated in HIV-infected children with CMV retinitis but is an option primarily for older children who weigh enough to receive the adult dose of valganciclovir (CIII). Intravitreal ganciclovir and combination therapy for non-responding, immunocompromised hosts; however, intravitreal injections may not be practical for most children.

6

Clinical Diagnosis	Therapy (evidence grade)	Comments
Bullous myringitis (See Otitis media, acute.)	Believed to be a clinical presentation of acute bacterial otitis media	
Mastoiditis, acute (pneumococcus, *Staphylococcus aureus*, including CA-MRSA; group A streptococcus; increasing *Pseudomonas* in adolescents, *Haemophilus* rare)[85-87]	Cefotaxime 150 mg/kg/day IV div q8h or ceftriaxone 50 mg/kg/day q24h AND clindamycin 40 mg/kg/day IV div q8h (BIII) For adolescents: cefepime 150 mg/kg/day IV div q8h AND clindamycin 40 mg/kg/day IV div q8h (BIII)	Rule out meningitis; surgery as needed for mastoid and middle ear drainage. Change to appropriate oral therapy after clinical improvement.
Mastoiditis, chronic (See also Otitis, chronic suppurative.) (anaerobes, *Pseudomonas*, *S aureus* [including CA-MRSA])[86]	Antibiotics only for acute superinfections (according to culture of drainage); for *Pseudomonas*: meropenem 60 mg/kg/day IV div q8h, OR pip/tazo 240 mg/kg/day IV div q4–6h for only 5–7 days after drainage stops (BIII)	Daily cleansing of ear important; if no response to antibiotics, surgery. Alternatives: cefepime IV or ceftazidime IV (poor anaerobic coverage with either antibiotic). Be alert for CA-MRSA.
Otitis externa		
Bacterial, swimmer's ear (*Pseudomonas aeruginosa*, *S aureus*, including CA-MRSA)[88,89]	Topical antibiotics: fluoroquinolone (ciprofloxacin or ofloxacin) with steroid, OR neomycin/polymyxin B/hydrocortisone (BII) Irrigation and cleaning canal of detritus important	Wick moistened with Burow (aluminum acetate topical) soln, used for marked swelling of canal; to prevent swimmer's ear, 2% acetic acid to canal after water exposure will restore acid pH.
– Bacterial, malignant otitis externa (*P aeruginosa*)[90]	Cefepime 150 mg/kg/day IV div q8h (AIII)	Other antipseudomonal antibiotics should also be effective: ceftazidime IV AND tobramycin IV, OR meropenem IV or imipenem IV, pip/tazo IV. For more mild infection, ciprofloxacin PO.
– Bacterial furuncle of canal (*S aureus*, including CA-MRSA)	Standard: oxacillin/nafcillin 150 mg/kg/day IV div q6h OR cefazolin 100 mg/kg/day IV div q8h (BIII) CA-MRSA: clindamycin 30 mg/kg/day IV div q8h or vancomycin 40 mg/kg/day IV div q8h (BIII)	I&D; antibiotics for cellulitis Oral therapy for mild disease, convalescent therapy: for MSSA: cephalexin; for CA-MRSA: clindamycin, TMP/SMX, OR linezolid (BIII)
– Candida	Fluconazole 6–12 mg/kg/day PO qd for 5–7 days (CIII)	May occur following antibiotic therapy of bacterial external otitis; debride canal.

Antimicrobial Therapy According to Clinical Syndromes

6

D. EAR AND SINUS INFECTIONS (continued)

Clinical Diagnosis	Therapy (evidence grade)	Comments
Otitis media, acute		
A note on AOM: The natural history of AOM in different age groups by specific pathogens has not been well defined; therefore, the actual contribution of antibiotic therapy on resolution of disease had also been poorly defined until 2 amox/clav vs placebo, prospective studies were published in 2011,[91,92] although neither study used tympanocentesis to define a pattern. The benefits and risks (including development of antibiotic resistance) of antibiotic therapy for AOM need to be further evaluated before the most accurate advice on the "best" antibiotic can be provided. However, based on available data, for most children, amoxicillin or amox/clav can be used initially. Considerations for the need for extended antimicrobial activity of amox/clav include severity of disease, young age of the child, previous antibiotic therapy within 6 months, and child care attendance, which address the issues of types of pathogens and antibiotic resistance patterns to expect. However, with universal PCV13 immunization, data suggest that the risk of antibiotic-resistant pneumococcal otitis has decreased but the percent of *Haemophilus* responsible for AOM have increased; therefore, some experts recommend use of amox/clav as first-line therapy for well-documented AOM. The most current AAP guidelines[93] and meta-analyses[94] suggest the greatest benefit with therapy occurs in children with bilateral AOM who are younger than 2 years; for other children, close observation is also an option. AAP guidelines provide an option to treatment in non-severe cases, particularly disease in older children, to provide a prescription to parents but have them only fill the prescription if the child deteriorates.[93] Although prophylaxis is only rarely indicated, amoxicillin or other antibiotics can be used in half the therapeutic dose once or twice daily to prevent infections if the benefits outweigh the risks of development of resistant organisms for that child.[93]		
– Newborns	See Chapter 5.	
– Infants and children (pneumococcus, *Haemophilus influenzae* non–type b, *Moraxella* most common)[95-97]	Usual therapy: amoxicillin 90 mg/kg/day PO div bid, with or without clavulanate; failures will be caused by highly pen-R pneumococcus or, if amoxicillin is used alone, by beta-lactamase–producing *Haemophilus* (or *Moraxella*). a) For *Haemophilus* strains that are beta-lactamase positive, the following oral antibiotics offer better in vitro activity than amoxicillin: amox/clav, cefdinir, cefpodoxime, cefuroxime, ceftriaxone IM, levofloxacin. b) For pen-R pneumococci: high-dosage amoxicillin achieves greater middle ear activity than oral cephalosporins. Options	See Chapter 11 for dosages. Published data suggest continued presence of penicillin resistance in pneumococci isolated in the post-PCV13 era,[98] high-dosage amoxicillin (90 mg/kg/day) should still be used for empiric therapy. The high serum and middle ear fluid concentrations achieved with 45 mg/kg/dose of amoxicillin, combined with a long half-life in middle ear fluid, allow for a therapeutic antibiotic exposure in the middle ear with only twice-daily dosing; high-dosage amoxicillin (90 mg/kg/day) with clavulanate (Augmentin ES) is also available. If published data subsequently document

	include ceftriaxone IM 50 mg/kg/day q24h for 1–3 doses; OR levofloxacin 20 mg/kg/day PO bid for children ≤5 y and 10 mg/kg PO qd for children >5 y; OR a macrolide-class antibiotic*: azithromycin PO at 1 of 3 dosages: (1) 10 mg/kg on day 1, followed by 5 mg/kg qd on days 2–5; (2) 10 mg/kg qd for 3 days; or (3) 30 mg/kg once. **Caution:** Up to 40% of pen-R pneumococci are also macrolide resistant.	decreasing resistance to amoxicillin, standard dosage (45 mg/kg/day) can again be recommended. Tympanocentesis should be performed in children who fail second-line therapy.
Otitis, chronic suppurative (*P aeruginosa, S aureus*, including CA-MRSA, and other respiratory tract/skin flora)[89,99,100]	Topical antibiotics: fluoroquinolone (ciprofloxacin, ofloxacin, besifloxacin) with or without steroid (BII) Cleaning of canal, view of tympanic membrane, for patency; cultures important	Presumed middle ear drainage through open tympanic membrane; possible aminoglycoside toxicity if neomycin-containing topical therapy used[101] Other topical fluoroquinolones with/without steroids available
Sinusitis, acute (*H influenzae* non–type b, pneumococcus, group A streptococcus, *Moraxella*)[102–106]	Same antibiotic therapy as for AOM as pathogens similar: amoxicillin 90 mg/kg/day PO div bid, OR for children at higher risk of *Haemophilus*, amox/clav 14:1 ratio, with amoxicillin component at 90 mg/kg/day PO div bid (BII). Therapy of 14 days may be necessary while mucosal swelling resolves and ventilation is restored.	IDSA sinusitis guidelines recommend amox/clav as first-line therapy,[105] while AAP guidelines (same pediatric authors) recommend amoxicillin.[103] Lack of data prevents a definitive evidence-based recommendation. The same antibiotic therapy considerations used for AOM apply to acute bacterial sinusitis. There is no controlled evidence to determine whether the use of antihistamines, decongestants, or nasal irrigation is efficacious in children with acute sinusitis.[104]

6

Antimicrobial Therapy According to Clinical Syndromes

Antimicrobial Therapy According to Clinical Syndromes

E. OROPHARYNGEAL INFECTIONS

Clinical Diagnosis	Therapy (evidence grade)	Comments
Dental abscess (mixed aerobic/anaerobic oral flora)[107,108]	Clindamycin 30 mg/kg/day PO, IV, IM div q6–8h OR penicillin G 100–200,000 U/kg/day IV div q6h (AIII)	Amox/clav PO; amoxicillin PO; ampicillin AND metronidazole IV are other options. Tooth extraction usually necessary. Erosion of abscess may occur into facial, sinusitis, deep head, and neck compartments.
Diphtheria[109]	Erythromycin 40–50 mg/kg/day PO div qid for 14 days OR penicillin G 150,000 U/kg/day IV div q6h; PLUS DAT (AIII)	DAT, a horse antisera, is investigational and only available from CDC Emergency Operations Center at 770/488-7100. The investigational protocol and dosages of DAT are provided on the CDC Web site at www.cdc.gov/diphtheria/downloads/protocol.pdf (protocol version September 21, 2016; accessed October 2, 2017).
Epiglottitis (supraglottitis; *Haemophilus influenzae* type b in an unimmunized child; rarely pneumococcus, *Staphylococcus aureus*)[110,111]	Ceftriaxone 50 mg/kg/day IV, IM q24h OR cefotaxime 150 mg/kg/day IV div q8h for 7–10 days	Emergency: provide airway. For *S aureus* (causes only 5% of epiglottitis), consider adding clindamycin 40 mg/kg/day IV div q8h.
Gingivostomatitis, herpetic[112–114]	Acyclovir 80 mg/kg/day PO div qid (max dose: 800 mg) for 7 days (for severe disease, use IV therapy at 30 mg/kg/day div q8h) (BIII); OR for infants ≥3 mo, valacyclovir 20 mg/kg/dose PO bid (max dose: 1,000 mg; instructions for preparing liquid formulation with 28-day shelf life included in package insert) (CIII)[114]	Early treatment is likely to be the most effective. Start treatment as soon as oral intake is compromised. Extended duration of therapy may be needed for immunocompromised children. The oral acyclovir (ACV) dose provided is safe and effective for varicella; 75 mg/kg/day div into 5 equal doses has been studied for HSV.[113]

6

Lemierre syndrome (*Fusobacterium necrophorum* primarily, new reports with MRSA)[115-119] (pharyngitis with internal jugular vein septic thrombosis, postanginal sepsis, necrobacillosis)	Empiric: meropenem 60 mg/kg/day div q8h (or 120 mg/kg/day div q8h for CNS metastatic foci) (AIII) OR ceftriaxone 100 mg/kg/day q24h AND metronidazole 40 mg/kg/day div q8h or clindamycin 40 mg/kg/day div q6h (BIII). ADD empiric vancomycin if MRSA suspected.	Anecdotal reports suggest metronidazole may be effective for apparent failures with other agents. Often requires anticoagulation. Metastatic and recurrent abscesses often develop while on active, appropriate therapy, requiring multiple debridements and prolonged antibiotic therapy. Treat until CRP and ESR are normal (AIII).
Peritonsillar cellulitis or abscess (group A streptococcus with mixed oral flora, including anaerobes, CA-MRSA)[120]	Clindamycin 30 mg/kg/day PO, IV, IM div q8h; for preschool infants with consideration of enteric bacilli, ADD cefotaxime 150 mg/kg/day IV div q8h or ceftriaxone 50 mg/kg/day IV q24h (BIII)	Consider incision and drainage for abscess. Alternatives: meropenem or imipenem; pip/tazo; amox/clav for convalescent oral therapy (BIII). No controlled prospective data on benefits/risks of steroids.[121]
Pharyngitis (group A streptococcus primarily)[7,122-124]	Amoxicillin 50–75 mg/kg/day PO, either qd, bid, or tid for 10 days OR penicillin V 50–75 mg/kg/day PO, either div, bid, or tid, OR benzathine penicillin 600,000 units IM for children <27 kg, 1.2 million units IM if >27 kg, as a single dose (AII) For penicillin-allergic children: erythromycin (estolate at 20–40 mg/kg/day PO div bid to qid; OR 40 mg/kg/day PO div bid to qid) for 10 days; OR azithromycin 12 mg/kg qd for 5 days (AII); OR clindamycin 30 mg/kg/day PO div tid	Although penicillin V is the treatment of choice of the AAP *Red Book* committee, amoxicillin displays better GI absorption than oral penicillin V; the suspension is better tolerated. These advantages should be balanced by the unnecessary increased spectrum of activity. Once-daily amoxicillin dosage: for children 50 mg/kg (max 1,000–1,200 mg).[7] Meta-analysis suggests that oral cephalosporins are more effective than penicillin for treatment of strep.[125] A 5-day treatment course is FDA approved for some oral cephalosporins (cefdinir, cefpodoxime), with rapid clinical response to treatment that can also be seen with other antibiotics; a 10-day course is preferred for the prevention of ARF, particularly areas where ARF is prevalent, as no data exist on efficacy of 5 days of therapy for prevention of ARF.[124,126]

6

Antimicrobial Therapy According to Clinical Syndromes

E. OROPHARYNGEAL INFECTIONS (continued)

Clinical Diagnosis	Therapy (evidence grade)	Comments
Retropharyngeal, parapharyngeal, or lateral pharyngeal cellulitis or abscess (mixed aerobic/anaerobic flora, now including CA-MRSA)[1],[20],[127-129]	Clindamycin 40 mg/kg/day IV div q8h AND cefotaxime 150 mg/kg/day IV div q8h or ceftriaxone 50 mg/kg/day IV q24h	Consider I&D; possible airway compromise, mediastinitis. Alternatives: meropenem or imipenem (BIII); pip/tazo. Amox/clav for convalescent oral therapy (BIII).
Tracheitis, bacterial (S aureus, including CA-MRSA; group A streptococcus; pneumococcus; H influenzae type b, rarely Pseudomonas)[130],[131]	Vancomycin 40 mg/kg/day IV div q8h or clindamycin 40 mg/kg/day IV div q8h AND ceftriaxone 50 mg/kg/day q24h or cefotaxime 150 mg/kg/day div q8h (BIII) OR ceftaroline: 2 mo–<2 y, 24 mg/kg/day IV div q8h; ≥2 y, 36 mg/kg/day IV div q8h (max single dose 400 mg); >33 kg, either 400 mg/dose IV q8h or 600 mg/dose IV q12h (BIII)	For susceptible S aureus, oxacillin/nafcillin or cefazolin. May represent bacterial superinfection of viral laryngotracheobronchitis, including influenza.

F. LOWER RESPIRATORY TRACT INFECTIONS

Clinical Diagnosis	Therapy (evidence grade)	Comments
Abscess, lung		
– Primary (severe, necrotizing community-acquired pneumonia caused by pneumococcus, *Staphylococcus aureus*, including CA-MRSA, group A streptococcus)[132-134]	Empiric therapy with ceftriaxone 50–75 mg/kg/day q24h or cefotaxime 150 mg/kg/day div q8h AND clindamycin 40 mg/kg/day div q8h or vancomycin 45 mg/kg/day IV div q8h for 14–21 days or longer (AIII) OR (for MRSA) ceftaroline: 2–<6 mo, 30 mg/kg/day IV div q8h (each dose given over 2 h); ≥6 mo, 45 mg/kg/day IV div q8h (each dose given over 2 h) (max single dose 600 mg) (BII)	For severe CA-MRSA infections, see Chapter 4. Bronchoscopy may be necessary if abscess fails to drain; surgical excision rarely necessary for pneumococcus but may be important for CA-MRSA and MSSA. Focus antibiotic coverage based on culture results. For MSSA: oxacillin/nafcillin or cefazolin.
– Secondary to aspiration (ie, foul smelling; polymicrobial infection with oral aerobes and anaerobes)[135]	Clindamycin 40 mg/kg/day IV div q8h or meropenem 60 mg/kg/day IV div q8h for 10 days or longer (AIII)	Alternatives: imipenem IV or pip/tazo IV or ticar/clav IV (BIII) Oral step-down therapy with clindamycin or amox/clav (BII)
Allergic bronchopulmonary aspergillosis[136]	Prednisone 0.5 mg/kg qd for 1–2 wk and then taper (BII) AND voriconazole 18 mg/kg/day PO div q12h load followed by 16 mg/kg/day PO div q12h (AIII) OR itraconazole 10 mg/kg/day PO div q12h (BII)	Not all allergic pulmonary disease is associated with true fungal infection. Additionally, not all allergic pulmonary disease is caused only by *Aspergillus*. Larger steroid dosages may lead to tissue invasion by *Aspergillus*. Voriconazole not as well studied in allergic bronchopulmonary aspergillosis but is more active than itraconazole. Voriconazole or itraconazole require trough concentration monitoring.

Antimicrobial Therapy According to Clinical Syndromes

F. LOWER RESPIRATORY TRACT INFECTIONS (continued)

Clinical Diagnosis	Therapy (evidence grade)	Comments
Aspiration pneumonia (polymicrobial infection with oral aerobes and anaerobes)[135]	Clindamycin 40 mg/kg/day IV div q8h; ADD ceftriaxone 50–75 mg/kg/day div q24h or cefotaxime 150 mg/kg/day div q8h for additional *Haemophilus* activity OR meropenem 60 mg/kg/day IV div q8h; for 10 days or longer (BIII).	Alternatives: imipenem IV or pip/tazo IV (BIII) Oral step-down therapy with clindamycin or amox/clav (BIII)
Atypical pneumonia (See *Mycobacterium pneumoniae*, Legionnaires disease.)		
Bronchitis (bronchiolitis), acute[137]	For bronchitis/bronchiolitis in children, no antibiotic needed for most cases, as disease is usually viral	Multicenter global studies with anti-RSV therapy are currently underway.
Community-acquired pneumonia (See Pneumonia: Community-acquired, bronchopneumonia; Pneumonia: Community-acquired, lobar consolidation.)		
Cystic fibrosis: Seek advice from those expert in acute and chronic management. Larger than standard dosages of beta-lactam antibiotics are required in most patients with cystic fibrosis.[138]		
– Acute exacerbation (*Pseudomonas aeruginosa* primarily; also *Burkholderia cepacia, Stenotrophomonas maltophilia, S aureus*, including CA-MRSA, nontuberculous mycobacteria)[139-144]	Ceftazidime 150–200 mg/kg/day div q6–8h or meropenem 120 mg/kg/day div q6h AND tobramycin 6–10 mg/kg/day IM, IV div q6–8h for treatment of acute exacerbation (AII); alternatives: imipenem, cefepime, or ciprofloxacin 30 mg/kg/day PO, IV div tid. May require vancomycin 60–80 mg/kg/day IV div q8h for MRSA, OR ceftaroline 45 mg/kg/day IV div q8h (each dose given over 2 h) (max single dose 600 mg) (BIII).	Monitor concentrations of aminoglycosides, vancomycin. Insufficient evidence to recommend routine use of inhaled antibiotics for acute exacerbations.[145] Cultures with susceptibility testing and synergy testing will help select antibiotics, as multidrug resistance is common, but synergy testing is not well standardized.[146,147] Combination therapy may provide synergistic killing and delay the emergence of resistance (BIII). Attempt at early eradication of new onset *Pseudomonas* may decrease progression of disease.[142,148]

	Duration of therapy not well defined: 10–14 days (BIII).[140]	Failure to respond to antibacterials should prompt evaluation for invasive/allergic fungal disease.
Chronic inflammation (Minimize long-term damage to lung.)	Inhaled tobramycin 300 mg bid, cycling 28 days on therapy, 28 days off therapy, is effective adjunctive therapy between exacerbation[146,149] (AI). Inhaled aztreonam[150] provides an alternative to inhaled tobramycin (AI). Azithromycin adjunctive chronic therapy, greatest benefit for those colonized with *Pseudomonas* (AII).[151,152]	Alternative inhaled antibiotics: aztreonam[152,]; colistin[145,153] (BII). Two newer powder preparations of inhaled tobramycin are available.
Pertussis[154-156]	Azithromycin 10 mg/kg/day for 5 days, or clarithromycin 15 mg/kg/day div bid for 7 days, or erythromycin (estolate preferable) 40 mg/kg/day PO div qid; for 7–10 days (AII) Alternative: TMP/SMX 8 mg/kg/day TMP div bid for 10 days (BIII)	Azithromycin and clarithromycin are better tolerated than erythromycin; azithromycin is preferred in young infants to reduce pyloric stenosis risk (see Chapter 5). The azithromycin dosage that is recommended for very young neonates with the highest risk of mortality (<1 mo) is 10 mg/kg/day for 5 days. This dose should be used up to 6 mo of age. Older children should receive 10 mg/kg on day 1, followed by 5 mg/kg on days 2–5.[154] Provide prophylaxis to family members. Unfortunately, no adjunctive therapy has been shown beneficial in decreasing the cough.[157]

6

Antimicrobial Therapy According to Clinical Syndromes

F. LOWER RESPIRATORY TRACT INFECTIONS (continued)

Clinical Diagnosis	Therapy (evidence grade)	Comments
Pneumonia: Community-acquired, bronchopneumonia		
- Mild to moderate illness (overwhelmingly viral, especially in preschool children)[158]	No antibiotic therapy unless epidemiologic, clinical, or laboratory reasons to suspect bacteria or *Mycoplasma*.	Broad-spectrum antibiotics may increase risk of subsequent infection with antibiotic-resistant pathogens.
- Moderate to severe illness (pneumococcus; group A streptococcus; *S aureus*, including CA-MRSA and for unimmunized children, *Haemophilus influenzae* type b; or *Mycoplasma pneumoniae*[132,133,159-161]; and for those with aspiration and underlying comorbidities; *Haemophilus influenzae*, non-typable)	Empiric therapy For regions with high PCV13 vaccine use or low pneumococcal resistance to penicillin: ampicillin 150–200 mg/kg/day div q6h. For regions with low rates of PCV13 use or high pneumococcal resistance to penicillin: ceftriaxone 50–75 mg/kg/day q24h or cefotaxime 150 mg/kg/day div q8h (AI). For suspected CA-MRSA: vancomycin 40–60 mg/kg/day (AIII)[2] OR ceftaroline: 2–<6 mo, 30 mg/kg/day IV div q8h (each dose given over 2 h); ≥6 mo, 45 mg/kg/day IV div q8h (each dose given over 2 h) (max single dose 600 mg) (BII).[134] For suspect *Mycoplasma*/atypical pneumonia agents, particularly in school-aged children, ADD azithromycin 10 mg/kg IV, PO on day 1, then 5 mg/kg qd for days 2–5 of treatment (AII).	Tracheal aspirate or bronchoalveolar lavage for Gram stain/culture for severe infection in intubated children. Check vancomycin serum concentrations and renal function, particularly at the higher dosage needed to achieve an AUC:MIC of 400 for CA-MRSA pneumonia. Alternatives to azithromycin for atypical pneumonia include erythromycin IV, PO, or clarithromycin PO, or doxycycline IV, PO for children >7 y, or levofloxacin. New data suggest that combination empiric therapy with a beta-lactam and a macrolide results in shorter hospitalization compared with a beta-lactam alone, but we are not ready to recommend routine empiric combination therapy yet.[162,163] Empiric oral outpatient therapy for less severe illness: high-dosage amoxicillin 80–100 mg/kg/day PO div tid (NOT bid) (BII).
Pneumonia: Community-acquired, lobar consolidation		
Pneumococcus (May occur with non-vaccine strains, even if immunized for pneumococcus.)[132,133,159-161]	Empiric therapy For regions with high PCV13 vaccine use or low pneumococcal resistance to penicillin: ampicillin 200 mg/kg/day div q6h.	Change to PO after improvement (decreased fever, no oxygen needed); treat until clinically asymptomatic and chest radiography significantly improved (7–21 days) (BII).

	For regions with low rates of PCV13 use or high pneumococcal resistance to penicillin: ceftriaxone 50–75 mg/kg/day div q24h or cefotaxime 150 mg/kg/day div q8h (AI); for more severe disease ADD clindamycin 40 mg/kg/day div q8h or vancomycin 40–60 mg/kg/day div q8h for suspect S aureus (AIII).[2] For suspect Mycoplasma/atypical pneumonia agents, particularly in school-aged children, ADD azithromycin 10 mg/kg IV, PO on day 1, then 5 mg/kg qd for days 2–5 of treatment (AII). Empiric oral outpatient therapy for less severe illness: high-dosage amoxicillin 80–100 mg/kg/day PO div tid (NOT bid); for Mycoplasma, ADD a macrolide as above (BIII).	No reported failures of ceftriaxone/cefotaxime for pen-R pneumococcus; no need to add empiric vancomycin for this reason (CIII). Oral therapy for pneumococcus and Haemophilus may also be successful with amox/clav, cefdinir, cefixime, cefpodoxime, or cefuroxime. Levofloxacin is an alternative, particularly for those with severe allergy to beta-lactam antibiotics (BI),[164] but, due to theoretical cartilage toxicity concerns for humans, should not be first-line therapy.
– Pneumococcal, pen-S	Penicillin G 250,000–400,000 U/kg/day IV div q4–6h for 10 days (BII) OR ampicillin 150–200 mg/kg/day IV div q6h	After improvement, change to PO amoxicillin 50–75 mg/kg/day PO div tid OR penicillin V 50–75 mg/kg/day div qid.
– Pneumococcal, pen-R	Ceftriaxone 75 mg/kg/day q24h, or cefotaxime 150 mg/kg/day q8h for 10–14 days (BIII)	Addition of vancomycin has not been required for eradication of pen-R strains. For oral convalescent therapy, high-dosage amoxicillin (100–150 mg/kg/day PO div tid), clindamycin (30 mg/kg/day PO div tid), linezolid (30 mg/kg/day PO div tid), or levofloxacin PO.

Antimicrobial Therapy According to Clinical Syndromes

F. LOWER RESPIRATORY TRACT INFECTIONS (continued)

Clinical Diagnosis	Therapy (evidence grade)	Comments
Staphylococcus aureus (including CA-MRSA)[26,132,159,165]	For MSSA: oxacillin/nafcillin 150 mg/kg/day IV div q6h or cefazolin 100 mg/kg/day IV div q8h (AII). For CA-MRSA: vancomycin 60 mg/kg/day IV div q6h; ≥6 mo, 30 mg/kg/day IV div q8h; OR ceftaroline: 2–<6 mo, 45 mg/kg/day IV div q8h; ≥6 mo, 45 mg/kg/day IV div q8h (max single dose 600 mg) (BII)[134]; may need addition of rifampin, clindamycin, or gentamicin (AIII) (see Chapter 4).	Check vancomycin serum concentrations and renal function, particularly at the higher dosage designed to attain an AUC:MIC of 400, or serum trough concentrations of 15 µg/mL for invasive CA-MRSA disease. For life-threatening disease, optimal therapy of CA-MRSA is not defined: add gentamicin and/or rifampin for combination therapy (CIII). Linezolid 30 mg/kg/day IV, PO div q8h is another option, more effective in adults than vancomycin for MRSA nosocomial pneumonia[166] (follow platelets and WBC count weekly).
Pneumonia: Immunosuppressed, neutropenic host[167] (P aeruginosa, other community-associated or nosocomial Gram-negative bacilli, S aureus, fungi, AFB, Pneumocystis, viral [adenovirus, CMV, EBV, influenza, RSV, others])	Cefepime 150 mg/kg/day IV div q8h and tobramycin 6.0–7.5 mg/kg/day IM, IV div q8h (AII), OR meropenem 60 mg/kg/day div q8h (AII) ± tobramycin (BIII); AND if S aureus (including MRSA) is suspected clinically, ADD vancomycin 40–60 mg/kg/day IV div q8h (AIII) OR ceftaroline: 2–<6 mo, 30 mg/kg/day IV div q8h; ≥6 mo, 45 mg/kg/day IV div q8h (max single dose 600 mg) (BIII).	Biopsy or bronchoalveolar lavage usually needed to determine need for antifungal, antiviral, antimycobacterial treatment. Antifungal therapy usually started if no response to antibiotics in 48–72 h (AmB, voriconazole, or caspofungin/micafungin—see Chapter 8). Amikacin 15–22.5 mg/kg/day as an alternative aminoglycoside. Use 2 active agents for definitive therapy for neutropenic hosts, as neutrophils cannot assist clearing the pathogen; may also decrease risk of emergence of resistance (BII).
– **Pneumonia: Interstitial pneumonia syndrome of early infancy**	If Chlamydia trachomatis suspected, azithromycin 10 mg/kg on day 1, followed by 5 mg/kg/day qd days 2–5 OR erythromycin 40 mg/kg/day PO div qid for 14 days (BII)	Most often respiratory viral pathogens, CMV, or chlamydial; role of Ureaplasma uncertain

– Pneumonia, nosocomial (health care–associated/ventilator-associated) (*P aeruginosa*, Gram-negative enteric bacilli [*Enterobacter, Klebsiella, Serratia, Escherichia coli*], *Acinetobacter, Stenotrophomonas*, and Gram-positive organisms including CA-MRSA and *Enterococcus*)[168-170]	Commonly used regimens Meropenem 60 mg/kg/day div q8h, OR pip/tazo 240–300 mg/kg/day div q6–8h, ± cefepime 150 mg/kg/day div q8h; ± gentamicin 6.0–7.5 mg/kg/day div q8h (AIII); ADD vancomycin 40–60 mg/kg/day div q8h for suspect CA-MRSA (AIII).	Empiric therapy should be institution specific, based on your hospital's nosocomial pathogens and susceptibilities. Pathogens that cause nosocomial pneumonia often have multidrug resistance. Cultures are critical. Empiric therapy also based on child's prior colonization/infection. For MDR Gram-negative bacilli, IV therapy options include ceftazidime/avibactam, ceftolozane/tazobactam, or colistin. Aerosol delivery of antibiotics may be required for MDR pathogens, but little high-quality controlled data are available for children.[171]
– Pneumonia: With pleural fluid/empyema (same pathogens as for community-acquired bronchopneumonia) (Based on extent of fluid and symptoms, may benefit from chest tube drainage with fibrinolysis or video-assisted thoracoscopic surgery.)[159,172-175]	Empiric therapy: ceftriaxone 50–75 mg/kg/day q24h or cefotaxime 150 mg/kg/day div q8h AND vancomycin 40–60 mg/kg/day IV div q8h (BIII) OR ceftaroline as single drug therapy: 2–<6 mo, 30 mg/kg/day IV div q8h (each dose given over 2 h); ≥6 mo, 45 mg/kg/day IV div q8h (each dose given over 2 h) (max single dose 600 mg) (BII)	Initial therapy based on Gram stain of empyema fluid; typically, clinical improvement is slow, with persisting but decreasing "spiking" fever for 2–3 wk.
– Group A streptococcal	Penicillin G 250,000 U/kg/day IV div q4–6h for 10 days (BII)	Change to PO amoxicillin 75 mg/kg/day div tid or penicillin V 50–75 mg/kg/day div qid to tid after clinical improvement (BIII).
– Pneumococcal	(See Pneumonia: Community-acquired, lobar consolidation.)	

Antimicrobial Therapy According to Clinical Syndromes

F. LOWER RESPIRATORY TRACT INFECTIONS (continued)

Clinical Diagnosis	Therapy (evidence grade)	Comments
S aureus (including CA-MRSA)[2,6,132,165]	For MSSA: oxacillin/nafcillin or cefazolin (AII). For CA-MRSA: use vancomycin 60 mg/kg/day (AIII) (designed to attain an AUC:MIC of 400, or serum trough concentrations of 15 µg/mL); follow serum concentrations and renal function; OR ceftaroline: 2–<6 mo, 30 mg/kg/day IV div q8h (each dose given over 2 h); ≥6 mo, 45 mg/kg/day IV div q8h (each dose given over 2 h) (max single dose 600 mg) (BII)[134]; may need additional antibiotics (see Chapter 4).	For life-threatening disease, optimal therapy of CA-MRSA is not defined; add gentamicin and/or rifampin. For MRSA nosocomial pneumonia in adults, linezolid was superior to vancomycin.[166] Oral convalescent therapy for MSSA: cephalexin PO; for CA-MRSA: clindamycin or linezolid PO. Total course for 21 days or longer (AIII). For children infected who do not tolerate high-dose vancomycin, alternatives include ceftaroline, clindamycin, and linezolid.

Pneumonias of other established etiologies (See Chapter 7 for treatment by pathogen.)

Clinical Diagnosis	Therapy (evidence grade)	Comments
– Chlamydophila[176] (formerly Chlamydia) pneumoniae, Chlamydophila psittaci, or Chlamydia trachomatis	Azithromycin 10 mg/kg on day 1, followed by 5 mg/kg/day qd days 2–5 or erythromycin 40 mg/kg/day PO div qid; for 14 days	Doxycycline (patients >7 y)
– CMV (immunocompromised host)[177,178] (See chapters 5 and 9 for CMV infection in newborns and older children, respectively.)	Ganciclovir IV 10 mg/kg IV div q12h for 2 wk (BIII); if needed, continue at 5 mg/kg/day q24h to complete 4–6 wk total (BII).	Some experts add CMV immune globulin to provide a possible small incremental benefit in bone marrow transplant patients[179] (BII). Oral valganciclovir may be used for convalescent therapy (BII). Foscarnet for ganciclovir-resistant strains.
– E coli	Ceftriaxone 50–75 mg/kg/day q24h or cefotaxime 150 mg/kg/day div q8h (AII)	For cephalosporin-resistant strains (ESBL producers), use meropenem, imipenem, or ertapenem (AIII).

6

– *Enterobacter* spp	Cefepime 100 mg/kg/day div q12h or meropenem 60 mg/kg/day div q8h; OR ceftriaxone 50–75 mg/kg/day q24h or cefotaxime 150 mg/kg/day div q8h AND gentamicin 6.0–7.5 mg/kg/day IM, IV div q8h (AIII)	Addition of aminoglycoside to 3rd-generation cephalosporins may retard the emergence of ampC-mediated constitutive high-level resistance, but concern exists for inadequate aminoglycoside concentration in airways[171]; not an issue with beta-lactams (cefepime, meropenem, or imipenem).
– *Francisella tularensis*[180]	Gentamicin 6.0–7.5 mg/kg/day IM, IV div q8h for 10 days or longer for more severe disease (AIII); for less severe disease, doxycycline PO for 14–21 days (AIII)	Alternatives for oral therapy of mild disease: ciprofloxacin or levofloxacin (BIII)
– Fungi (See Chapter 8.) Community-associated pathogens, vary by region (eg, *Coccidioides*,[181,182] *Histoplasma*)[183,184] *Aspergillus*, mucormycosis, other mold infections in immunocompromised hosts (See Chapter 8.)	For detailed pathogen-specific recommendations, see Chapter 8. For suspected endemic fungi or mucormycosis in immunocompromised host, treat empirically with a lipid AmB and not voriconazole; biopsy needed to guide therapy. For suspected invasive aspergillosis, treat with voriconazole (AI) (load 18 mg/kg/day div q12h on day 1, then continue 16 mg/kg/day div q12h).[144]	For normal hosts, triazoles (fluconazole, itraconazole, voriconazole, posaconazole, isavuconazole) are better tolerated than AmB and equally effective for many community-associated pathogens (see Chapter 2). For dosage, see Chapter 8. Check voriconazole trough concentrations; need to be at least >2 µg/mL. For refractory *Coccidioides* infection, posaconazole or combination therapy with voriconazole and caspofungin may be effective[181] (AIII).

Antimicrobial Therapy According to Clinical Syndromes (continued)

F. LOWER RESPIRATORY TRACT INFECTIONS (continued)

Clinical Diagnosis	Therapy (evidence grade)	Comments
– Influenza virus[185,186] – Recent seasonal influenza A and influenza B strains continue to be resistant to adamantanes.	Empiric therapy, or documented influenza A or influenza B Oseltamivir[186,187] (AII): <12 mo: Term infants 0–8 mo: 3 mg/kg/dose bid 9–11 mo: 3.5 mg/kg/dose bid ≥12 mo: ≤15 kg: 30 mg PO bid >15–23 kg: 45 mg PO bid >23–40 kg: 60 mg PO bid >40 kg: 75 mg PO bid Zanamivir inhaled (AII): for those ≥7 y 10 mg (two 5-mg inhalations) bid	Check for antiviral susceptibility each season at www.cdc.gov/flu/professionals/antivirals/index.htm (updated January 11, 2017; accessed October 2, 2017). For children 12–23 mo, the unit dose of 30 mg/dose may provide inadequate drug exposure. 3.5 mg/kg/dose PO bid has been studied,[187] but sample sizes have been inadequate to recommend weight-based dosing at this time. The adamantanes (amantadine and rimantadine) had activity against influenza A prior to the late 1990s, but all circulating A strains of influenza have been resistant for many years. Influenza B is intrinsically resistant to adamantanes. Limited data for preterm neonates.[186] <38 wk PMA (gestational plus chronologic age): 1.0 mg/kg/dose, PO bid 38–40 wk PMA: 1.5 mg/kg/dose, PO bid Parenteral peramivir and parenteral zanamivir being evaluated in clinical trials in children.
– *Klebsiella pneumoniae*[188,189]	Ceftriaxone 50–75 mg/kg/day IV, IM q24h OR cefotaxime 150 mg/kg/day IV, IM q8h (AIII); for ceftriaxone-resistant strains (ESBL strains), use meropenem 60 mg/kg/day IV div q8h (AIII) or other carbapenem.	For *K pneumoniae* that contain ESBLs, pip/tazo and fluoroquinolones are other options. For KPC-producing strains that are resistant to meropenem: alternatives include ceftazidime/avibactam (FDA-approved for adults, pediatric studies in progress), fluoroquinolones, or colistin (BII).
– Legionnaires disease (*Legionella pneumophila*)	Azithromycin 10 mg/kg IV, PO q24h for 5 days (AIII)	Alternatives: clarithromycin, erythromycin, ciprofloxacin, levofloxacin, doxycycline
– Mycobacteria, nontuberculous (*Mycobacterium avium* complex most common)[11,190]	In a normal host: azithromycin PO or clarithromycin PO for 6–12 wk if susceptible	Highly variable susceptibilities of different nontuberculous mycobacterial species

6

	For more extensive disease: a macrolide AND rifampin AND ethambutol; ± amikacin or streptomycin (AIII)	Check if immunocompromised: HIV or gamma-interferon receptor deficiency
– *Mycobacterium tuberculosis* (See Tuberculosis.)		
– *Mycobacterium pneumoniae*[159,191]	Azithromycin 10 mg/kg on day 1, followed by 5 mg/kg/day qd days 2–5, or clarithromycin 15 mg/kg/day div bid for 7–14 days, or erythromycin 40 mg/kg/day PO div qid for 14 days	*Mycoplasma* often causes self-limited infection and does not routinely require treatment (AIII). Little prospective, well-controlled data exist for treatment of documented mycoplasma pneumonia specifically in children.[191] Doxycycline (patients >7 y), or levofloxacin. Macrolide-resistant strains have recently appeared worldwide.[192]
– *Paragonimus westermani*	See Chapter 10.	
– *Pneumocystis jiroveci* (formerly *Pneumocystis carinii*)[193], disease in immunosuppressed children and those with HIV	Severe disease: preferred regimen is TMP/SMX, 15–20 mg TMP component/kg/day IV div q8h for 3 wk (AI). Mild–moderate disease: may start with IV therapy, then after acute pneumonitis is resolving, TMP/SMX 20 mg of TMP/kg/day PO div qid for 21 days (AII). Use steroid adjunctive treatment for more severe disease (AII).	Alternatives for TMP/SMX intolerant, or clinical failure: pentamidine 3–4 mg IV qd, infused over 60–90 min (AII); TMP AND dapsone; OR primaquine AND clindamycin; OR atovaquone. Prophylaxis: TMP/SMX as 5 mg TMP/kg/day PO, divided in 2 doses, q12h, daily or 3 times/wk on consecutive days (AI); OR TMP/SMX 5 mg TMP/kg/day PO as a single dose, once daily, given 3 times/wk on consecutive days (AII); once-weekly regimens have also been successful[194], OR dapsone 2 mg/kg (max 100 mg) PO qd, or 4 mg/kg (max 200 mg) once weekly; OR atovaquone: 30 mg/kg/day for infants 1–3 mo, 45 mg/kg/day for infants 4–24 mo, and 30 mg/kg/day for children >24 mo.
– *P aeruginosa*[171,195,196]	Cefepime 150 mg/kg/day IV div q8h ± tobramycin 6.0–7.5 mg/kg/day IM, IV div q8h (AII). Alternatives: meropenem 60 mg/kg/day div q8h, OR pip/tazo 240–300 mg/kg/day div q6–8h (AII) ± tobramycin (BIII).	Ciprofloxacin IV, or colistin IV for MDR strains[197]

Antimicrobial Therapy According to Clinical Syndromes

6

Antimicrobial Therapy According to Clinical Syndromes

6

F. LOWER RESPIRATORY TRACT INFECTIONS (continued)

Clinical Diagnosis	Therapy (evidence grade)	Comments
RSV infection (bronchiolitis, pneumonia)[198]	For immunocompromised hosts, the only FDA-approved treatment is ribavirin aerosol: 6-g vial (20 mg/mL in sterile water), by SPAG-2 generator, over 18–20 h daily for 3–5 days, although questions remain regarding efficacy. Two RSV antivirals, ALS-008176 by Alios/J&J and GS-5806 by Gilead, are currently under investigation in children.	Treat only for severe disease, immunocompromised, severe underlying cardiopulmonary disease, as aerosol ribavirin only provides a small benefit. Airway reactivity with inhalation precludes routine use. Palivizumab (Synagis) is not effective for treatment of an active RSV infection, only effective for prevention of hospitalization in high-risk patients.
— Tuberculosis		
— Primary pulmonary disease[13,14]	INH 10–15 mg/kg/day (max 300 mg) PO qd for 6 mo AND rifampin 10–20 mg/kg/day (max 600 mg) PO qd for 6 mo AND PZA 30–40 mg/kg/day (max 2 g) PO qd for first 2 mo therapy only (AII). If risk factors present for multidrug resistance, ADD ethambutol 20 mg/kg/day PO qd OR streptomycin 30 mg/kg/day IV, IM q12h initially.	It is common to have mildly elevated liver transaminase concentrations (2–3 times normal) that do not further increase during the entire treatment interval. Obese children may have mild elevation when started on therapy. Contact TB specialist for therapy of drug-resistant TB. Fluoroquinolones may play a role in treating MDR strains. Bedaquiline, in a new drug class for TB therapy, was recently approved for adults with MDR TB, when used in combination therapy. Toxicities and lack of pediatric data preclude routine use in children. Directly observed therapy preferred; after 2 wk of daily therapy, can change to twice-weekly dosing double dosage of INH (max 900 mg). PZA (max 2 g), and ethambutol (max 2.5 g); rifampin remains same dosage (10–20 mg/kg/day, max 600 mg) (AII). LP ± CT of head for children ≤2 y to rule out occult, concurrent CNS infection; consider testing for HIV infection (AIII).

Mycobacterium bovis infection from unpasteurized dairy products is also called "tuberculosis" but rarely causes pulmonary disease; all strains of *M bovis* are PZA resistant.

– Latent TB infection[14] (skin test conversion)	INH 10–15 mg/kg/day (max 300 mg) PO daily for 9 mo (12 mo for immunocompromised patients) (AIII); treatment with INH at 20–30 mg/kg twice weekly for 9 mo is also effective (AIII). Alternative[199] (BII): for children ≥2 y, once-weekly DOT for 12 wk: INH (15 mg/kg/dose, max 900 mg), AND rifapentine: 10.0–14.0 kg: 300 mg 14.1–25.0 kg: 450 mg 25.1–32.0 kg: 600 mg 32.1–49.9 kg: 750 mg ≥50.0 kg: 900 mg (max)	Obtain baseline LFTs. Consider monthly LFTs or as needed for symptoms. Stop INH-rifapentine if AST or ALT ≥5 times the ULN even in the absence of symptoms or ≥3 times the ULN in the presence of symptoms. For children ≥2–12 y, 12 wk of INH and rifapentine may be used, but less data on safety and efficacy. Insufficient data for children <2 y. For exposure to known INH-R but rifampin-S strains, use rifampin 6 mo (AIII).
– Exposed child <4 y, or immunocompromised patient (high risk of dissemination)	INH 10–15 mg/kg PO daily for 2–3 mo after last exposure with repeated skin test or interferon-gamma release assay test negative at that time (AIII)	If PPD remains negative at 2–3 mo and child well, consider stopping empiric therapy. PPD may not be reliable in immunocompromised patients. Not much data to assess reliability of interferon-gamma release assays in very young infants or immunocompromised hosts, but not likely to be much better than the PPD skin test.

G. CARDIOVASCULAR INFECTIONS

Clinical Diagnosis	Therapy (evidence grade)	Comments
Bacteremia		
– Occult bacteremia (late-onset neonatal sepsis; fever without focus), infants <2 mo (group B streptococcus, *Escherichia coli*, *Listeria*, pneumococcus, meningococcus)[200–204]	In general, hospitalization for late-onset neonatal sepsis, with cultures of blood, urine, and CSF; start ampicillin 200 mg/kg/day IV div q6h AND cefotaxime 150 mg/kg/day IV div q8h (AII); higher dosages if meningitis is documented.	Current data document the importance of ampicillin-resistant *E coli* in bacteremia in infants <90 days.[202,203,205] For a nontoxic, febrile infant with good access to medical care: cultures may be obtained of blood, urine, and CSF; ceftriaxone 50 mg/kg IM (lacks *Listeria* activity) given with outpatient follow-up the next day (Boston criteria) (BII); alternative is home without antibiotics if evaluation is negative (Rochester; Philadelphia criteria)[200,204] (BI).
– Occult bacteremia (fever without focus) in age 2–3 mo to 36 mo (*Haemophilus influenzae* type B, pneumococcus, meningococcus; increasingly *Staphylococcus aureus*)[203–205]	Empiric therapy: if unimmunized, febrile, mild-moderate toxic: after blood culture: ceftriaxone 50 mg/kg IM (BII). If fully immunized (*Haemophilus* and *Pneumococcus*) and nontoxic, routine empiric therapy of fever with antibiotics is no longer recommended, but follow closely in case of vaccine failure or meningococcal bacteremia (BII).	Oral convalescent therapy is selected by susceptibility of blood isolate, following response to IM/IV treatment, with CNS and other foci ruled out by examination ± laboratory tests ± imaging.
– *H influenzae* type b, non-CNS infections	Ceftriaxone IM/IV OR, if beta-lactamase negative, ampicillin IV, followed by oral convalescent therapy (AII)	If beta-lactamase negative: amoxicillin 75–100 mg/kg/day PO tid (AII) If positive: high-dosage cefixime, ceftibuten, cefdinir PO, or levofloxacin PO (CIII)
– Meningococcus	Ceftriaxone IM/IV or penicillin G IV, followed by oral convalescent therapy (AII)	Amoxicillin 75–100 mg/kg/day PO div tid (AIII)

– Pneumococcus, non-CNS infections	Ceftriaxone IM/IV or penicillin G IV (if pen-S), followed by oral convalescent therapy (AII). Ampicillin IM/IV or penicillin G IV are other options (AII).	If pen-S: amoxicillin 75–100 mg/kg/day PO div tid (AII). If pen-R: continue ceftriaxone IM, or switch to clindamycin if susceptible (CIII); linezolid or levofloxacin may also be options (CIII).
– S aureus[2,6,206–209] usually associated with focal infection	MSSA: nafcillin or oxacillin/nafcillin IV 150–200 mg/kg/day div q6h ± gentamicin 6 mg/kg/day div q8h (AII). MRSA: vancomycin 40–60 mg/kg/day IV div q8h OR ceftaroline: 2 mo–<2 y, 24 mg/kg/day IV div q8h; ≥2 y, 36 mg/kg/day IV div q8h (max single dose 400 mg) (BIII) ± gentamicin 6 mg/kg/day div q8h ± rifampin 20 mg/kg/day div q12h (AIII). Treat for 2 wk (IV plus PO) from negative blood cultures unless endocarditis/endovascular thrombus present, which may require 6 wk of therapy (BIII).	For persisting bacteremia caused by MRSA, consider adding gentamicin, or changing from vancomycin to ceftaroline or daptomycin (but will not treat pneumonia), particularly for MRSA with vancomycin MIC of >2 µg/mL. For toxic shock syndrome, clindamycin should be added for the initial 48–72 h of therapy to decrease toxin production (linezolid may also act in this way); IVIG may be added to bind circulating toxin (linezolid may also act in this way); no controlled data exist for these measures. Watch for the development of metastatic foci of infection, including endocarditis. If catheter-related, remove catheter.

Endocarditis: Surgical indications: intractable heart failure; persistent infection; large mobile vegetations; peripheral embolism; and valve dehiscence, perforation, rupture or fistula, or a large perivalvular abscess.[210–214] Consider community versus nosocomial pathogens based on recent surgeries, prior antibiotic therapy, and possible entry sites for bacteremia (skin, oropharynx and respiratory tract, gastrointestinal tract). Children with congenital heart disease are more likely to have more turbulent cardiovascular blood flow, which increases risk of endovascular infection. Immune-compromised hosts may become bacteremic with a wide range of bacteria, fungi, and mycobacteria. Prospective, controlled data on therapy for endocarditis in neonates, infants, and children is quite limited, and many recommendations provided are extrapolations from adults, where some level of evidence exists, or from current invasive bacteremia infections.

G. CARDIOVASCULAR INFECTIONS (continued)

Clinical Diagnosis	Therapy (evidence grade)	Comments
– Native valve[210–213]		
– Empiric therapy for presumed endocarditis (viridans streptococci, *S aureus*, HACEK group)	Ceftriaxone IV 100 mg/kg q24h AND gentamicin IV, IM 6 mg/kg/day div q8h (AII). For more acute, severe infection, ADD vancomycin 40–60 mg/kg/day IV div q8h to cover *S aureus* (AII).	Combination (ceftriaxone + gentamicin) provides bactericidal activity against most strains of viridans streptococci, the more common pathogens in infective endocarditis. Cefepime is recommended for adults,[214] but resistance data in enteric bacilli in children suggest that ceftriaxone remains a reasonable choice. May administer gentamicin with a qd regimen (CIII). For beta-lactam allergy, use vancomycin 45 mg/kg/day IV div q8h AND gentamicin 6 mg/kg/day IV div q8h.
Culture-negative native valve endocarditis: treat 4–6 wk (please obtain advice from an infectious diseases specialist for an appropriate regimen that is based on likely pathogens).[210]		
– Viridans streptococci: Follow echocardiogram for resolution of vegetation (BIII); for beta-lactam allergy: vancomycin.		
Fully susceptible to penicillin	Ceftriaxone 50 mg/kg IV, IM q24h for 4 wk OR penicillin G 200,000 U/kg/day IV div q4–6h for 4 wk (BII); OR penicillin G or ceftriaxone AND gentamicin 6 mg/kg/day IM, IV div q8h (AII) for 14 days for adults (4 wk for children per AHA guidelines due to lack of data in children)	AHA recommends higher dosage of ceftriaxone similar to that for penicillin nonsusceptible strains.
Relatively resistant to penicillin	Penicillin G 300,000 U/kg/day IV div q4–6h for 4 wk, or ceftriaxone 100 mg/kg IV q24h for 4 wk; AND gentamicin 6 mg/kg/day IM, IV div q8h for the first 2 wk (AII)	Gentamicin is used for the first 2 wk of a total of 4 wk of therapy for relatively resistant strains. Vancomycin-containing regimens should use at least a 4-wk treatment course, with gentamicin used for the entire course.
– Enterococcus (dosages for native or prosthetic valve infections)		

Organism	Dosing	Comments
Ampicillin-susceptible (gentamicin-S)	Ampicillin 300 mg/kg/day IV, IM div q6h or penicillin G 300,000 U/kg/day IV div q4–6h; AND gentamicin 6.0 mg/kg/day IV div q8h; for 4–6 wk (AII)	Combined treatment with cell-wall active antibiotic plus aminoglycoside used to achieve bactericidal activity. For beta-lactam allergy: vancomycin. Little data exist in children for daptomycin or linezolid. For gentamicin-R strains, use streptomycin or other aminoglycoside if susceptible.
Ampicillin-resistant (gentamicin-S)	Vancomycin 40 mg/kg/day IV div q8h AND gentamicin 6.0 mg/kg/day IV div q8h; for 6 wk (AII)	
Vancomycin-resistant (gentamicin-S)	Daptomycin IV if also ampicillin-resistant (dose is age-dependent; see Chapter 11) AND gentamicin 6.0 mg/kg/day IV div q8h; for 4–6 wk (AIII)	
– Staphylococci: S aureus, including CA-MRSA; S epidermidis[6,207] Consider continuing therapy at end of 6 wk if vegetations persist on echocardiogram. The risk of persisting organisms in deep venous thromboses that occurred during bacteremia is not defined.	MSSA or MSSE: nafcillin or oxacillin/nafcillin 150–200 mg/kg/day IV div q6h for 4–6 wk AND gentamicin 6 mg/kg/day div q8h for first 14 days. CA-MRSA or MRSE: vancomycin 40–60 mg/kg/day IV div q8h AND gentamicin for 6 wk; consider for slow response, ADD rifampin 20 mg/kg/day IV div q8–12h. For vancomycin-resistant MRSA, please consult an infectious diseases specialist.	Surgery may be necessary in acute phase; avoid 1st-generation cephalosporins (conflicting data on efficacy). AHA suggests gentamicin for only the first 3–5 days for MSSA or MSSE and optional gentamicin for MRSA. For failures on therapy, or vancomycin-resistant MRSA, consider daptomycin (dose is age-dependent; see Chapter 11) AND gentamicin 6 mg/kg/day div q8h.
– Pneumococcus, gonococcus, group A streptococcus	Penicillin G 200,000 U/kg/day IV div q4–6h for 4 wk (BII); alternatives: ceftriaxone or vancomycin	Ceftriaxone plus azithromycin for suspected gonococcus until susceptibilities known. For penicillin non-susceptible strains of pneumococcus, use high-dosage penicillin G 300,000 U/kg/day IV div q4–6h or high-dosage ceftriaxone 100 mg/kg IV q24h for 4 wk.
HACEK (Haemophilus, Aggregatibacter [formerly Actinobacillus], Cardiobacterium, Eikenella, Kingella spp)	Usually susceptible to ceftriaxone 100 mg/kg IV q24h for 4 wk (BII)	Some organisms will be ampicillin-susceptible. Usually do not require the addition of gentamicin.

6

Antimicrobial Therapy According to Clinical Syndromes

Antimicrobial Therapy According to Clinical Syndromes

6

G. CARDIOVASCULAR INFECTIONS (continued)

Clinical Diagnosis	Therapy (evidence grade)	Comments
– Enteric Gram-negative bacilli	Antibiotics specific to pathogen (usually ceftriaxone plus gentamicin); duration at least 6 wk (AIII)	For ESBL organisms, carbapenems or beta-lactam/beta-lactamase inhibitor combinations PLUS gentamicin, should be effective.
– *Pseudomonas aeruginosa*	Antibiotic specific to susceptibility: cefepime or meropenem PLUS tobramycin	Cefepime and meropenem are both more active against *Pseudomonas* and less likely to allow beta-lactamase–resistant pathogens to emerge than ceftazidime.
– **Prosthetic valve/material**[210,214]	Follow echocardiogram for resolution of vegetation. For beta-lactam allergy: vancomycin.	
– Viridans streptococci		
Fully susceptible to penicillin	Ceftriaxone 100 mg/kg IV, IM q24h for 6 wk OR penicillin G 300,000 U/kg/day IV div q4–6h for 6 wk (AIII); OR penicillin G or ceftriaxone AND gentamicin 6.0 mg/kg/day IM, IV div q8h for first 2 wk of 6 wk course (AII)	Gentamicin is optional for the first 2 wk of a total of 6 wk of therapy for prosthetic valve/material endocarditis.
Relatively resistant to penicillin	Penicillin G 300,000 U/kg/day IV div q4–6h for 6 wk, or ceftriaxone 100 mg/kg IV q24h for 6 wk; AND gentamicin 6 mg/kg/day IM, IV div q8h for 6 wk (AIII)	Gentamicin is used for all 6 wk of therapy for prosthetic valve/material endocarditis caused by relatively resistant strains.
– Enterococcus (See dosages under native valve.) Treatment course is at least 6 wk, particularly if vancomycin is used.[210,214]		
– Staphylococci: *S aureus*, including CA-MRSA;[6-210] *S epidermidis*[6-210] Consider continuing therapy at end of 6 wk if vegetations persist on echocardiogram.	MSSA or MSSE: nafcillin or oxacillin/nafcillin 150–200 mg/kg/day IV div q6h for ≥6 wk AND gentamicin 6 mg/kg/day div q8h for first 14 days. CA-MRSA or MRSE: vancomycin 40–60 mg/kg/day IV div q8h AND gentamicin for ≥6 wk; ADD rifampin 20 mg/kg/day IV div q8–12h.	For failures on therapy, consider daptomycin (dose is age-dependent; see Chapter 11) AND gentamicin 6 mg/kg/day div q8h.

– *Candida*[81,214,215]	AmB preparations have more experience (no comparative trials against echinocandins), OR caspofungin 70 mg/m² load on day 1, then 50 mg/m²/day or micafungin 2–4 mg/kg/day (BIII).	Poor prognosis; please obtain advice from an infectious diseases specialist. Surgery may be required to resect infected valve. Long-term suppressive therapy with fluconazole. Suspect *Candida* vegetations when lesions are large on echocardiography.

– Culture negative prosthetic valve endocarditis: treat at least 6 wk.

Endocarditis prophylaxis[208,212,216]. Given that (1) endocarditis is rarely caused by dental/GI procedures and (2) prophylaxis for procedures prevents an exceedingly small number of cases, the risks of antibiotics outweigh the benefits. Highest risk conditions currently recommended for prophylaxis: (1) prosthetic heart valve (or prosthetic material used to repair a valve); (2) previous endocarditis; (3) cyanotic congenital heart disease that is unrepaired (or palliatively repaired with shunts and conduits); (4) congenital heart disease that is repaired but with defects at the site of repair adjacent to prosthetic material; (5) completely repaired congenital heart disease using prosthetic material, for the first 6 mo after repair; or (6) cardiac transplant patients with valvulopathy. Routine prophylaxis no longer is required for children with native valve abnormalities. Assessment of new prophylaxis guidelines documents a possible increase in viridans streptococcal endocarditis in children 10–17 y old but not 0–9 y old.[217] However, no changes in prophylaxis recommendations are being made at this time.

– In highest risk patients: dental procedures that involve manipulation of the gingival or periodontal region of teeth	Amoxicillin 50 mg/kg PO 60 min before procedure OR ampicillin or ceftriaxone or cefazolin, all at 50 mg/kg IM/IV 30–60 min before procedure	If penicillin allergy: clindamycin 20 mg/kg PO (60 min before) or IV (30 min before); OR azithromycin 15 mg/kg or clarithromycin 15 mg/kg, 60 min before
– Genitourinary and GI procedures	None	No longer recommended
Lemierre syndrome (*Fusobacterium necrophorum* primarily, new reports with MRSA)[115–119] (pharyngitis with internal jugular vein septic thrombosis, postanginal sepsis, necrobacillosis)	Empiric: meropenem 60 mg/kg/day div q8h (or 120 mg/kg/day div q8h for CNS metastatic foci [AIII]) OR ceftriaxone 100 mg/kg/day q24h AND metronidazole 40 mg/kg/day div q8h or clindamycin 40 mg/kg/day div q6h (BIII). ADD empiric vancomycin if MRSA suspected.	Anecdotal reports suggest metronidazole may be effective for apparent failures with other agents. Often requires anticoagulation. Metastatic and recurrent abscesses often develop while on active, appropriate therapy, requiring multiple debridements and prolonged antibiotic therapy. Treat until CRP and ESR are normal (AIII).

G. CARDIOVASCULAR INFECTIONS (continued)

Clinical Diagnosis	Therapy (evidence grade)	Comments
Purulent pericarditis		
– Empiric (acute, bacterial: S aureus [including MRSA], group A streptococcus, pneumococcus, meningococcus, H influenzae type b)[218,219]	Vancomycin 40 mg/kg/day IV div q8h AND ceftriaxone 50–75 mg/kg/day q24h (AIII), OR cefaroline: 2–<6 mo, 30 mg/kg/day IV div q8h; ≥6 mo, 45 mg/kg/day IV div q8h (max single dose 600 mg) (BIII)	For presumed staphylococcal infection, ADD gentamicin (AIII). Increasingly uncommon with immunization against pneumococcus and H influenzae type b.[219] Pericardiocentesis is essential to establish diagnosis. Surgical drainage of pus with pericardial window or pericardiectomy is important to prevent tamponade.
– S aureus	For MSSA: oxacillin/nafcillin 150–200 mg/kg/day IV div q6h OR cefazolin 100 mg/kg/day IV div q8h. Treat for 2–3 wk after drainage (BIII). For CA-MRSA: continue vancomycin or ceftaroline. Treat for 3–4 wk after drainage (BIII).	Continue therapy with gentamicin; consider use of rifampin in severe cases due to tissue penetration characteristics.
– H influenzae type b in unimmunized children	Ceftriaxone 50 mg/kg/day q24h or cefotaxime 150 mg/kg/day div q8h; for 10–14 days (AIII)	Ampicillin for beta-lactamase–negative strains
– Pneumococcus, meningococcus, group A streptococcus	Penicillin G 200,000 U/kg/day IV, IM div q6h for 10–14 days OR ceftriaxone 50 mg/kg qd for 10–14 days (AIII)	Ceftriaxone or cefotaxime for penicillin non-susceptible pneumococci
– Coliform bacilli	Ceftriaxone 50–75 mg/kg/day q24h or cefotaxime 150 mg/kg/day div q8h for 3 wk or longer (AIII)	Alternative drugs depending on susceptibilities; for Enterobacter, Serratia, or Citrobacter, use cefepime or meropenem. For ESBL E coli or Klebsiella, use a carbapenem.
– Tuberculous[13,14]	INH 10–15 mg/kg/day (max 300 mg) PO, IV qd, for 6 mo AND rifampin 10–20 mg/kg/day (max 600 mg) PO qd, IV for 6 mo. ADD PZA 20–40 mg/kg/day PO qd for first 2 mo therapy; if suspected multidrug resistance, also add ethambutol 20 mg/kg/day PO qd (AIII).	Current guidelines do not suggest a benefit from routine use of corticosteroids. However, for those at highest risk of restrictive pericarditis, steroid continues to be recommended.[13] For children: prednisone 2 mg/kg/day for 4 wk, then 0.5 mg/kg/day for 4 wk, then 0.25 mg/kg/day for 2 wk, then 0.1 mg/kg/day for 1 wk.

H. GASTROINTESTINAL INFECTIONS (See Chapter 10 for parasitic infections.)

Clinical Diagnosis	Therapy (evidence grade)	Comments

Diarrhea/Gastroenteritis

Note on *Escherichia coli* and diarrheal disease: Antibiotic susceptibility of *E coli* varies considerably from region to region. For mild to moderate disease, TMP/SMX may be started as initial therapy, but for more severe disease and for locations with rates of TMP/SMX resistance greater than 10% to 20%, azithromycin, an oral 3rd-generation cephalosporin (eg, cefixime, cefdinir, ceftibuten), or ciprofloxacin should be used (AIII). Cultures and antibiotic susceptibility testing are recommended for significant disease (AIII).

Clinical Diagnosis	Therapy (evidence grade)	Comments
– Empiric therapy of community-associated diarrhea in the United States (*E coli* [STEC], including O157:H7 strains, and ETEC], *Salmonella, Campylobacter,* and *Shigella* predominate; *Yersinia* and parasites causing <5%; however, viral pathogens are far more common, especially for children <3 y.)[220,221]	Azithromycin 10 mg/kg qd for 3 days (BII), OR cefixime 8 mg/kg/day PO qd (BII) for 5 days; OR ciprofloxacin 30 mg/kg/day PO div bid for 3 days	Alternatives: other oral 3rd-generation cephalosporins (eg, cefdinir, ceftibuten); or rifaximin 600 mg/day div tid for 3 days (for nonfebrile, non-bloody diarrhea for children >11 y). Controversy exists regarding treatment of O157:H7 strains and the prevention or increased incidence of HUS, with retrospective data to support either treatment, or withholding treatment. Some experts treat with antimicrobials and others prefer to use supportive care.[221–226]

Antimicrobial Therapy According to Clinical Syndromes

H. GASTROINTESTINAL INFECTIONS (continued) (See Chapter 10 for parasitic infections.)

Clinical Diagnosis	Therapy (evidence grade)	Comments
– Traveler's diarrhea: empiric therapy (E coli, Campylobacter, Salmonella, Shigella, plus many other pathogens, including protozoa)[221,227-234]	Azithromycin 10 mg/kg qd for 1–3 days (AII); OR rifaximin 200 mg PO tid for 3 days (age ≥12 y) (BII); OR ciprofloxacin (BII); OR rifaximin 200 mg tid for 3 days for age ≥12 y (BII).	Susceptibility patterns of E coli, Campylobacter, Salmonella, and Shigella vary widely by country; check country-specific data for departing or returning travelers. Azithromycin preferable to ciprofloxacin for travelers to Southeast Asia given high prevalence of quinolone-resistant Campylobacter.

Rifaximin is less effective than ciprofloxacin for invasive bloody bacterial enteritis; rifaximin may also not be as effective for Shigella, Salmonella, and Campylobacter as other agents.

Interestingly, for adults who travel and take antibiotics (mostly fluoroquinolones), colonization with ESBL-positive E coli is more frequent on return home.[235] Adjunctive therapy with loperamide (antimotility) is not recommended for children <2 y and should be used only in nonfebrile, non-bloody diarrhea.[221,236,237] May shorten symptomatic illness by about 24 h. |
– Traveler's diarrhea: prophylaxis[227,228]	– Prophylaxis: Early self-treatment with agents listed previously is preferred over long-term prophylaxis, but may use prophylaxis for a short-term (<14 days) visit to very high-risk region: rifaximin (for older children), azithromycin, or bismuth subsalicylate (BII).	
– Aeromonas hydrophila[238]	Ciprofloxacin 30 mg/kg/day PO div bid for 5 days OR azithromycin 10 mg/kg qd for 3 days OR cefixime 8 mg/kg/day PO qd (BIII)	Not all strains produce enterotoxins and diarrhea; role in diarrhea questioned.[238] Resistance to TMP/SMX about 10%–15%. Choose narrowest spectrum agent based on in vitro susceptibilities.
– Campylobacter jejuni[239-241]	Azithromycin 10 mg/kg/day for 3 days (BII) or erythromycin 40 mg/kg/day PO div qid for 5 days (BII)	Alternatives: doxycycline or ciprofloxacin (high rate of fluoroquinolone resistance in Thailand, India, and now the United States).

	Single-dose azithromycin (1 g, once) is effective in adults.	Ciprofloxacin or TMP/SMX (if susceptible)
– Cholera[232,242]	Azithromycin 20 mg/kg once; OR erythromycin 50 mg/kg/day PO div qid for 3 days; OR doxycycline 4 mg/kg/day (max 200 mg/day) PO div bid, for all ages	
– Clostridium difficile (antibiotic-associated colitis)[243–248]	Metronidazole 30 mg/kg/day PO div qid OR vancomycin 40 mg/kg/day PO div qid for 7 days; for relapsing C difficile enteritis, consider pulse therapy (1 wk on/1 wk off for 3–4 cycles) or prolonged tapering therapy.[243]	Vancomycin is more effective for severe infection.[245] Fidaxomicin approved for adults; pediatric studies successfully completed with similar results to those in adults.[247] Many infants and children may have asymptomatic colonization with C difficile.[245] Higher risk of relapse in children with multiple comorbidities.
– E coli		
Enterotoxigenic (etiology of most traveler's diarrhea)[221,228–231]	Azithromycin 10 mg/kg qd for 3 days; OR cefixime 8 mg/kg/day PO qd for 3 days; OR ciprofloxacin 30 mg/kg/day PO bid for 3 days	Most illnesses brief and self-limited. Alternatives: rifaximin 600 mg/day div tid for 3 days (for nonfebrile, non-bloody diarrhea for children >11 y, as rifaximin is not absorbed systemically); OR TMP/SMX. Resistance increasing worldwide; check country-specific rates, if possible.[231]
Enterohemorrhagic (O157:H7; STEC, etiology of HUS)[221–225]	Controversy on whether treatment of O157:H7 diarrhea results in more or less toxin-mediated renal damage.[221–225] For severe infection, treat as for enterotoxigenic strains above, preferably with azithromycin that is associated with decreased toxin production in animal models.[225]	Injury to colonic mucosa may lead to invasive bacterial colitis.
Enteropathogenic	Neomycin 100 mg/kg/day PO div q6–8h for 5 days	Most traditional "enteropathogenic" strains are not toxigenic or invasive. Postinfection diarrhea may be problematic.

6

Antimicrobial Therapy According to Clinical Syndromes

Antimicrobial Therapy According to Clinical Syndromes

H. GASTROINTESTINAL INFECTIONS (continued) (See Chapter 10 for parasitic infections.)

Clinical Diagnosis	Therapy (evidence grade)	Comments
– Gastritis, peptic ulcer disease (*Helicobacter pylori*)[249–252]	Either triple agent therapy in areas of low clarithromycin resistance: clarithromycin 7.5 mg/kg/dose 2–3 times each day, AND amoxicillin 40 mg/kg/dose (max 1 g) PO bid AND omeprazole 0.5 mg/kg/dose PO bid 14 days (BII), OR quadruple therapy that includes metronidazole (15 mg/kg/day div bid) added to the regimen above.[253]	New pediatric guidelines recommend some restriction of testing for those at high risk of complications. Resistance to clarithromycin is as high as 20% in some regions.[249,251,254] Current approach for empiric therapy if clarithromycin resistance may be present: high-dose triple therapy is recommended with proton pump inhibitor, amoxicillin, and metronidazole for 14 days ± bismuth to create quadruple therapy.[249]
– Giardiasis (See Chapter 10.) (*Giardia intestinalis*, formerly *lamblia*)[255]	Metronidazole 30–40 mg/kg/day PO div tid for 7–10 days (BII); OR tinidazole 50 mg/kg/day (max 2 g) for 1 day (BII); OR nitazoxanide PO (take with food), age 12–47 mo, 100 mg/dose bid for 7 days; age 4–11 y, 200 mg/dose bid for 7 days; age ≥12 y, 1 tab (500 mg)/dose bid for 7 days (BII)	If therapy is inadequate, another course of the same agent is usually curative. Alternatives: paromomycin OR albendazole (CII). Prolonged or combination drug courses may be needed for immunocompromised conditions (eg, hypogammaglobulinemia). Treatment of asymptomatic carriers not usually recommended.
– Salmonellosis[256–258] (See Chapter 10 for discussion of traveler's diarrhea for typhoid infection outside of North America.)		
Non-typhoid strains[256–258]	Usually none for self-limited diarrhea in immunocompetent child (eg, diarrhea is often much improved by the time culture results are available). Treat those with persisting symptomatic infection and infants <3 mo who demonstrate an increased risk of bacteremia: azithromycin 10 mg/kg PO qd for 3 days (AII); OR ceftriaxone 75 mg/kg/day IV, IM q24h for 5 days (AII); OR cefixime 20–30 mg/kg/day PO for 5–7 days (BII); OR for susceptible strains: TMP/SMX 8 mg/kg/day of TMP PO div bid for 14 days (AI).	Alternatives: ciprofloxacin 30 mg/kg/day PO div bid for 5 days (AI). Carriage of strains may be prolonged in treated children.

Typhoid fever[258-262]	Azithromycin 10 mg/kg qd for 5 days (AII); OR ceftriaxone 75 mg/kg/day IV, IM q24h for 5 days (AII); OR cefixime 20–30 mg/kg/day PO, div q12h for 14 days (BII); OR for susceptible strains: TMP/SMX 8 mg/kg/day of TMP PO div bid for 10 days (AI)	Increasing cephalosporin resistance. For newly emergent MDR strains, may require prolonged IV therapy. Longer treatment courses for focal invasive disease (eg, osteomyelitis). Alternative: ciprofloxacin 30 mg/kg/day PO div bid for 5–7 days (AI).
— Shigellosis[263-265]	Cefixime 8 mg/kg/day PO qd for 5 days (AII); OR azithromycin 10 mg/kg/day PO for 3 days (AII); OR ciprofloxacin 30 mg/kg/day PO div bid for 3–5 days (BII)	Alternatives for susceptible strains: TMP/SMX 8 mg/kg/day of TMP PO div bid for 5 days; OR ampicillin (not amoxicillin). Ceftriaxone 50 mg/kg/day IM, IV if parenteral therapy necessary, for 2–5 days. Avoid antiperistaltic drugs. Treatment for the improving child is not usually necessary to hasten recovery, but some experts would treat to decrease communicability.
— Yersinia enterocolitica[266-268]	Antimicrobial therapy probably not of value for mild disease in normal hosts. TMP/SMX PO, IV; OR ciprofloxacin PO, IV (BIII).	Alternatives: ceftriaxone or gentamicin. High rates of resistance to ampicillin. May mimic appendicitis in older children. Limited clinical data exist on oral therapy.

Antimicrobial Therapy According to Clinical Syndromes

6

H. GASTROINTESTINAL INFECTIONS (continued) (See Chapter 10 for parasitic infections.)

Clinical Diagnosis	Therapy (evidence grade)	Comments
Intra-abdominal infection (abscess, peritonitis secondary to bowel/appendix contents)		
– Appendicitis; bowel-associated (enteric Gram-negative bacilli, Bacteroides spp, Enterococcus spp, increasingly Pseudomonas)[269-274]	Source control is critical to curing this infection. Meropenem 60 mg/kg/day IV div q8h or imipenem 60 mg/kg/day IV div q6h; OR pip/tazo 240 mg pip/kg/day div q6h; for 4–5 days for patients with adequate source control,[273] 7–10 days or longer if suspicion of persisting intra-abdominal abscess (AII).	Recent studies of the microbiology of appendicitis indicate Pseudomonas as a common pathogen (found in up to 30% of children),[269,271,275] documenting the need for empiric use of an antipseudomonal drug, such as a carbapenem or pip/tazo, **unless the surgery was highly effective at drainage/source control** (gentamicin is not active in an abscess), which may explain successful outcomes in retrospective studies that did not include antipseudomonal coverage.[276-278] Many other regimens may be effective, including ampicillin 150 mg/kg/day div q8h AND gentamicin 6–7.5 mg/kg/day IV, IM div q8h AND metronidazole 40 mg/kg/day IV div q8h; OR ceftriaxone 50 mg/kg q24h AND metronidazole 40 mg/kg/day IV div q8h.
	Data support IV outpatient therapy or oral step-down therapy[274] when clinically improved, particularly when oral therapy can be focused on the most prominent, invasive cultured pathogens.	
– Tuberculosis, abdominal (Mycobacterium bovis, from unpasteurized dairy products)[13,14,279,280]	INH 10–15 mg/kg/day (max 300 mg) PO qd for 6 mo AND rifampin 10–20 mg/kg/day (max 600 mg) PO qd for 6 mo (AII). Some experts recommend routine use of ethambutol in the empiric regimen. M bovis is resistant to PZA.	Corticosteroids are routinely used as adjunctive therapy to decrease morbidity from inflammation.[281] Directly observed therapy preferred; after 2+ wk of daily therapy, can change to twice-weekly dosing double dosage of INH (max 900 mg); rifampin remains same dosage (10–20 mg/kg/day, max 600 mg) (AII). LP ± CT of head for children ≤2 y with active disease to rule out occult, concurrent CNS infection (AIII).

	If risk factors are present for multidrug resistance (eg, poor adherence to previous therapy), add ethambutol 20 mg/kg/day PO qd OR a fluoroquinolone (moxifloxacin or levofloxacin).	
Perirectal abscess (*Bacteroides* spp, other anaerobes, enteric bacilli, and *S aureus* predominate)[282]	Clindamycin 30–40 mg/kg/day IV div q8h AND cefotaxime or ceftriaxone or gentamicin (BIII)	Surgical drainage alone may be curative. Obtaining cultures and susceptibilities is increasingly important with rising resistance to cephalosporins in community *E coli* isolates.
Peritonitis — Peritoneal dialysis indwelling catheter infection (staphylococcal; enteric Gram-negatives; yeast)[283,284]	Antibiotic added to dialysate in concentrations approximating those attained in serum for systemic disease (eg, 4 μg/mL for gentamicin, 25 μg/mL for vancomycin, 125 μg/mL for cefazolin, 25 μg/mL for ciprofloxacin) after a larger loading dose (AII)[284]	Selection of antibiotic based on organism isolated from peritoneal fluid; systemic antibiotics if there is accompanying bacteremia/fungemia
— Primary (pneumococcus or group A streptococcus)[285]	Ceftriaxone 50 mg/kg/day q24h, or cefotaxime 150 mg/kg/day div q8h; if pen-S, then penicillin G 150,000 U/kg/day IV div q6h; for 7–10 days (AII)	Other antibiotics according to culture and susceptibility tests, as peritonitis with nephrotic syndrome or with some chronic liver disease is not apparently more common than spontaneous peritonitis. A review of the current literature suggests spontaneous pneumococcal peritonitis has become a disease of the past in immune-competent children with the widespread use of conjugate pneumococcal vaccine.

Antimicrobial Therapy According to Clinical Syndromes

6

I. GENITAL AND SEXUALLY TRANSMITTED INFECTIONS

Clinical Diagnosis	Therapy (evidence grade)	Comments
Consider testing for HIV and other STIs in a child with one documented STI; consider sexual abuse in prepubertal children. The most recent CDC STI treatment guidelines are posted online at www.cdc.gov/std/treatment (accessed October 2, 2017).		
Chancroid (Haemophilus ducreyi)[55]	Azithromycin 1 g PO as single dose OR ceftriaxone 250 mg IM as single dose	Alternative: erythromycin 1.5 g/day PO div tid for 7 days OR ciprofloxacin 1,000 mg PO qd, div bid for 3 days
Chlamydia trachomatis (cervicitis, urethritis)[55,286]	Azithromycin 20 mg/kg (max 1 g) PO for 1 dose; OR doxycycline (patients >7 y) 4 mg/kg/day (max 200 mg/day) PO div bid for 7 days	Alternatives: erythromycin 2 g/day PO div qid for 7 days; OR levofloxacin 500 mg PO q24h for 7 days
Epididymitis (associated with positive urine cultures and STIs)[55,287,288]	Ceftriaxone 50 mg/kg/day q24h for 7–10 days AND (for older children) doxycycline 200 mg/day div bid for 10 days	Microbiology not well studied in children; in infants, also associated with urogenital tract anomalies. Treat infants for Staphylococcus aureus and Escherichia coli; may resolve spontaneously; in STI, caused by Chlamydia and gonococcus.
Gonorrhea[55,286,289–291]	Antibiotic resistance is an ongoing problem, with new data to suggest the emergence of azithromycin resistance being tracked closely by the CDC.[291]	
– Newborns	See Chapter 5.	
– Genital infections (uncomplicated vulvovaginitis, cervicitis, urethritis, or proctitis)[55,286,289,290]	Ceftriaxone 250 mg IM for 1 dose (regardless of weight) AND azithromycin 1 g PO for 1 dose or doxycycline 200 mg/day div q12h for 7 days	Cefixime no longer recommended due to increasing cephalosporin resistance.[290] Fluoroquinolones are no longer recommended due to resistance. Dual therapy has not been evaluated yet in children but should be effective.
– Pharyngitis[55,290,291]	Ceftriaxone 250 mg IM for 1 dose (regardless of weight) AND azithromycin 1 g PO for 1 dose or doxycycline 200 mg/day div q12h for 7 days	

– Conjunctivitis[55]	Ceftriaxone 1 g IM for 1 dose AND azithromycin 1 g PO for 1 dose	Lavage the eye with saline.
– Disseminated gonococcal infection[55,290,291]	Ceftriaxone 50 mg/kg/day IM, IV q24h (max: 1 g) AND azithromycin 1 g PO for 1 dose; total course for 7 days	No studies in children: increase dosage for meningitis.
Granuloma inguinale (donovanosis, *Klebsiella granulomatis*, formerly *Calymmatobacterium*)[55]	Azithromycin 1 g orally once per week or 500 mg daily for at least 3 weeks and until all lesions have completely healed	Primarily in tropical regions of India, Pacific, and Africa. Options: Doxycycline 4 mg/kg/day div bid (max 200 mg/day) PO for at least 3 wk OR ciprofloxacin 750 mg PO bid for at least 3 wk OR erythromycin base 500 mg PO qid for at least 3 wk OR TMP/SMX 1 double-strength (160 mg/800 mg) tablet PO bid for at least 3 wk; all regimens continue until all lesions have completely healed.
Herpes simplex virus, genital infection[55,292,293]	Acyclovir 20 mg/kg/dose (max 400 mg) PO tid for 7–10 days (first episode) (AI); OR valacyclovir 20 mg/kg/dose of extemporaneous suspension (directions on package label), max 1 g PO bid for 7–10 days (first episode) (AI); OR famciclovir 250 mg PO tid for 7–10 days (AI); for more severe infection: acyclovir 15 mg/kg/day IV div q8h as 1-h infusion for 7–10 days (AII)	For recurrent episodes: treat with acyclovir PO, valacyclovir PO, or famciclovir PO, immediately when symptoms begin, for 5 days. For suppression: acyclovir 20 mg/kg/dose (max 400 mg) PO bid; OR valacyclovir 20 mg/kg/dose PO qd (little long-term safety data in children; no efficacy data in children). Prophylaxis is recommended in pregnant women.[294]
Lymphogranuloma venereum (*C trachomatis*)[55]	Doxycycline 4 mg/kg/day (max 200 mg/day) PO (patients >7 y) div bid for 21 days	Alternatives: erythromycin 2 g/day PO qid for 21 days; OR azithromycin 1 g PO once weekly for 3 wk

6

Antimicrobial Therapy According to Clinical Syndromes

6

I. GENITAL AND SEXUALLY TRANSMITTED INFECTIONS (continued)

Clinical Diagnosis	Therapy (evidence grade)	Comments
Pelvic inflammatory disease (*Chlamydia*, gonococcus, plus anaerobes)[55,295]	Cefoxitin 2 g IV q6h; AND doxycycline 200 mg/day PO or IV div bid; OR cefotetan 2 g IV q12h AND doxycycline 100 mg orally or IV q12h, OR clindamycin 900 mg IV q8h AND gentamicin 1.5 mg/kg IV, IM q8h until clinical improvement for 24 h, followed by doxycycline 200 mg/day PO div bid (AND clindamycin 1,800 mg/day PO div qid for tubo-ovarian abscess) to complete 14 days of therapy	Optional regimen: ceftriaxone 250 mg IM for 1 dose AND doxycycline 200 mg/day PO div bid; WITH/WITHOUT metronidazole 1 g/day PO div bid; for 14 days
Syphilis[55,296] (Test for HIV.)		
– Congenital	See Chapter 5.	
– Neurosyphilis (positive CSF VDRL or CSF pleocytosis with serologic diagnosis of syphilis)	Crystalline penicillin G 200–300,000 U/kg/day (max 24,000,000 U/day) div q6h for 10–14 days (AIII)	
– Primary, secondary	Benzathine penicillin G 50,000 U/kg (max 2,400,000 U) IM as a single dose (AIII); do not use benzathine-procaine penicillin mixtures.	Follow-up serologic tests at 6, 12, and 24 mo; 15% may remain seropositive despite adequate treatment. If allergy to penicillin: doxycycline (patients >7 y) 4 mg/kg/day (max 200 mg) PO div bid for 14 days. CSF examination should be obtained for children being treated for primary or secondary syphilis to rule out asymptomatic neurosyphilis. Test for HIV.
– Syphilis of <1 y duration, without clinical symptoms (early latent syphilis)	Benzathine penicillin G 50,000 U/kg (max 2,400,000 U) IM as a single dose (AIII)	Alternative if allergy to penicillin: doxycycline (patients >7 y) 4 mg/kg/day (max 200 mg/day) PO div bid for 14 days
– Syphilis of >1 y duration, without clinical symptoms	Benzathine penicillin G 50,000 U/kg (max 2,400,000 U) IM weekly for 3 doses (AIII)	Alternative if allergy to penicillin: doxycycline (patients >7 y) 4 mg/kg/day (max 200 mg/day) PO div bid for 28 days

Condition	Therapy	Comments
(late latent syphilis) or syphilis of unknown duration		Look for neurologic, eye, and aortic complications of tertiary syphilis.
Trichomoniasis[55]	Tinidazole 50 mg/kg (max 2 g) PO for 1 dose (BII) OR metronidazole 2 gm PO for 1 dose OR metronidazole 500 mg PO bid for 7 days (BII)	
Urethritis, nongonococcal (See Gonorrhea for gonorrhea therapy.)[55,297]	Azithromycin 20 mg/kg (max 1 g) PO for 1 dose, OR doxycycline (patients >7 y) 40 mg/kg/day (max 200 mg/day) PO div bid for 7 days (AII)	Erythromycin, levofloxacin, or ofloxacin Increasing resistance noted in *Mycoplasma genitalium*[297]
Vaginitis[55]		
— Bacterial vaginosis[55,298]	Metronidazole 500 mg PO twice daily for 7 days OR metronidazole vaginal gel (0.75%) qd for 5 days, OR clindamycin vaginal cream for 7 days	Alternative: tinidazole 1 g PO qd for 5 days, OR clindamycin 300 mg PO bid for 7 days Relapse common Caused by synergy of *Gardnerella* with anaerobes
— Candidiasis, vulvovaginal[55,299]	Topical vaginal cream/tabs/suppositories (alphabetic order): butoconazole, clotrimazole, econazole, fenticonazole, miconazole, sertaconazole, terconazole, or tioconazole for 3–7 days (AII); OR fluconazole 10 mg/kg (max 150 mg) as a single dose (AII)	For uncomplicated vulvovaginal candidiasis, no topical agent is clearly superior. Avoid azoles during pregnancy. For recurring disease, consider 10–14 days of induction with topical agent or fluconazole, followed by fluconazole once weekly for 6 mo (AI).
— Prepubertal vaginitis[299,300]	No prospective studies	Cultures from symptomatic prepubertal girls are statistically more likely to yield *E coli*, enterococcus, coagulase-negative staphylococci, and streptococci (viridans strep and group A strep), but these organisms may also be present in asymptomatic girls.
— *Shigella*[301]	Cefixime 8 mg/kg/day PO qd for 5 days OR ciprofloxacin 30 mg/kg/day PO div bid for 5 days	50% have bloody discharge; usually not associated with diarrhea.
— *Streptococcus*, group A[302]	Penicillin V 50–75 mg/kg/day PO tid for 10 days	Amoxicillin 50–75 mg/kg/day PO div tid

Antimicrobial Therapy According to Clinical Syndromes

J. CENTRAL NERVOUS SYSTEM INFECTIONS

Clinical Diagnosis	Therapy (evidence grade)	Comments
Abscess, brain (respiratory tract flora, skin flora, or bowel flora, depending on the pathogenesis of infection based on underlying comorbid disease and origin of bacteremia)[303,304]	Until etiology established, use empiric therapy for presumed mixed-flora infection with origins from the respiratory tract, skin, and/or bowel, based on individual patient evaluation and risk for brain abscess (see Comments for MRSA considerations): meropenem 120 mg/kg/day div q8h (AIII); OR nafcillin 150–200 mg/kg/day IV div q6h AND cefotaxime 200–300 mg/kg/day IV div q6h or ceftriaxone 100 mg/kg/day IV q24h AND metronidazole 30 mg/kg/day IV div q8h (BIII); for 2–3 wk after successful drainage (depending on pathogen, size of abscess, and response to therapy); longer course if no surgery (3–6 wk) (BIII). For single pathogen abscess, use a single agent in doses that will achieve effective CNS exposure. The blood-brain barrier is not intact in brain abscesses.	Surgery for abscesses ≥2 cm diameter. If CA-MRSA suspected, ADD vancomycin 60 mg/kg/day IV div q8h ± rifampin 20 mg/kg/day IV div q12h, pending culture results. We have successfully treated MRSA intracranial infections with ceftaroline, but no prospective data exist: ceftaroline: 2–<6 mo, 30 mg/kg/day IV div q8h (each dose given over 2 h); ≥6 mo, 45 mg/kg/day IV div q8h (each dose given over 2 h) (max single dose 600 mg) (BII). If secondary to chronic otitis, include meropenem or cefepime in regimen for anti-*Pseudomonas* activity. For enteric Gram-negative bacilli, consider ESBL-producing *Escherichia coli* and *Klebsiella* that require meropenem and are resistant to cefotaxime. Follow resolution of abscess size by CT for difficult-to-treat pathogens.
Encephalitis[305]		
— Amebic (*Naegleria fowleri, Balamuthia mandrillaris,* and *Acanthamoeba*)	See Chapter 10, Amebiasis.	
— CMV	See Chapter 9, CMV. Not well studied in children. Consider ganciclovir 10 mg/kg/day IV div q12h; for severe immunocompromised, ADD foscarnet 180 mg/kg/day IV div q8h for 3 wk; follow quantitative PCR for CMV.	Reduce dose for renal insufficiency. Watch for neutropenia.
— Enterovirus	Supportive therapy; no antivirals currently FDA approved.	Pocapavir PO is currently under investigation for enterovirus (poliovirus).

		Pleconaril PO is currently under consideration for approval at the FDA for treatment of neonatal enteroviral sepsis syndrome.[306,307]
– EBV[308]	Not studied in a controlled comparative trial. Consider ganciclovir 10 mg/kg/day IV div q12h or acyclovir 60 mg/kg/day IV div q8h for 3 wk; follow quantitative PCR in CSF for EBV.	Efficacy of antiviral therapy not well defined
– Herpes simplex virus[309] See Chapter 5 for neonatal infection.	Acyclovir 60 mg/kg/day IV as 1–2 h infusion div q8h for 21 days for infants ≤4 mo; for older infants and children, 30–45 mg/kg/day IV for 21 days (AIII)	Perform CSF HSV PCR near end of 21 days of therapy and continue acyclovir until PCR negative. Safety of high-dose acyclovir (60 mg/kg/day) not well defined beyond the neonatal period; can be used, but monitor for neurotoxicity and nephrotoxicity; FDA has approved acyclovir at this dosage for encephalitis for children up to 12 y.
– *Toxoplasma* See Chapter 5 for neonatal congenital infection.	See Chapter 10.	
– Arbovirus (flavivirus—Zika, West Nile, St. Louis encephalitis, tick-borne encephalitis; togavirus— western equine encephalitis, eastern equine encephalitis; bunyavirus—La Crosse encephalitis, California encephalitis)[305]	Supportive therapy	Investigational only (antiviral, interferon, immune globulins). No specific antiviral agents are yet commercially available for any of the arboviruses, including Zika or West Nile.

6

Antimicrobial Therapy According to Clinical Syndromes

Antimicrobial Therapy According to Clinical Syndromes

6

J. CENTRAL NERVOUS SYSTEM INFECTIONS (continued)

Clinical Diagnosis	Therapy (evidence grade)	Comments
Meningitis, bacterial, community-associated		

NOTES
- In areas where pen-R pneumococci exist (>5% of invasive strains), initial empiric therapy for suspect pneumococcal meningitis should be with vancomycin AND cefotaxime or ceftriaxone until susceptibility test results are available. Although ceftaroline is more active than ceftriaxone against pneumococci and, as a beta-lactam, should be expected to achieve therapeutic CSF concentrations, no substantial pediatric data yet exist on CNS infections.
- Dexamethasone 0.6 mg/kg/day IV div q6h for 2 days as an adjunct to antibiotic therapy decreases hearing deficits and other neurologic sequelae in adults and children (for Haemophilus and pneumococcus; not prospectively studied in children for meningococcus or E coli). The first dose of dexamethasone is given before or concurrent with the first dose of antibiotic; probably little benefit if given ≥1 h after the antibiotic.[310,311]

– Empiric therapy[312]	Cefotaxime 200–300 mg/kg/day IV div q6h, or ceftriaxone 100 mg/kg/day IV q24h; AND vancomycin 60 mg/kg/day IV div q8h (AII)	If Gram stain or cultures demonstrate a pathogen other than pneumococcus, vancomycin is not needed; vancomycin used empirically for possible pen-R pneumococcus and possible MRSA; high-dose ceftaroline (MRSA dosing) should also prove effective, but no data exist currently for CNS infections.
– Haemophilus influenzae type b[312]	Cefotaxime 200–300 mg/kg/day IV div q6h, or ceftriaxone 100 mg/kg/day IV q24h; for 10 days (AI)	Alternative: ampicillin 200–400 mg/kg/day IV div q6h (for beta-lactamase–negative strains)
– Meningococcus (Neisseria meningitidis)[312]	Penicillin G 250,000 U/kg/day IV div q4h; or ceftriaxone 100 mg/kg/day IV q24h; or cefotaxime 200 mg/kg/day IV div q6h; treatment course for 7 days (AI)	Meningococcal prophylaxis: rifampin 10 mg/kg PO q12h for 4 doses OR ceftriaxone 125–250 mg IM once OR ciprofloxacin 500 mg PO once (adolescents and adults)
– Neonatal	See Chapter 5.	
– Pneumococcus (Streptococcus pneumoniae)[312]	For pen-S and cephalosporin-susceptible strains: penicillin G 250,000 U/kg/day IV div q4–6h, OR ceftriaxone 100 mg/kg/day IV q24h or	Some pneumococci may be resistant to penicillin but susceptible to cefotaxime and ceftriaxone and may be treated with the cephalosporin alone.

	cefotaxime 200–300 mg/kg/day IV div q6h; for 10 days (AI). For pen-R pneumococci: continue the combination of vancomycin and cephalosporin IV for total course (AIII).	With the efficacy of current pneumococcal conjugate vaccines, primary bacterial meningitis is uncommon, and penicillin resistance has decreased substantially. Test-of-cure LP may be helpful in those with pen-R pneumococci.
Meningitis, TB (Mycobacterium tuberculosis; Mycobacterium bovis)[13,14]	For non-immunocompromised children: INH 15 mg/kg/day PO, IV div q12–24h AND rifampin 15 mg/kg/day PO, IV div q12–24h for 12 mo AND PZA 30 mg/kg/day PO div q12–24h for first 2 mo of therapy, AND streptomycin 30 mg/kg/day IV, IM div q12h or ethionamide for first 4–8 wk of therapy; followed by INH and rifampin combination therapy to complete at least 12 mo for the total course.	Hyponatremia from inappropriate ADH secretion is common; ventricular drainage may be necessary for obstructive hydrocephalus. Corticosteroids (can use the same dexamethasone dose as for bacterial meningitis, 0.6 mg/kg/day IV div q6h) for 4 wk until neurologically stable, then taper dose for 1–3 mo to decrease neurologic complications and improve prognosis by decreasing the incidence of infarction.[313] Watch for rebound inflammation during taper; increase dose to previously effective level, then taper more slowly. For recommendations for drug-resistant strains and treatment of TB in HIV-infected patients, visit the CDC Web site for TB: www.cdc.gov/tb (accessed October 2, 2017).

Shunt infections: The use of antibiotic-impregnated shunts has decreased the frequency of this infection.[314] Shunt removal is usually necessary for cure, with placement of a new external ventricular drain; intraventricular injection of antibiotics should be considered in children who are responding poorly to systemic antibiotic therapy. Duration of therapy varies by pathogen and response to treatment.[315]

– Empiric therapy pending Gram stain and culture[312,315]	Vancomycin 60 mg/kg/day IV div q8h, AND ceftriaxone 100 mg/kg IV q24h (AII)	If Gram stain shows only Gram-positive cocci, can use vancomycin alone. Cefepime, meropenem, or ceftazidime should be used instead of ceftriaxone if Pseudomonas is suspected. For ESBL-containing Gram-negative bacilli, meropenem should be used.

6

Antimicrobial Therapy According to Clinical Syndromes

Antimicrobial Therapy According to Clinical Syndromes

J. CENTRAL NERVOUS SYSTEM INFECTIONS

Clinical Diagnosis	Therapy (evidence grade)	Comments
– Staphylococcus epidermidis or Staphylococcus aureus[312,315]	Vancomycin (for S epidermidis and CA-MRSA) 60 mg/kg/day IV div q6h; OR nafcillin (if organisms susceptible) 150–200 mg/kg/day AND rifampin; for 10–14 days (AIII)	For children who cannot tolerate vancomycin, ceftaroline has anecdotally been successful: ceftaroline: 2–<6 mo, 30 mg/kg/day IV div q8h (each dose given over 2 h); ≥6 mo, 45 mg/kg/day IV div q8h (each dose given over 2 h) (max single dose 600 mg) (BIII). Linezolid, daptomycin, and trimethoprim-sulfamethoxazole are other options.
– Gram-negative bacilli[312,315]	Empiric therapy with meropenem 120 mg/kg/day IV div q8h OR cefepime 150 mg/kg/day IV div q8h (AIII). For E coli (without ESBLs): ceftriaxone 100 mg/kg/day IV q12h OR cefotaxime 200–300 mg/kg/day IV div q6h; for at least 10–14 days, preferably 21 days.	Remove shunt. Select appropriate therapy based on in vitro susceptibilities. Meropenem, ceftriaxone, cefotaxime, and cefepime have all been studied in pediatric meningitis. Systemic gentamicin as combination therapy is not routinely recommended. Intrathecal therapy with aminoglycosides not routinely necessary with highly active beta-lactam therapy and shunt removal.

K. URINARY TRACT INFECTIONS

Clinical Diagnosis	Therapy (evidence grade)	Comments

NOTE: Antibiotic susceptibility profiles of *Escherichia coli*, the most common cause of UTI, vary considerably. For mild disease, TMP/SMX may be started as initial therapy if local susceptibility ≥80% and a 20% failure rate is acceptable. For moderate to severe disease (possible pyelonephritis), obtain cultures and begin an oral 2nd- or 3rd-generation cephalosporin (cefuroxime, cefaclor, cefprozil, cefixime, ceftibuten, cefdinir, cefpodoxime), ciprofloxacin PO, or ceftriaxone IM. Antibiotic susceptibility testing will help direct your therapy to the narrowest spectrum agent.

Cystitis, acute (*E coli*)[316,317]	For mild disease: TMP/SMX, 8 mg/kg/day of TMP PO div bid for 3 days (See NOTE about resistance to TMP/SMX.)	Alternative: amoxicillin 30 mg/kg/day PO div tid OR amoxicillin/clavulanate PO if susceptible (BII); ciprofloxacin 15–20 mg/kg/day PO div bid for suspected or documented resistant organisms

	For moderate to severe disease: cefixime 8 mg/kg/day PO qd; OR ceftriaxone 50 mg/kg IM q24h for 3–5 days (with normal anatomy) (BII); follow-up culture after 36–48 h treatment ONLY if still symptomatic	
Nephronia, lobar *E coli* and other enteric rods (also called focal bacterial nephritis)[318,319]	Ceftriaxone 50 mg/kg/day IV, IM q24h. Duration depends on resolution of cellulitis vs development of abscess (10–21 days) (AIII). For ESBL-positive *E coli*, carbapenems and fluoroquinolones are often active agents.	Invasive, consolidative parenchymal infection; complication of pyelonephritis, can evolve into renal abscess. Step-down therapy with oral cephalosporins once cellulitis/abscess has initially responded to therapy.
Pyelonephritis, acute (*E coli*)[316,317,320-323]	Ceftriaxone 50 mg/kg/day IV, IM q24h OR gentamicin 5–6 mg/kg/day IV, IM q24h. For documented or suspected ceftriaxone-resistant ESBL-positive strains, use meropenem IV, imipenem IV, or ertapenem IV; OR gentamicin IV, IM, OR pip/tazo. Switch to oral therapy following clinical response (BII). If organism resistant to amoxicillin and TMP/SMX, use an oral 2nd- or 3rd-generation cephalosporin (BII); if cephalosporin-R, can use ciprofloxacin PO 30 mg/kg/day div q12h (BII); for 7–14 days total (depending on response to therapy).	For mild to moderate infection, oral therapy is likely to be as effective as IV/IM therapy for susceptible strains, down to 3 mo of age.[320] If bacteremia documented and infant is <2–3 mo, rule out meningitis and treat 14 days IV + PO (AIII). Aminoglycosides at any dose are more nephrotoxic than beta-lactams but represent effective therapy (AI). Once-daily dosing of gentamicin is preferred to tid.[321]
Recurrent urinary tract infection, prophylaxis[316,324-327]	Only for those with grade III–V reflux or with recurrent febrile UTI: TMP/SMX 2 mg/kg/dose of TMP PO qd OR nitrofurantoin 1–2 mg/kg PO qd at bedtime; more rapid resistance may develop using beta-lactams (BII).	Prophylaxis not recommended for patients with grade I–II reflux and no evidence of renal damage (although the RIVUR study[326] included these children, and they may also benefit, but early treatment of new infections is recommended for these children). *Resistance eventually develops to every antibiotic;* follow resistance patterns for each patient. The use of periodic urine cultures is controversial, as there are no comparative data to guide management of asymptomatic bacteriuria in a child at high risk of recurrent UTI.

L. MISCELLANEOUS SYSTEMIC INFECTIONS

Clinical Diagnosis	Therapy (evidence grade)	Comments
Actinomycosis[328–330]	Penicillin G 250,000 U/kg/day IV div q6h, OR ampicillin 150 mg/kg/day IV div q8h until improved (often up to 6 wk); then long-term convalescent therapy with penicillin V 100 mg/kg/day (up to 4 g/day) PO for 6–12 mo (AII)	Surgery as indicated Alternatives: amoxicillin, clindamycin, erythromycin; ceftriaxone IM/IV, doxycycline for children >7 y
Anaplasmosis[331,332] (human granulocytotropic anaplasmosis, *Anaplasma phagocytophilum*)	Doxycycline 4 mg/kg/day IV, PO (max 200 mg/day) div bid for 7–10 days (regardless of age) (AII)	For mild disease, consider rifampin 20 mg/kg/day PO div bid for 7–10 days (BIII).
Anthrax, sepsis/pneumonia, community vs bioterror exposure (inhalation, cutaneous, gastrointestinal, meningoencephalitis)[15]	For community-associated anthrax infection, amoxicillin 75 mg/kg/day div q8h or doxycycline for children >7 y should be effective. For bioterror-associated exposure (regardless of age): ciprofloxacin 20–30 mg/kg/day IV div q12h, OR levofloxacin 16 mg/kg/day IV div q12h not to exceed 250 mg/dose (AIII); OR doxycycline 4 mg/kg/day PO (max 200 mg/day) div bid (regardless of age).	For invasive infection after bioterror exposure, 2 or 3 antibiotics may be required.[15] For oral step-down therapy, can use oral ciprofloxacin or doxycycline; if susceptible, can use penicillin, amoxicillin, or clindamycin.

Appendicitis (See Table 6H, Gastrointestinal Infections, Intra-abdominal infection, Appendicitis.)

Brucellosis[333–336]	Doxycycline 4 mg/kg/day PO (max 200 mg/day) div bid (for children >7 y) AND rifampin (15–20 mg/kg/day div q12h) (BIII); OR for children <8 y: TMP/SMX 10 mg/kg/day TMP IV, PO div q12h AND rifampin 15–20 mg/kg/day div q12h (BIII); for at least 6 wk	Combination therapy with rifampin will decrease the risk of relapse. ADD gentamicin 6–7.5 mg/kg/day IV, IM div q8h for the first 1–2 wk of therapy to further decrease risk of relapse[336] (BIII), particularly for endocarditis, osteomyelitis, or meningitis. Prolonged treatment for 4–6 mo and surgical debridement may be necessary for deep infections (AIII).

Cat-scratch disease (*Bartonella henselae*)[337-339]	Supportive care for adenopathy (I&D of infected lymph node); azithromycin 12 mg/kg/day PO qd for 5 days shortens the duration of adenopathy (AIII). No prospective data exist for invasive CSD: gentamicin (for 14 days) AND TMP/SMX AND rifampin for hepatosplenic disease and osteomyelitis (AIII). For CNS infection, use cefotaxime AND gentamicin ± TMP/SMX (AIII). Alternatives: ciprofloxacin, doxycycline.	This dosage of azithromycin has been documented to be safe and effective for streptococcal pharyngitis and may offer greater deep tissue exposure than the dosage studied by Bass et al[8] and used for otitis media.
Chickenpox/shingles (varicella-zoster virus) See Chapter 9, Varicella virus.		
Ehrlichiosis (human monocytic ehrlichiosis, caused by *Ehrlichia chaffeensis*, and *Ehrlichia ewingii*)[331,340-342]	Doxycycline 4 mg/kg/day IV, PO div bid (max 100 mg/dose) for 7–10 days (regardless of age) (AIII)	For mild disease, consider rifampin 20 mg/kg/day PO div bid (max 300 mg/dose) for 7–10 days (BIII).
Febrile neutropenic patient (empiric therapy of invasive infection: *Pseudomonas*, enteric Gram-negative bacilli, staphylococci, streptococci, yeast, fungi)[343,344]	Cefepime 150 mg/kg/day div q8h (AI); or meropenem 60 mg/kg/day div q8h (AIII); OR pip/tazo (300-mg pip component/kg/day div q8h for 9 mo; 240 mg/kg/day div q8h for 2–9 mo), OR ceftazidime 150 mg/kg/day IV div q8h AND tobramycin 6 mg/kg/day IV q8h (AII). ADD vancomycin 40 mg/kg/day IV q8h if MRSA or coagulation-negative staph suspected (eg, central catheter infection) (AIII). ADD metronidazole to ceftazidime or cefepime if colitis or other deep anaerobic infection suspected (AIII).	Alternatives: other anti-*Pseudomonas* beta-lactams (imipenem) AND antistaphylococcal antibiotics. If no response in 2–3 days and no alternative etiology demonstrated, begin additional empiric therapy with antifungals (BII); dosages and formulations outlined in Chapter 8. Increasingly resistant pathogens (ESBL *Escherichia coli* and *Klebsiella*, KPC) will require alternative empiric therapy if MDR organisms are colonizing or present on the child's hospital unit. For low-risk patients with close follow-up, alternative management strategies are being explored: oral therapy with amox/clav and ciprofloxacin may be used, or early hospital discharge.[345]

Antimicrobial Therapy According to Clinical Syndromes

6

L. MISCELLANEOUS SYSTEMIC INFECTIONS (continued)

Clinical Diagnosis	Therapy (evidence grade)	Comments
Human immunodeficiency virus infection	See Chapter 9.	
Infant botulism[346]	Botulism immune globulin for infants (BabyBIG) 50 mg/kg IV for 1 dose (AI); BabyBIG can be obtained from the California Department of Public Health at www.infantbotulism.org, through your state health department.	www.infantbotulism.org provides information for physicians and parents. Web site organized by the California Department of Public Health (accessed October 2, 2017). Aminoglycosides should be avoided because they potentiate the neuromuscular effect of botulinum toxin.
Kawasaki syndrome[347-350]	No antibiotics; IVIG 2 g/kg as single dose (AI); may need to repeat dose in up to 15% of children for persisting fever that lasts 24 h after completion of the IVIG infusion (AII). For subsequent relapse, many children will respond to a second IVIG infusion, otherwise consult an infectious diseases physician or pediatric cardiologist. Adjunctive therapy with corticosteroids for those at high risk for the development of aneurysms.[333]	Aspirin 80–100 mg/kg/day div qid in acute, febrile phase; once afebrile for 24–48 h, initiate low-dosage (3–5 mg/kg/day) aspirin therapy for 6–8 wk (assuming echocardiogram is normal). Role of corticosteroids, infliximab, calcineurin inhibitors, and anti-thrombotic therapy, as well as methotrexate and cyclosporin, for IVIG-resistant Kawasaki syndrome under investigation and may improve outcome in severe cases.[350]
Leprosy (Hansen disease)[351]	Dapsone 1 mg/kg/day PO qd AND rifampin 10 mg/kg/day PO qd; ADD (for multibacillary disease) clofazimine 1 mg/kg/day PO qd; for 12 mo for paucibacillary disease; for 24 mo for multibacillary disease (AII).	Consult Health Resources and Services Administration National Hansen's Disease (Leprosy) Program at www.hrsa.gov/hansens-disease (accessed October 2, 2017) for advice about treatment and free antibiotics: 800/642-2477.

Leptospirosis[352,353]	Penicillin G 250,000 U/kg/day IV div q6h, or ceftriaxone 50 mg/kg/day IV, IM q24h; for 7 days (BII) For mild disease, doxycycline (>7 y) 4 mg/kg/day (max 200 mg/day) PO bid for 7–10 days and for those ≤7 y or intolerant of doxycycline, azithromycin 20 mg/kg on day 1, 10 mg/kg on days 2 and 3 (BII)	Alternative: amoxicillin for children ≤7 y of age with mild disease
Lyme disease (*Borrelia burgdorferi*)[342,354-356]	Neurologic evaluation, including LP, if there is clinical suspicion of CNS involvement	
– Early localized disease	>7 y: doxycycline 4 mg/kg/day (max 200 mg/day) PO div bid for 14 days (AII) ≤7 y: amoxicillin 50 mg/kg/day (max 1.5 g/day) PO div tid for 14 days (AII)	Alternative: cefuroxime, 30 mg/kg/day (max 1,000 mg/day) PO, in 2 div doses (or 1 g/day) for 14 days
– Arthritis (no CNS disease)	Oral therapy as outlined previously, but for 28 days (AIII). Alternative: ceftriaxone 50–75 mg/kg/day IV q24h OR penicillin 300,000 U/kg/day IV div q4h; either for 14–28 days.	Persistent or recurrent joint swelling after treatment: repeat a 4-wk course of oral antibiotics or give ceftriaxone 50–75 mg/kg IV q24h OR penicillin 300,000 U/kg/day IV div q4h; either for 14–28 days. For persisting arthritis after 2 defined antibiotic treatment courses, use symptomatic therapy.
– Erythema migrans	Oral therapy as outlined previously; for 14 days (AIII)	
– Isolated facial (Bell) palsy	Oral therapy as outlined previously; for 21–28 days (AIII)	LP is not routinely required unless CNS symptoms present. Treatment to prevent late sequelae; will not provide a quick response for palsy.
– Carditis	Ceftriaxone 50–75 mg/kg IV q24h OR penicillin 300,000 U/kg/day IV div q4h; for 14–21 days (AIII)	For asymptomatic disease, treat with oral regimen as for early localized disease.
– Neuroborreliosis	Ceftriaxone 50–75 mg/kg IV q24h OR penicillin G 300,000 U/kg/day IV div q4h; for 14–28 days (AIII)	

6

Antimicrobial Therapy According to Clinical Syndromes

Antimicrobial Therapy According to Clinical Syndromes

6

L. MISCELLANEOUS SYSTEMIC INFECTIONS (continued)

Clinical Diagnosis	Therapy (evidence grade)	Comments
Melioidosis (Burkholderia pseudomallei)[357,358]	Acute sepsis: meropenem 75 mg/kg/day IV q8h; OR ceftazidime 150 mg/kg/day IV div q8h; followed by TMP/SMX (10 mg/kg/day of TMP) PO bid for 3–6 mo	Alternative convalescent therapy: amox/clav (90 mg/kg/day amox div tid, not bid) for children ≤7 y; or doxycycline for children >7 y; for 20 wk (AII)
Mycobacteria, nontuberculous[9,11,12,359]		
– Adenitis in normal host (See Adenitis entries in this table and Table 6A.)	Excision usually curative (BII); azithromycin PO OR clarithromycin PO for 6–12 wk (with or without rifampin) if susceptible (BII)	Antibiotic susceptibility patterns are quite variable; cultures should guide therapy; medical therapy 60%–70% effective. Newer data suggest toxicity of antimicrobials may not be worth the small clinical benefit.
– Pneumonia or disseminated infection in compromised hosts (HIV or gamma-interferon receptor deficiency)[11,359–362]	Usually treated with 3 or 4 active drugs (eg, clarithromycin OR azithromycin, AND amikacin, cefoxitin, meropenem). Also test for ciprofloxacin, TMP/SMX, ethambutol, rifampin, linezolid, clofazimine, and doxycycline (BII).	See Chapter 11 for dosages; cultures are essential, as the susceptibility patterns of nontuberculous mycobacteria are varied.
Nocardiosis (Nocardia asteroides and Nocardia brasiliensis)[363,364]	TMP/SMX 8 mg/kg/day TMP div bid or sulfisoxazole 120–150 mg/kg/day PO div qid for 6–12 wk or longer. For severe infection, particularly in immunocompromised hosts, use ceftriaxone or imipenem AND amikacin 15–20 mg/kg/day IM, IV div q8h (AIII).	Wide spectrum of disease from skin lesions to brain abscess Surgery when indicated Alternatives: doxycycline (for children >7 y), amox/clav, or linezolid
Plague (Yersinia pestis)[365–367]	Gentamicin 7.5 mg/kg/day IV div q8h (AII)	Doxycycline 4 mg/kg/day (max 200 mg/day) PO div bid or ciprofloxacin 30 mg/kg/day PO div bid
Q fever (Coxiella burnetii)[368,369]	Acute stage: doxycycline 4.4 mg/kg/day (max 200 mg/day) PO div bid for 14 days (All) for children of any age.	Follow doxycycline and hydroxychloroquine serum concentrations during endocarditis/chronic disease therapy.

Endocarditis and chronic disease (ongoing symptoms for 6–12 mo): doxycycline for children >7 y AND hydroxychloroquine for 18–36 mo (AIII). Seek advice from pediatric infectious diseases specialist for children ≤7 y: may require TMP-SMX, 8–10 mg TMP/kg/day div q12h with doxycycline; or levofloxacin with rifampin for 18 mo.	CNS: Use fluoroquinolone (no prospective data) (BIII). Clarithromycin may be an alternative based on limited data (CIII).
Rocky Mountain spotted fever (fever, petechial rash with centripetal spread; *Rickettsia rickettsii*)[370,371]	Doxycycline 4.4 mg/kg/day (max 200 mg/day) PO div bid for 7–10 days (AI) for children of any age	Start empiric therapy early.
Tetanus (*Clostridium tetani*)[372,373]	Metronidazole 30 mg/kg/day IV, PO div q8h or penicillin G 100,000 U/kg/day IV div q6h for 10–14 days AND TIG 3,000–6,000 U IM (AII)	Wound debridement essential; IVIG may provide antibody to toxin if TIG not available. Immunize with Td or Tdap. See Chapter 14 for prophylaxis recommendations.
Toxic shock syndrome (toxin-producing strains of *S aureus* [including MRSA] or group A streptococcus)[1,6,7,374,375]	Empiric: vancomycin 45 mg/kg/day IV div q8h AND oxacillin/nafcillin 150 mg/kg/day IV div q6h, AND clindamycin 30–40 mg/kg/day div q8h ± gentamicin for 7–10 days (AIII)	Clindamycin added for the initial 48–72 h of therapy to decrease toxin production. Ceftaroline is an option for MRSA treatment, particularly with renal insufficiency from shock and vancomycin (BIII). IVIG may provide additional benefit by binding circulating toxin (CIII). For MSSA: oxacillin/nafcillin AND clindamycin ± gentamicin. For CA-MRSA: vancomycin AND clindamycin ± gentamicin. For group A streptococcus: penicillin G AND clindamycin.
Tularemia (*Francisella tularensis*)[180,376]	Gentamicin 6–7.5 mg/kg/day IM, IV div q8h; for 10–14 days (AII)	Alternatives: ciprofloxacin (for 10 days); doxycycline no longer recommended due to higher relapse rate.

6

Antimicrobial Therapy According to Clinical Syndromes

7. Preferred Therapy for Specific Bacterial and Mycobacterial Pathogens

NOTES

- For fungal, viral, and parasitic infections, see chapters 8, 9, and 10, respectively.

- Limitations of space do not permit listing of all possible alternative antimicrobials.

- **Abbreviations:** amox/clav, amoxicillin/clavulanate (Augmentin); amp/sul, ampicillin/sulbactam (Unasyn); CA-MRSA, community-associated methicillin-resistant *Staphylococcus aureus;* CDC, Centers for Disease Control and Prevention; CNS, central nervous system; ESBL, extended spectrum beta-lactamase; FDA, US Food and Drug Administration; HRSA, Health Resources and Services Administration; IM, intramuscular; IV, intravenous; IVIG, intravenous immunoglobulin; KPC, *Klebsiella pneumoniae* carbapenemase; MDR, multidrug resistant; MIC, minimal inhibitory concentration; MRSA, methicillin-resistant *S aureus;* MSSA, methicillin-susceptible *S aureus;* NARMS, National Antimicrobial Resistance Monitoring System for Enteric Bacteria; NDM, New Delhi metallo-beta-lactamase; pen-S, penicillin-susceptible; pip/tazo, piperacillin/tazobactam (Zosyn); PO, oral; PZA, pyrazinamide; spp, species; ticar/clav, ticarcillin/clavulanate (Timentin); TIG, tetanus immune globulin; TMP/SMX, trimethoprim/sulfamethoxazole; UTI, urinary tract infection.

A. COMMON BACTERIAL PATHOGENS AND USUAL PATTERN OF SUSCEPTIBILITY TO ANTIBIOTICS (GRAM POSITIVE)

	Commonly Used Antibiotics (One Agent per Class Listed) Scale − to ++			
	Penicillin	**Ampicillin/ Amoxicillin**	**Amoxicillin/ Clavulanate**	**Methicillin/ Oxacillin**
Enterococcus faecalis[a]	+	+	+	−
Enterococcus faecium[a]	+	+	+	−
Staphylococcus, coagulase negative	−	−	−	+/−
Staphylococcus aureus, methicillin-resistant	−	−	−	−
Staphylococcus aureus, methicillin-susceptible	−	−	−	++
Streptococcus pneumoniae	++	++	++	+
Streptococcus pyogenes	++	++	++	++

NOTE: ++ = very active (>90% of isolates are susceptible in most locations); + = some decreased susceptibility (substantially less active in vitro or resistance in isolates between 10% and 30% in some locations); +/− = significant resistance (30%–80% in some locations); − = not likely to be effective.
[a] Need to add gentamicin or other aminoglycoside to ampicillin/penicillin or vancomycin for in vitro bactericidal activity.

Commonly Used Antibiotics (One Agent per Class Listed)

Cefazolin/ Cephalexin	Vancomycin	Clindamycin	Linezolid	Daptomycin	Ceftaroline
−	+	−	+	++	−
−	+	−	+	+	−
+/−	++	+	++	++	++
−	++	+	++	++	++
++	++	+	++	++	++
++	++	++	++	++	++
++	++	++	++	++	++

B. COMMON BACTERIAL PATHOGENS AND USUAL PATTERN OF SUSCEPTIBILITY TO ANTIBIOTICS (GRAM NEGATIVE)[a]

	Commonly Used Antibiotics (One Agent per Class Listed) Scale 0 to ++				
	Ampicillin/ Amoxicillin	Amoxicillin/ Clavulanate	Cefazolin/ Cephalexin	Cefuroxime	Ceftriaxone/ Cefotaxime
Acinetobacter spp	−	−	−	−	+
Citrobacter spp	−	−	−	+	+
Enterobacter spp[b]	−	−	−	+/−	+
Escherichia coli[c]	+/−	+	+	++[d]	++[d]
Haemophilus influenzae[f]	++	++	++	++	++
Klebsiella spp[c]	−	−	+	++	++
Neisseria meningitidis	++	++	0	++	++
Pseudomonas aeruginosa	−	−	−	−	−
Salmonella, non-typhoid spp	+	++	0	0	++
Serratia spp[b]	−	−	−	+/−	+
Shigella spp	+	+	0	+	++
Stenotrophomonas maltophilia	−	−	−	−	−

NOTE: ++ = very active (>90% of isolates are susceptible in most locations); + = some decreased susceptibility (substantially less active in vitro or resistance in isolates between 10% and 30% in some locations); +/− = significant resistance (30%–80% in some locations); − = not likely to be effective; 0 = not usually tested for treatment of infections (resistant or has not previously been considered for routine therapy, so little data exist).

[a] CDC (NARMS) statistics and SENTRY surveillance system (JMI Laboratories) as primary references; also using current antibiograms from Children's Medical Center, Dallas, TX, and Rady Children's Hospital San Diego, CA, to assess pediatric trends. When sufficient data are available, pediatric community isolate susceptibility data are used. Nosocomial resistance patterns may be quite different, usually with increased resistance, particularly in adults; please check your local/regional hospital antibiogram for your local susceptibility patterns.

[b] AmpC will be constitutively produced in low frequency in every population of organisms and will be selected out during therapy with third-generation cephalosporins if used as single agent therapy.

[c] Rare carbapenem-resistant isolates in pediatrics (KPC, NDM strains).

[d] Will be resistant to virtually all current cephalosporins if ESBL producing.

[e] Follow the MIC, and not the report for susceptible (S), intermediate (I), or resistant (R), as some ESBL producers will have low MICs and can be effectively treated with higher dosages.

[f] Will be resistant to ampicillin/amoxicillin if beta-lactamase producing.

Commonly Used Antibiotics (One Agent per Class Listed)

Ceftazidime	Cefepime	Meropenem/ Imipenem	Piperacillin/ Tazobactam	TMP/ SMX	Ciprofloxacin	Gentamicin
+	+	++	+	+	+	++
+	++	++	+	++	++	++
+	++	++	+	+	++	++
++[d]	++[e]	++	++	+	++	++
++	++	++	++	++	++	+/−
++	++[e]	++	++	++	++	++
+	++	++	++	0	++	0
+	++	++	++	−	++	+
++	++	++	++	++	++	0
+	++	++	+	++	++	++
++	++	++	++	+/−	++	0
+	+/−	+/−	+	++	++	+/−

C. COMMON BACTERIAL PATHOGENS AND USUAL PATTERN OF SUSCEPTIBILITY TO ANTIBIOTICS (ANAEROBES)

	Commonly Used Antibiotics (One Agent per Class Listed) Scale 0 to ++				
	Penicillin	Ampicillin/ Amoxicillin	Amoxicillin/ Clavulanate	Cefazolin	Cefoxitin
Anaerobic streptococci	++	++	++	++	++
Bacteroides fragilis	+/−	+/−	++	−	+
Clostridia (eg, *tetani, perfringens*)	++	++	++	0	+
Clostridium difficile	−	−	−	0	−

NOTE: ++ = very active (>90% of isolates are susceptible in most locations); + = some decreased susceptibility (substantially less active in vitro or resistance in isolates between 10% and 30% in some locations); +/− = significant resistance (30%–80% in some locations); − = not likely to be effective; 0 = not usually tested for susceptibility for treatment of infections (resistant or has not previously been considered for routine therapy, so little data exist).

Commonly Used Antibiotics (One Agent per Class Listed)					
Ceftriaxone/ Cefotaxime	Meropenem/ Imipenem	Piperacillin/ Tazobactam	Metronidazole	Clindamycin	Vancomycin
++	++	++	++	++	++
−	++	++	++	+	0
+/−	++	++	++	+	++
−	++	0	++	−	++

Preferred Therapy for Specific Bacterial and Mycobacterial Pathogens

D. PREFERRED THERAPY FOR SPECIFIC BACTERIAL AND MYCOBACTERIAL PATHOGENS

Organism	Clinical Illness	Drug of Choice (evidence grade)	Alternatives
Acinetobacter baumannii[1-4]	Sepsis, meningitis, nosocomial pneumonia, wound infection	Meropenem (BIII) or other carbapenem	Use culture results to guide therapy: ceftazidime, amp/sul; pip/tazo; TMP/SMX; ciprofloxacin; tigecycline; colistin. Watch for emergence of resistance during therapy, including to colistin. Consider combination therapy for life-threatening infection. Inhaled colistin for pneumonia caused by MDR strains (BIII).
Actinomyces israelii[5]	Actinomycosis (cervicofacial, thoracic, abdominal)	Penicillin G; ampicillin (CIII)	Amoxicillin; doxycycline; clindamycin; ceftriaxone; imipenem
Aeromonas hydrophila[6]	Diarrhea	Ciprofloxacin (CIII)	Azithromycin, cefepime, TMP/SMX
	Sepsis, cellulitis, necrotizing fasciitis	Cefepime (BIII)	Meropenem; ciprofloxacin
Aggregatibacter (formerly Actinobacillus) actinomycetemcomitans[7]	Periodontitis, abscesses (including brain), endocarditis	Ceftriaxone (CIII)	Ampicillin (amoxicillin or amox/clav); doxycycline; TMP/SMX; ciprofloxacin; ceftriaxone
Anaplasma (formerly Ehrlichia) phagocytophilum[8,9]	Human granulocytic anaplasmosis	Doxycycline (all ages) (AII)	Rifampin, levofloxacin
Arcanobacterium haemolyticum[10]	Pharyngitis, cellulitis, Lemierre syndrome	Erythromycin; penicillin (BIII)	Azithromycin, amoxicillin, clindamycin, doxycycline; vancomycin
Bacillus anthracis[11]	Anthrax (cutaneous, gastrointestinal, inhalational, meningoencephalitis)	Ciprofloxacin (regardless of age) (AIII). For invasive, systemic infection, use combination therapy.	Doxycycline; amoxicillin, levofloxacin, clindamycin; penicillin G; vancomycin, meropenem. Bioterror strains may be antibiotic resistant.

7

Organism	Clinical Syndrome		
Bacillus cereus or *subtilis*[12,13]	Sepsis; toxin-mediated gastroenteritis	Vancomycin (BIII)	Ciprofloxacin, linezolid, daptomycin, clindamycin
Bacteroides fragilis[14,15]	Peritonitis, sepsis, abscesses	Metronidazole (AI)	Meropenem or imipenem (AI); ticar/clav; pip/tazo (AI); amox/clav (BII). Recent surveillance suggests resistance of up to 25% for clindamycin.
Bacteroides, other spp[14,15]	Pneumonia, sepsis, abscesses	Metronidazole (BII)	Meropenem or imipenem; penicillin G or ampicillin if beta-lactamase negative
Bartonella henselae[16,17]	Cat-scratch disease	Azithromycin for lymph node disease (BII); gentamicin in combination with TMP/SMX AND rifampin for invasive disease (BIII)	Cefotaxime; ciprofloxacin; doxycycline
Bartonella quintana[17,18]	Bacillary angiomatosis, peliosis hepatis	Gentamicin plus doxycycline (BIII); erythromycin; ciprofloxacin (BIII)	Azithromycin; doxycycline
Bordetella pertussis, parapertussis[19,20]	Pertussis	Azithromycin (AIII); erythromycin (BII)	Clarithromycin; TMP/SMX; ampicillin
Borrelia burgdorferi, Lyme disease[21–23]	Treatment based on stage of infection (See Lyme disease in Chapter 6.)	Doxycycline if >7 y (AIII); amoxicillin or cefuroxime in children ≤7 y (AIII); ceftriaxone IV for CNS/meningitis (AII)	Penicillin or erythromycin in children intolerant of doxycycline (BIII)
Borrelia hermsii, turicatae, parkeri, tick-borne relapsing fever[24,25]	Relapsing fever	Doxycycline for all ages (AIII)	Penicillin or erythromycin in children intolerant of doxycycline (BIII)
Borrelia recurrentis, louse-borne relapsing fever[24,25]	Relapsing fever	Single-dose doxycycline for all ages (AIII)	
Brucella spp[26–28]	Brucellosis (See Chapter 6.)	Doxycycline AND rifampin (BIII); OR, for children ≤7 y: TMP/SMX AND rifampin (BII)	For serious infection: doxycycline AND gentamicin AND rifampin; or TMP/SMX AND gentamicin AND rifampin (AIII). May require extended therapy (months).

Preferred Therapy for Specific Bacterial and Mycobacterial Pathogens

7

Preferred Therapy for Specific Bacterial and Mycobacterial Pathogens

7

D. PREFERRED THERAPY FOR SPECIFIC BACTERIAL AND MYCOBACTERIAL PATHOGENS (continued)

Organism	Clinical Illness	Drug of Choice (evidence grade)	Alternatives
Burkholderia cepacia complex[29-31]	Pneumonia, sepsis in immunocompromised children; pneumonia in children with cystic fibrosis[32]	Meropenem (BIII); for severe disease, ADD tobramycin AND TMP/SMX (AIII).	Imipenem, doxycycline; ceftazidime; pip/tazo; ciprofloxacin. Aerosolized antibiotics may provide higher concentrations in lung.[31]
Burkholderia pseudomallei[33-35]	Melioidosis	Meropenem (AIII) or ceftazidime (BIII), followed by prolonged TMP/SMX for 12 wk (AII)	TMP/SMX, doxycycline, or amox/clav for chronic disease
Campylobacter fetus[36,37]	Sepsis, meningitis in the neonate	Meropenem (BIII)	Cefotaxime; gentamicin; erythromycin
Campylobacter jejuni[38,39]	Diarrhea	Azithromycin (BII); erythromycin (BII)	Doxycycline; ciprofloxacin (very high rates of ciprofloxacin-resistant strains in Thailand, Hong Kong, and Spain)
Capnocytophaga canimorsus[40,41]	Sepsis after dog bite (increased risk with asplenia)	Pip/tazo OR meropenem; amox/clav (BIII)	Clindamycin; linezolid; penicillin G; ciprofloxacin
Capnocytophaga ochracea[42]	Sepsis, abscesses	Clindamycin (BIII); amox/clav (BIII)	Meropenem; pip/tazo
Chlamydia trachomatis[43-45]	Lymphogranuloma venereum	Doxycycline (AII)	Azithromycin; erythromycin
	Urethritis, cervicitis	Doxycycline (AII)	Azithromycin; erythromycin; ofloxacin
	Inclusion conjunctivitis of newborn	Azithromycin (AIII)	Erythromycin
	Pneumonia of infancy	Azithromycin (AIII)	Erythromycin; ampicillin
	Trachoma	Azithromycin (AI)	Doxycycline; erythromycin

Organism	Infection	Preferred therapy	Alternative/comments
Chlamydophila (formerly *Chlamydia*) *pneumoniae*[43,44,46,47]	Pneumonia	Azithromycin (AIII); erythromycin (AII)	Doxycycline; ciprofloxacin
Chlamydophila (formerly *Chlamydia*) *psittaci*[48]	Psittacosis	Doxycycline for >7 y; azithromycin (AIII) OR erythromycin (AIII) for ≤7 y	Doxycycline, levofloxacin
Chromobacterium violaceum[49,50]	Sepsis, pneumonia, abscesses	Meropenem AND ciprofloxacin (AIII)	Imipenem, TMP/SMX
Citrobacter koseri (formerly *diversus*) and *freundii*[51,52]	Meningitis, sepsis	Meropenem (AIII) for ampC beta-lactamase resistance	Cefepime; ciprofloxacin; pip/tazo; ceftriaxone AND gentamicin; TMP/SMX. Carbapenem-resistant strains now reported
Clostridium botulinum[53-55]	Botulism: foodborne; wound; potentially bioterror related	Botulism antitoxin heptavalent (equine) types A–G FDA approved in 2013 (www.fda.gov/downloads/BiologicsBloodVaccines/BloodBloodProducts/ApprovedProducts/LicensedProductsBLAs/FractionatedPlasmaProducts/UCM345147.pdf; accessed October 3, 2017). No antibiotic treatment	For more information, call your state health department or the CDC Emergency Operations Center, 770/488-7100 (https://www.cdc.gov/botulism/health-professional.html; accessed October 3, 2017).
	Infant botulism	Human botulism immune globulin for infants (BabyBIG) (AII) No antibiotic treatment	BabyBIG available nationally from the California Department of Public Health at 510/231-7600 (www.infantbotulism.org; accessed October 3, 2017)
Clostridium difficile[56-58]	Antibiotic-associated colitis (See Chapter 6, Table 6H, Gastrointestinal Infections, *Clostridium difficile*.)	Metronidazole PO (AI)	Vancomycin PO for metronidazole failures; stop the predisposing antimicrobial therapy, if possible. New pediatric data on fidaxomicin PO.[59] No pediatric data on fecal transplantation for recurrent disease.

Preferred Therapy for Specific Bacterial and Mycobacterial Pathogens

7

Preferred Therapy for Specific Bacterial and Mycobacterial Pathogens

D. PREFERRED THERAPY FOR SPECIFIC BACTERIAL AND MYCOBACTERIAL PATHOGENS (continued)

Organism	Clinical Illness	Drug of Choice (evidence grade)	Alternatives
Clostridium perfringens[60,61]	Gas gangrene/necrotizing fasciitis/sepsis (also caused by Clostridium sordellii, Clostridium septicum, Clostridium novyi) Food poisoning	Penicillin G AND clindamycin for invasive infection (BII); no antimicrobials indicated for foodborne illness	Meropenem, metronidazole, clindamycin monotherapy
Clostridium tetani[62,63]	Tetanus	Tetanus immune globulin 3,000–6,000 U IM, with part injected directly into the wound (IVIG if TIG not available) Metronidazole (AIII) OR penicillin G (BIII)	Prophylaxis for contaminated wounds: 250 U IM for those with <3 tetanus immunizations. Start/continue immunization for tetanus. Alternative antibiotics: meropenem; doxycycline, clindamycin.
Corynebacterium diphtheriae[64]	Diphtheria	Diphtheria equine antitoxin (available through CDC under an investigational protocol [www.cdc.gov/diphtheria/dat.html; accessed October 3, 2017]) AND erythromycin or penicillin G (AIII)	Antitoxin from the CDC Emergency Operations Center, 770/488-7100; protocol: www.cdc.gov/diphtheria/downloads/protocol.pdf (accessed October 3, 2017)
Corynebacterium jeikeium[65,66]	Sepsis, endocarditis	Vancomycin (AIII)	Penicillin G AND gentamicin, tigecycline, linezolid, daptomycin
Corynebacterium minutissimum[67,68]	Erythrasma; bacteremia in compromised hosts	Erythromycin PO for erythrasma (BIII); vancomycin IV for bacteremia (BIII)	Topical clindamycin for cutaneous infection
Coxiella burnetii[69,70]	Q fever (See Chapter 6, Table 6L, Miscellaneous Systemic Infections, Q fever.)	Acute infection: doxycycline (all ages) (AII) Chronic infection: TMP/SMX AND doxycycline (BII); OR levofloxacin AND if...	Alternative for acute infection: TMP/SMX

7

Ehrlichia chaffeensis[8,9] *Ehrlichia muris*-like[71]	Human monocytic ehrlichiosis	Doxycycline (all ages) (AII)	Rifampin
E ewingii[8,9]	*E ewingii* ehrlichiosis	Doxycycline (all ages) (AII)	Rifampin
Eikenella corrodens[72]	Human bite wounds; abscesses, meningitis, endocarditis	Ampicillin; penicillin G (BIII)	Amox/clav; ticar/clav; pip/tazo; amp/sul; ceftriaxone; ciprofloxacin; imipenem Resistant to clindamycin, cephalexin, erythromycin
Elizabethkingia (formerly *Chryseobacterium*) *meningoseptica*[73,74]	Sepsis, meningitis	Levofloxacin; TMP/SMX (BIII)	Add rifampin to another active drug; pip/tazo.
Enterobacter spp[52,75,76]	Sepsis, pneumonia, wound infection, UTI	Cefepime; meropenem; pip/tazo (BII)	Ertapenem; imipenem; cefotaxime or ceftriaxone AND gentamicin; TMP/SMX; ciprofloxacin Newly emerging carbapenem-resistant strains worldwide[76,77]
Enterococcus spp[78-80]	Endocarditis, UTI, intra-abdominal abscess	Ampicillin AND gentamicin (AI)	Vancomycin AND gentamicin. For strains that are resistant to gentamicin on synergy testing, use streptomycin or other active aminoglycoside for invasive infections. For vancomycin-resistant strains that are also ampicillin resistant: daptomycin OR linezolid.
Erysipelothrix rhusiopathiae[81]	Cellulitis (erysipeloid), sepsis, abscesses, endocarditis[82]	Ampicillin (BIII); penicillin G (BIII)	Ceftriaxone; clindamycin, meropenem; amoxicillin, ciprofloxacin, erythromycin Resistant to vancomycin, daptomycin, TMP/SMX

7

Preferred Therapy for Specific Bacterial and Mycobacterial Pathogens

Preferred Therapy for Specific Bacterial and Mycobacterial Pathogens

7

D. PREFERRED THERAPY FOR SPECIFIC BACTERIAL AND MYCOBACTERIAL PATHOGENS (continued)

Organism	Clinical Illness	Drug of Choice (evidence grade)	Alternatives
Escherichia coli See Chapter 6 for specific infection entities and references. *Increasing resistance to 3rd-generation cephalosporins due to ESBLs.*	UTI, community acquired, not hospital acquired	A 2nd- or 3rd-generation cephalosporin PO, IM as empiric therapy (BI)	Amoxicillin; TMP/SMX if susceptible. Ciprofloxacin if resistant to other options. For hospital-acquired UTI, review hospital antibiogram for choices.
	Traveler's diarrhea	Azithromycin (AII)	Rifaximin (for nonfebrile, non-bloody diarrhea for children >11 y); cefixime
	Sepsis, pneumonia, hospital-acquired UTI	A 2nd- or 3rd-generation cephalosporin IV (BI)	For ESBL-producing strains: meropenem (AIII) or other carbapenem; pip/tazo and ciprofloxacin if resistant to other antibiotics
	Meningitis	Ceftriaxone; cefotaxime (AIII)	For ESBL-producing strains: meropenem (AIII)
Francisella tularensis[83,84]	Tularemia	Gentamicin (AII)	Doxycycline; ciprofloxacin
Fusobacterium spp[85,86]	Sepsis, soft tissue infection, Lemierre syndrome	Metronidazole (AIII); clindamycin (BIII)	Penicillin G; meropenem; pip/tazo
Gardnerella vaginalis[45,87]	Bacterial vaginosis	Metronidazole (BII)	Tinidazole; clindamycin; metronidazole gel; clindamycin cream
Haemophilus (now *Aggregatibacter*) *aphrophilus*[88]	Sepsis, endocarditis, abscesses (including brain abscess)	Ceftriaxone (AII); OR ampicillin AND gentamicin (BII)	Ciprofloxacin, amox/clav (for strains resistant to ampicillin)
Haemophilus ducreyi[45]	Chancroid	Azithromycin (AIII); ceftriaxone (BIII)	Erythromycin; ciprofloxacin
Haemophilus influenzae[89]	Nonencapsulated strains: upper respiratory tract infections	Beta-lactamase negative: ampicillin IV (AI); amoxicillin PO (AI) Beta-lactamase positive: ceftriaxone IV, IM (AI) or cefotaxime IV (AI); amox/clav (AI) OR 2nd- or 3rd-generation cephalosporins PO (AI)	Levofloxacin; azithromycin; TMP/SMX

	Type b strains: meningitis, arthritis, cellulitis, epiglottitis, pneumonia	Beta-lactamase negative: ampicillin IV (AI); amoxicillin PO (AI) Beta-lactamase positive: ceftriaxone IV, IM (AI) or cefotaxime IV (AI); amox/clav (AI) OR 2nd- or 3rd-generation cephalosporins PO (AI)	Full IV course (10 days) for meningitis, but oral step-down therapy well documented after response to treatment for non-CNS infections Levofloxacin PO for step-down therapy
Helicobacter pylori[90,91]	Gastritis, peptic ulcer	Clarithromycin (susceptible strains) AND amoxicillin AND omeprazole (AII)	Other regimens include metronidazole (especially for concerns of clarithromycin resistance) and bismuth[92] in addition to other proton-pump inhibitors.
Kingella kingae[93,94]	Osteomyelitis, arthritis	Ampicillin; penicillin G (AII)	Ceftriaxone; TMP/SMX; cefuroxime; ciprofloxacin
Klebsiella spp (_K pneumoniae_, _K oxytoca_)[95-97]	UTI	A 2nd- or 3rd-generation cephalosporin (AII)	Use most narrow spectrum agent active against pathogen: TMP/SMX; ciprofloxacin, gentamicin. ESBL producers should be treated with a carbapenem (meropenem, ertapenem, imipenem), but KPC (carbapenemase)-containing bacteria may require ciprofloxacin, colistin.[97]
	Sepsis, pneumonia, meningitis	Ceftriaxone; cefotaxime, cefepime (AIII)	Carbapenem or ciprofloxacin if resistant to other routine antibiotics. Meningitis caused by ESBL producer: meropenem. KPC (carbapenemase) producers: ciprofloxacin, colistin, OR ceftazidime/avibactam, approved by FDA for adults in 2015 and should be active against current strains of KPC.
Klebsiella granulomatis[45]	Granuloma inguinale	Azithromycin (AII)	Doxycycline; TMP/SMX; ciprofloxacin

Preferred Therapy for Specific Bacterial and Mycobacterial Pathogens

7

Preferred Therapy for Specific Bacterial and Mycobacterial Pathogens

D. PREFERRED THERAPY FOR SPECIFIC BACTERIAL AND MYCOBACTERIAL PATHOGENS (continued)

Organism	Clinical Illness	Drug of Choice (evidence grade)	Alternatives
Legionella spp[98]	Legionnaires disease	Azithromycin (AI) OR levofloxacin (AI)	Erythromycin, TMP/SMX, doxycycline
Leptospira spp[99]	Leptospirosis	Penicillin G IV (AII); ceftriaxone IV (AII)	Amoxicillin; doxycycline; azithromycin
Leuconostoc[100]	Bacteremia	Penicillin G (AIII); ampicillin (BIII)	Clindamycin; erythromycin; doxycycline (resistant to vancomycin)
Listeria monocytogenes[101]	Sepsis, meningitis in compromised host; neonatal sepsis	Ampicillin (ADD gentamicin for severe infection.) (AII)	Ampicillin AND TMP/SMX; ampicillin AND linezolid
Moraxella catarrhalis[102]	Otitis, sinusitis, bronchitis	Amox/clav (AI)	TMP/SMX; a 2nd- or 3rd-generation cephalosporin
Morganella morganii[103,104]	UTI, neonatal sepsis, wound infection	Cefepime (AIII); meropenem (AIII)	Pip/tazo; ceftriaxone AND gentamicin; ciprofloxacin
Mycobacterium abscessus[105-107]	Skin and soft tissue infections; pneumonia in cystic fibrosis	Clarithromycin or azithromycin (AIII); ADD amikacin ± cefoxitin for invasive disease (AIII).	Also test for susceptibility to meropenem, tigecycline, linezolid. May need pulmonary resection.
Mycobacterium avium complex[105,108,109]	Cervical adenitis	Clarithromycin (AII); azithromycin (AII)	Surgical excision is more likely to lead to cure than sole medical therapy. May increase cure rate with addition of rifampin or ethambutol.
	Pneumonia	Clarithromycin (AII) or azithromycin (AII) AND ethambutol ± rifampin	Depending on susceptibilities and the severity of illness, ADD amikacin ± ciprofloxacin.

7

	Disseminated disease in competent host, or disease in immunocompromised host	Clarithromycin or azithromycin AND ethambutol AND rifampin (AIII)	Depending on susceptibilities and the severity of illness, ADD amikacin ± ciprofloxacin.
Mycobacterium bovis[110,111]	Tuberculosis (adenitis; abdominal tuberculosis; meningitis)	Isoniazid AND rifampin (AII); ADD ethambutol for suspected resistance (AIII).	ADD streptomycin for severe infection. *M bovis* is always resistant to PZA.
Mycobacterium chelonae[105,108,112,113]	Abscesses; catheter infection	Clarithromycin or azithromycin (AIII); ADD amikacin ± cefoxitin for invasive disease (AIII).	Also test for susceptibility to cefoxitin; TMP/SMX; doxycycline; tobramycin, imipenem; moxifloxacin, linezolid.
Mycobacterium fortuitum complex[105,108,113]	Skin and soft tissue infections; catheter infection	Amikacin AND meropenem (AIII) ± ciprofloxacin (AIII)	Also test for susceptibility to clarithromycin, cefoxitin; sulfonamides; doxycycline; linezolid.
Mycobacterium leprae[114]	Leprosy	Dapsone AND rifampin for paucibacillary (1–5 patches) (AII). ADD clarithromycin (or clofazimine) for lepromatous, multibacillary (>5 patches) disease (AII).	Consult HRSA (National Hansen's Disease [Leprosy] Program) at www.hrsa.gov/hansens-disease for advice about treatment and free antibiotics: 800/642-2477 (accessed October 3, 2017).
Mycobacterium marinum/balnei[105,115]	Papules, pustules, abscesses (swimming pool granuloma)	Clarithromycin ± rifampin (AIII)	TMP/SMX AND rifampin; doxycycline

7

Preferred Therapy for Specific Bacterial and Mycobacterial Pathogens

Preferred Therapy for Specific Bacterial and Mycobacterial Pathogens

D. PREFERRED THERAPY FOR SPECIFIC BACTERIAL AND MYCOBACTERIAL PATHOGENS (continued)

Organism	Clinical Illness	Drug of Choice (evidence grade)	Alternatives
Mycobacterium tuberculosis[110,116] See Tuberculosis in Chapter 6, Table 6F, Lower Respiratory Tract Infections, for detailed recommendations for active infection, latent infection, and exposures in high-risk children.	Tuberculosis (pneumonia; meningitis; cervical adenitis; mesenteric adenitis; osteomyelitis)	For active infection: isoniazid AND rifampin AND PZA (AI) For latent infection: isoniazid daily, biweekly, or in combination with rifapentine once weekly (AII)	Add ethambutol for suspect resistance; add streptomycin for severe infection. For MDR tuberculosis, bedaquiline is now FDA approved for adults and available for children. Corticosteroids should be added to regimens for meningitis, mesenteric adenitis, and endobronchial infection (AII).
Mycoplasma hominis[117,118]	Nongonococcal urethritis; neonatal infection including meningitis	Clindamycin (AIII); fluoroquinolones	Doxycycline Usually erythromycin resistant
Mycoplasma pneumoniae[119,120]	Pneumonia	Azithromycin (AI); erythromycin (BI); macrolide resistance emerging worldwide[121]	Doxycycline and fluoroquinolones are active against macrolide-susceptible and macrolide-resistant strains.
Neisseria gonorrhoeae[45]	Gonorrhea; arthritis	Ceftriaxone AND azithromycin or doxycycline (AIII)	Oral cefixime as single drug therapy no longer recommended due to increasing resistance[122] Spectinomycin IM
Neisseria meningitidis[123,124]	Sepsis, meningitis	Ceftriaxone (AI); cefotaxime (AI)	Penicillin G or ampicillin if susceptible. For prophylaxis following exposure: rifampin or ciprofloxacin (ciprofloxacin-resistant strains have now been reported). Azithromycin may be less effective.
Nocardia asteroides or brasiliensis[125,126]	Nocardiosis	TMP/SMX (AII); sulfisoxazole (BII); imipenem AND amikacin for severe infection (AII)	Linezolid, ceftriaxone; clarithromycin; minocycline, levofloxacin, tigecycline, amox/clav

7

Organism	Infection	Preferred therapy	Alternatives/comments
Oerskovia (now known as *Cellulosimicrobium cellulans*)[127]	Wound infection; catheter infection	Vancomycin ± rifampin (AIII)	Linezolid: resistant to beta-lactams, macrolides, clindamycin, aminoglycosides
Pasteurella multocida[128]	Sepsis, abscesses, animal bite wound	Penicillin G (AIII); ampicillin (AIII); amoxicillin (AIII)	Amox/clav; ticar/clav; pip/tazo; doxycycline; ceftriaxone; cefpodoxime; cefuroxime, TMP/SMX. Cephalexin may not demonstrate adequate activity. Not usually susceptible to clindamycin.
Peptostreptococcus[129]	Sepsis, deep head/neck space and intra-abdominal infection	Penicillin G (AII); ampicillin (AII)	Clindamycin; vancomycin; meropenem, imipenem, metronidazole
Plesiomonas shigelloides[130,131]	Diarrhea, neonatal sepsis, meningitis	Antibiotics may not be necessary to treat diarrhea: 2nd- and 3rd-generation cephalosporins (AIII); azithromycin (BIII); ciprofloxacin (CIII). For meningitis/sepsis: ceftriaxone.	Meropenem; TMP/SMX, amox/clav
Prevotella (formerly *Bacteroides*) spp.[132] *melaninogenica*	Deep head/neck space abscess; dental abscess	Metronidazole (AII); meropenem or imipenem (AII)	Pip/tazo; clindamycin
Propionibacterium acnes[133,134]	In addition to acne, invasive infection: sepsis, post-op wound infection	Penicillin G (AIII); vancomycin (AIII)	Cefotaxime; ceftriaxone, doxycycline; clindamycin; linezolid, daptomycin
Proteus mirabilis[135]	UTI, sepsis, meningitis	Ceftriaxone (AII) or cefotaxime (AIII); cefepime; ciprofloxacin; gentamicin	Carbapenem; pip/tazo; increasing resistance to ampicillin, TMP/SMX, and fluoroquinolones, particularly in nosocomial isolates Colistin resistant

Preferred Therapy for Specific Bacterial and Mycobacterial Pathogens

D. PREFERRED THERAPY FOR SPECIFIC BACTERIAL AND MYCOBACTERIAL PATHOGENS (continued)

Organism	Clinical Illness	Drug of Choice (evidence grade)	Alternatives
Proteus vulgaris, other spp (indole-positive strains)[52]	UTI, sepsis, meningitis	Cefepime; ciprofloxacin; gentamicin (BII)	Meropenem or other carbapenem; pip/tazo; TMP/SMX Colistin resistant
Providencia spp[52,73,136]	Sepsis	Cefepime; ciprofloxacin, gentamicin (BII)	Meropenem or other carbapenem; pip/tazo; TMP/SMX Colistin resistant
Pseudomonas aeruginosa[73,137–141]	UTI	Cefepime (AII); other antipseudomonal beta-lactams	Tobramycin; amikacin; ciprofloxacin
	Nosocomial sepsis, pneumonia	Cefepime (AI) or meropenem (AI); OR pip/tazo AND tobramycin (BII); ceftazidime AND tobramycin (BII)	Ciprofloxacin AND tobramycin. Controversy regarding additional clinical benefit in outcomes using newer, more potent beta-lactams over aminoglycoside combinations, but combinations may decrease emergence of resistance. Ceftolozane/tazobactam was approved by FDA for adults in 2015 and may be active against otherwise resistant strains.
	Pneumonia in cystic fibrosis[142–145] See Cystic Fibrosis in Chapter 6, Table 6F, Lower Respiratory Tract Infections.	Cefepime (AII) or meropenem (AI); OR ceftazidime AND tobramycin (BII); ADD aerosol tobramycin (AI). Azithromycin provides benefit in prolonging interval between exacerbations.	Inhalational antibiotics for prevention of acute exacerbations: tobramycin, aztreonam, colistin. Many organisms are MDR; consider ciprofloxacin or colistin parenterally; in vitro synergy testing may suggest effective combinations.[137] For MDR organisms, colistin aerosol (AIII).
Pseudomonas cepacia, mallei, or pseudomallei (See Burkholderia.)			
Rhodococcus equi[146]	Necrotizing pneumonia	Imipenem AND vancomycin (AIII)	Combination therapy with ciprofloxacin AND azithromycin or rifampin

Rickettsia[67,147,148]	Rocky Mountain spotted fever, Q fever, typhus, rickettsialpox	Doxycycline (all ages) (AII)	Chloramphenicol is less effective than doxycycline.
Salmonella, non-*typhi*[149–151]	Gastroenteritis (may not require therapy if clinically improving and not immunocom- promised or <1 y [or, at highest risk, those <3 mo]); focal infections; bacteremia	Ceftriaxone (AII); cefixime (AII); azithromycin (AII)	For susceptible strains: ciprofloxacin; TMP/SMX; ampicillin; resistance to fluoroquinolones detected by nalidixic acid testing
Salmonella typhi[149,152]	Typhoid fever	Azithromycin (AII); ceftriaxone (AII); ciprofloxacin (AII)	For susceptible strains: TMP/SMX; ampicillin
Serratia marcescens[52,73]	Nosocomial sepsis, pneumonia	A carbapenem (AII)	Pip/tazo; cefepime if susceptible; ceftriaxone or cefotaxime AND gentamicin; or ciprofloxacin Resistant to colistin
Shewanella spp[153]	Wound infection, nosocomial pneumonia, peritoneal-dialysis peritonitis, ventricular shunt infection, neonatal sepsis	Ceftazidime (AIII); gentamicin (AIII)	Ampicillin, meropenem, pip/tazo, ciprofloxacin
Shigella spp[154,155]	Enteritis, UTI, prepubertal vaginitis	Ceftriaxone (AII); azithromycin[156] (AII); cefixime (AII); ciprofloxacin[157] (AII)	Resistance to azithromycin now reported. Use most narrow spectrum agent active against pathogen: ampicillin (not amoxicillin for enteritis); TMP/SMX.
Spirillum minus[158,159]	Rat-bite fever (sodoku)	Penicillin G IV (AII); for endocarditis, ADD gentamicin or streptomycin (AIII).	Ampicillin; doxycycline; cefotaxime, vancomycin, streptomycin

7

Preferred Therapy for Specific Bacterial and Mycobacterial Pathogens

Preferred Therapy for Specific Bacterial and Mycobacterial Pathogens

7

D. PREFERRED THERAPY FOR SPECIFIC BACTERIAL AND MYCOBACTERIAL PATHOGENS (continued)

Organism	Clinical Illness	Drug of Choice (evidence grade)	Alternatives
Staphylococcus aureus (See chapters 4 and 6 for specific infections.)[160–162]			
– Mild–moderate infections	Skin infections, mild–moderate	MSSA: a 1st-generation cephalosporin (cefazolin IV, cephalexin PO) (AI); oxacillin/nafcillin IV (AI), dicloxacillin PO (AI) MRSA: vancomycin IV, or clindamycin IV or PO (if susceptible), or TMP/SMX PO (AII)	For MSSA: amox/clav For CA-MRSA: linezolid IV, PO; daptomycin IV[163]
– Moderate–severe infections, treat empirically for CA-MRSA.	Pneumonia, sepsis, myositis, osteomyelitis, etc	MSSA: oxacillin/nafcillin IV (AI); a 1st-generation cephalosporin (cefazolin IV) (AI) ± gentamicin (AIII) MRSA: vancomycin (AII) OR clindamycin (AII) OR ceftaroline (AII); ± gentamicin ± rifampin (AIII)	For CA-MRSA: linezolid (AII); OR daptomycin for non-pulmonary infection (AII) (studies published in children); ceftaroline IV (studies published in children) Approved for adults in 2015: dalbavancin, oritavancin, tedizolid (See Chapter 4.)
Staphylococcus, coagulase negative[164,165]	Nosocomial bacteremia (neonatal bacteremia), infected intravascular catheters, CNS shunts, UTI	Vancomycin (AII)	If susceptible: nafcillin (or other anti-staph beta-lactam); rifampin (in combination); clindamycin, linezolid; ceftaroline IV (studies published in children)
Stenotrophomonas maltophilia[166,167]	Sepsis	TMP/SMX (AII)	Ceftazidime; ticar/clav; doxycycline; levofloxacin
Streptobacillus moniliformis[158,159]	Rat-bite fever (Haverhill fever)	Penicillin G (AIII); ampicillin (AIII); for endocarditis, ADD gentamicin or streptomycin (AIII).	Doxycycline; ceftriaxone; carbapenems; clindamycin; vancomycin
Streptococcus, group A[168]	Pharyngitis, impetigo, adenitis, cellulitis, necrotizing fasciitis	Penicillin (AI); amoxicillin (AI)	A 1st-generation cephalosporin (cefazolin or cephalexin) (AI); clindamycin (AII); a macrolide (AII), vancomycin (AIII)

		For recurrent streptococcal pharyngitis, clindamycin or amox/clav, or the addition of rifampin to the last 4 days of therapy (AIII)
Streptococcus, group B[169]	Neonatal sepsis, pneumonia, meningitis	Penicillin (AII) or ampicillin (AII)
		Gentamicin is used initially until group B strep has been identified as the cause of infection and a clinical/microbiologic response has been documented (AIII).
Streptococcus, milleri/ anginosus group (S intermedius, anginosus, and constellatus; includes some beta-hemolytic group C and group G streptococci)[170-172]	Pneumonia, sepsis, skin and soft tissue infection, sinusitis,[173] arthritis, brain abscess, meningitis	Ceftriaxone; clindamycin; vancomycin
Streptococcus pneumoniae[174-177] With widespread use of conjugate pneumococcal vaccines, antibiotic resistance in pneumococci has decreased.[177]	Pneumonia, sepsis, skin and soft tissue infection, sinusitis,[173] arthritis, brain abscess, meningitis	Penicillin G (AIII); ampicillin (AIII); ADD gentamicin for serious infection (AIII). Many strains show decreased susceptibility to penicillin, requiring higher dosages.
	Sinusitis, otitis[174]	Amoxicillin, high-dose (90 mg/kg/day) (AIII); new data suggest that standard dose (40–45 mg/kg/day) may again be effective.[177] Amox/clav; cefdinir; cefpodoxime; cefuroxime; clindamycin; OR ceftriaxone IM
	Meningitis	Ceftriaxone (AI) or cefotaxime (AI); AND vancomycin for possible ceftriaxone-resistant strains (AIII) Penicillin G alone for pen-S strains; ceftriaxone alone for ceftriaxone-susceptible strains
	Pneumonia, osteomyelitis/arthritis, sepsis	Ampicillin (AII); ceftriaxone (AI); cefotaxime (AI) Penicillin G alone for pen-S strains; ceftriaxone alone for ceftriaxone-susceptible strains
Streptococcus, viridans group (alpha-hemolytic streptococci, most commonly S sanguis, S oralis [mitis], S salivarius, S mutans, S morbillorum)[178]	Endocarditis	Penicillin G ± gentamicin (AII) OR ceftriaxone ± gentamicin (AII) Vancomycin

Preferred Therapy for Specific Bacterial and Mycobacterial Pathogens

7

Preferred Therapy for Specific Bacterial and Mycobacterial Pathogens

D. PREFERRED THERAPY FOR SPECIFIC BACTERIAL AND MYCOBACTERIAL PATHOGENS (continued)

Organism	Clinical Illness	Drug of Choice (evidence grade)	Alternatives
Treponema pallidum[48,179]	Syphilis	Penicillin G (AII)	Desensitize to penicillin preferred to alternate therapies. Doxycycline; ceftriaxone.
Ureaplasma urealyticum[45,180]	Genitourinary infections	Azithromycin (AII)	Erythromycin; doxycycline, ofloxacin (for adolescent genital infections)
	Neonatal pneumonia (Therapy may not be effective.)	Azithromycin (AIII)	
Vibrio cholerae[181,182]	Cholera	Azithromycin (AII) OR doxycycline (AI)	If susceptible: ciprofloxacin
Vibrio vulnificus[183,184]	Sepsis, necrotizing fasciitis	Doxycycline AND ceftazidime (AII)	Ciprofloxacin AND cefotaxime or ceftriaxone
Yersinia enterocolitica[185,186]	Diarrhea, mesenteric enteritis, reactive arthritis, sepsis	TMP/SMX for enteritis (AIII); ciprofloxacin or ceftriaxone for invasive infection (AIII)	Gentamicin, doxycycline
Yersinia pestis[187,188]	Plague	Gentamicin (AIII)	Levofloxacin; doxycycline; ciprofloxacin
Yersinia pseudotuberculosis[185,186,189]	Mesenteric adenitis; Far East scarlet-like fever; reactive arthritis	TMP/SMX (AIII) or ciprofloxacin (AIII)	Ceftriaxone; gentamicin, doxycycline

7

8. Preferred Therapy for Specific Fungal Pathogens

NOTES

- See Chapter 2 for discussion of the differences between polyenes, azoles, and echinocandins.

- **Abbreviations:** ABLC, amphotericin B lipid complex (Abelcet); AmB, amphotericin B; AmB-D, amphotericin B deoxycholate, the conventional standard AmB (original trade name Fungizone); bid, twice daily; CNS, central nervous system; CSF, cerebrospinal fluid; CT, computed tomography; div, divided; ECMO, extracorporeal membrane oxygenation; HAART, highly active antiretroviral therapy; HIV, human immuno-deficiency virus; IV, intravenous; L-AmB, liposomal amphotericin B (AmBisome); PO, orally; qd, once daily; qid, 4 times daily; spp, species; TMP/SMX, trimethoprim/sulfamethoxazole.

Preferred Therapy for Specific Fungal Pathogens

A. OVERVIEW OF MORE COMMON FUNGAL PATHOGENS AND THEIR USUAL PATTERN OF ANTIFUNGAL SUSCEPTIBILITIES

Fungal Species	Amphotericin B Formulations	Fluconazole	Itraconazole	Voriconazole	Posaconazole	Isavuconazole	Flucytosine	Caspofungin, Micafungin, or Anidulafungin
Aspergillus calidoustus	++	–	–	–	–	–	–	++
Aspergillus fumigatus	+	–	+/–	++	+	++	–	+
Aspergillus terreus	–	–	+	++	+	++	–	+
Blastomyces dermatitidis	++	+	++	+	+	+	–	–
Candida albicans	+	++	+	+	+	+	+	++
Candida auris	+/–	–	+/–	+/–	+	+	+/–	++
Candida glabrata	+	–	+/–	+/–	+/–	+/–	+	+/–
Candida guilliermondii	+	+/–	+	+	+	+	+	+/–
Candida krusei	+	–	–	+	+	+	+	++
Candida lusitaniae	–	++	+	+	+	+	+	+
Candida parapsilosis	++	++	+	+	+	+	+	+
Candida tropicalis	+	+	+	+	+	+	+	++

Coccidioides immitis	++	++	++	+	+	++	+	–
Cryptococcus spp	++	+	+	+	+	+	+	++
Fusarium spp	+/–	–	–	–	+	++	+	–
Histoplasma capsulatum	++	+	++	++	+	+	+	–
Mucor spp	++	–	+/–	–	+	–	+	–
Paracoccidioides spp	+	+	++	+	+	+	+	–
Penicillium spp	+/–	–	++	++	+	+	+	–
Rhizopus spp	++	–	–	–	+	–	+	–
Scedosporium apiospermum	–	–	+/–	+/–	+	+	+	+/–
Scedosporium prolificans	–	–	+/–	+/–	+/–	+/–	+/–	+/–
Sporothrix spp	+	+	++	+	+	+	+	–
Trichosporon spp	–	+	+	++	+	++	+	–

NOTE: ++ = preferred therapy(ies); + = usually active; +/– = variably active; – = usually not active.

8

Preferred Therapy for Specific Fungal Pathogens

Preferred Therapy for Specific Fungal Pathogens

8

B. SYSTEMIC INFECTIONS

Infection	Therapy (evidence grade)	Comments
Prophylaxis		
Prophylaxis of invasive fungal infection in patients with hematologic malignancies[1-11]	Fluconazole 6 mg/kg/day for prevention of infection (AII). Posaconazole for prevention of infection has been well studied in adults (AI) and offers anti-mold coverage.[4]	Fluconazole is not effective against molds and some strains of Candida. Posaconazole PO, voriconazole PO, and micafungin IV are effective in adults in preventing yeast and mold infections but are not well studied in children for this indication.[12]
Prophylaxis of invasive fungal infection in patients with solid organ transplants[13-17]	Fluconazole 6 mg/kg/day for prevention of infection (AII)	AmB, caspofungin, micafungin, voriconazole, or posaconazole may be effective in preventing infection.
Treatment		
Aspergillosis[1,18-28]	Voriconazole (AI) 18 mg/kg/day IV q12h for a loading dose on the first day, then 16 mg/kg/day IV div q12h as a maintenance dose for children 2-12 y or 12-14 y and weighing <50 kg. In children ≥15 y or 12-14 y and weighing >50 kg, use adult dosing (load 12 mg/kg/day IV div q12h on the first day, then 8 mg/kg/day div q12h as a maintenance dose) (AII). When stable, may switch from voriconazole IV to voriconazole PO at a dose of 18 mg/kg/day div bid for children 2-12 y and at least 400 mg/day div bid for children >12 y (AII). Dosing in children <2 y is less clear, but doses are generally higher (AIII). These are only initial dosing recommendations; continued dosing in all ages is guided by close monitoring of trough serum voriconazole concentrations in individual patients (AII). Unlike in adults, voriconazole PO bioavailability in children is only approximately 50%-60%, so trough levels are crucial when using PO.[29]	Voriconazole is the preferred primary antifungal therapy for all clinical forms of aspergillosis. Early initiation of therapy in patients with strong suspicion of disease is important while a diagnostic evaluation is conducted. Optimal voriconazole trough serum concentrations (generally thought to be 2-5 μg/mL) are important for success. It is critical to monitor trough concentrations to guide therapy due to high inter-patient variability.[30] Low voriconazole concentrations are a leading cause of clinical failure. Younger children (especially <3 y) often have lower voriconazole levels and need much higher dosing. Total treatment course is for a minimum of 6-12 wk, largely dependent on the degree and duration of immunosuppression and evidence of disease improvement.

Alternatives for primary therapy when voriconazole cannot be administered: L-AmB 5 mg/kg/day (AII) or isavuconazole (AI). Dosing of isavuconazole in children is unknown. ABLC is another possible alternative. Echinocandin primary monotherapy should not be used for treating invasive aspergillosis (CII). AmB deoxycholate should be used only in resource-limited settings in which no alternative agent is available (AII).

Salvage antifungal therapy options after failed primary therapy include a change of antifungal class (using L-AmB or an echinocandin), switching to isavuconazole, switching to posaconazole (serum trough concentrations ≥1 μg/mL), or using combination antifungal therapy.

Careful consideration has to be used before beginning azole therapy after a patient has failed azole prophylaxis.

Combination antifungal therapy with voriconazole plus an echinocandin may be considered in select patients. The addition of anidulafungin to voriconazole as combination therapy found some statistical benefit to the combination over voriconazole monotherapy in only certain patients.[31] In vitro data suggest some synergy with 2 (but not 3) drug combinations: an azole plus an echinocandin is the most well studied. If combination therapy is employed, this is likely best done initially when voriconazole trough concentrations may not be appropriate yet.

Routine antifungal susceptibility testing is not recommended but is suggested for patients suspected of having an azole-resistant isolate or who are unresponsive to therapy.

Azole-resistant Aspergillus fumigatus is increasing. If local epidemiology suggests >10% azole resistance, empiric initial therapy should be voriconazole + echinocandin OR with L-AmB, and subsequent therapy guided based on antifungal susceptibilities.[32]

Micafungin likely has equal efficacy to caspofungin against aspergillosis.[33]

Return of immune function is paramount to treatment success; for children receiving corticosteroids, decreasing the corticosteroid dosage or changing to steroid-sparing protocols is important.

Preferred Therapy for Specific Fungal Pathogens

8

B. SYSTEMIC INFECTIONS (continued)

Infection	Therapy (evidence grade)	Comments
Bipolaris, Cladophialophora, Exophiala, Curvularia, Alternaria, and other agents of **phaeohyphomycosis** (dematiaceous, pigmented molds)[32–41]	Voriconazole (AI) 18 mg/kg/day IV q12h for a loading dose on the first day, then 16 mg/kg/day IV div q12h as a maintenance dose for children 2–12 y or 12–14 y and weighing <50 kg. In children ≥15 y or 12–14 y and weighing >50 kg, use adult dosing (load 12 mg/kg/day IV div q12h on the first day, then 8 mg/kg/day div q12h as a maintenance dose) (AII). When stable, may switch from voriconazole IV to voriconazole PO at a dose of 18 mg/kg/day div bid for children 2–12 y and at least 400 mg/day div bid for children >12 y (AII). Dosing in children <2 y is less clear, but doses are generally higher (AIII). These are only initial dosing recommendations; continued dosing in all ages is guided by close monitoring of trough serum voriconazole concentrations in individual patients (AII). Unlike in adults, voriconazole PO bioavailability in children is only approximately 50%–60%, so trough levels are crucial.[29] Alternatives could include posaconazole (trough concentrations >0.7 µg/mL) or combination therapy with an echinocandin + azole or an echinocandin + L-AmB (BIII).	Aggressive surgical debulking/excision is essential for CNS lesions. These can be highly resistant infections, so strongly recommend antifungal susceptibility testing to guide therapy and consultation with a pediatric infectious diseases expert. Antifungal susceptibilities are often variable, but empiric therapy with voriconazole is the best start. Optimal voriconazole trough serum concentrations (generally thought to be 2–5 µg/mL) are important for success. It is critical to monitor trough concentrations to guide therapy due to high inter-patient variability.[30] Low voriconazole concentrations are a leading cause of clinical failure. Younger children (especially <3 y) often have lower voriconazole levels and need much higher dosing.
Blastomycosis (North American)[42–48]	For moderate–severe pulmonary disease: ABLC or L-AmB 5 mg/kg IV daily for 1–2 wk or until improvement noted, followed by itraconazole oral solution 10 mg/kg/day div bid (max 400 mg/day) PO for a total of 6–12 mo (AIII). Itraconazole loading dose (double dose for first 2 days) is recommended in adults but has not been studied in children (but likely helpful).	Itraconazole oral solution provides greater and more reliable absorption than capsules and only the oral solution should be used (on an empty stomach); serum concentrations of itraconazole should be determined 2 wk after start of therapy to ensure adequate drug exposure. For blastomycosis, maintain trough itraconazole concentrations 1–2 µg/mL (values for both itraconazole and hydroxyl-itraconazole are added together). If only itraconazole capsules are

For mild–moderate pulmonary disease: itraconazole oral solution 10 mg/kg/day div bid (max 400 mg/day) PO for a total of 6–12 mo (AIII). Itraconazole loading dose (double dose for first 2 days) recommended in adults but has not been studied in children (but likely helpful).

For CNS blastomycosis: ABLC/L-AmB for 4–6 wk, followed by an azole (fluconazole is preferred, at 12 mg/kg/day after a loading dose of 25 mg/kg; alternatives for CNS disease are voriconazole or itraconazole), for a total of at least 12 mo and until resolution of CSF abnormalities (AII). Some experts suggest combination therapy with L-AmB plus high-dose fluconazole as induction therapy in CNS blastomycosis until clinical improvement (BIII).

available, use 20 mg/kg/day div q12h and take with cola product to increase gastric acidity and bioavailability.

Alternative to itraconazole: 12 mg/kg/day fluconazole (BIII) after a loading dose of 25 mg/kg/day.

Patients with extrapulmonary blastomycosis should receive at least 12 mo of total therapy.

If induction with L-AmB alone is failing, add itraconazole or high-dose fluconazole until clinical improvement. Lifelong itraconazole if immunosuppression cannot be reversed.

Candidiasis[49–53] (See Chapter 2.)		
– Cutaneous	Topical therapy (alphabetic order): ciclopirox, clotrimazole, econazole, haloprogin, ketoconazole, miconazole, oxiconazole, sertaconazole, sulconazole	Fluconazole 6 mg/kg/day PO qd for 5–7 days Relapse common in cases of chronic mucocutaneous disease, and antifungal susceptibilities critical to drive appropriate therapy

8

Preferred Therapy for Specific Fungal Pathogens

B. SYSTEMIC INFECTIONS (continued)

Infection	Therapy (evidence grade)	Comments
– Disseminated, acute (including candle catheter fungemia) infection	For neutropenic patients: An echinocandin is recommended as initial therapy. Caspofungin 70 mg/m² IV loading dose on day 1 (max dose 70 mg), followed by 50 mg/m² IV (max dose 70 mg) on subsequent days (AII); OR micafungin 2 mg/kg/day q24h (children weighing <40 kg), up to max dose 100 mg/day (AII),[54] ABLC or L-AmB 5 mg/kg/day IV q24h (BII) is an effective but less attractive alternative due to potential toxicity (AII). Fluconazole (12 mg/kg/day) is an alternative for patients who are not critically ill and have had no prior azole exposure (CIII). A fluconazole loading dose is standard of care in adult patients but has only been studied in infants[55]—it is likely that the beneficial effect of a loading dose extends to children. Fluconazole can be used as step-down therapy in stable neutropenic patients with susceptible isolates and documented bloodstream clearance (CIII). For children on ECMO, 35 mg/kg load on day 1 followed by 12 mg/kg/day (BII).[56] For non-neutropenic patients: An echinocandin is recommended as initial therapy. Caspofungin 70 mg/m² IV loading dose on day 1 (max dose 70 mg), followed by 50 mg/m² IV (max dose 70 mg) on subsequent days (AII); OR micafungin 2 mg/kg/day q24h (children weighing <40 kg), up to max dose 100 mg/day (AI).[42] Fluconazole (12 mg/kg/day IV or PO q24h, after a load of 25 mg/kg/day) is an acceptable alternative to an echinocandin as initial therapy in selected patients,	Prompt removal of infected IV catheter or any infected devices is absolutely critical to success (AII). For infections with *Candida krusei* or *Candida glabrata*, an echinocandin is preferred; however, there are increasing reports of some *C glabrata* resistance to echinocandins (treatment would, therefore, be lipid formulation AmB) (BIII). There are increasing reports of some *Candida tropicalis* resistance to fluconazole. Lipid formulation AmB (5 mg/kg daily) is a reasonable alternative if there is intolerance, limited availability, or resistance to other antifungal agents (AI). Transition from lipid AmB to fluconazole is recommended after 5–7 days among patients who have isolates that are susceptible to fluconazole, who are clinically stable, and in whom repeat cultures on antifungal therapy are negative (AI). Voriconazole (18 mg/kg/day div q12h load, followed by 16 mg/kg/day div q12h) is effective for candidemia but offers little advantage over fluconazole as initial therapy. Voriconazole is recommended as step-down oral therapy for selected cases of candidemia due to *C krusei* or if mold coverage is needed. Follow-up blood cultures should be performed every day or every other day to establish the time point at which candidemia has been cleared (AIII). Duration of therapy is for 2 wk AFTER negative cultures in pediatric patients without obvious metastatic complications and after symptom resolution (AII). In neutropenic patients, ophthalmologic findings of choroidal and vitreal infection are minimal until recovery from neutropenia; therefore, dilated funduscopic

including those who are not critically ill and who are considered unlikely to have a fluconazole-resistant *Candida* spp (AI). For children on ECMO, use 35 mg/kg load followed by 12 mg/kg/day (BII).[56] Transition from an echinocandin to fluconazole (usually within 5–7 days) is recommended for non-neutropenic patients who are clinically stable, have isolates that are susceptible to fluconazole (eg, *Candida albicans*), and have negative repeat blood cultures following initiation of antifungal therapy (AII).

For CNS infections: AmB-D (1 mg/kg/day) or L-AmB/ABLC (5 mg/kg/day) with or without flucytosine 100 mg/kg/day PO div q6h (AII) until initial clinical response, followed by step-down therapy with fluconazole (12 mg/kg/day q24h, after a load of 25 mg/kg/day); echinocandins do not achieve therapeutic concentrations in CSF.

examinations should be performed within the first week after recovery from neutropenia (AII).
All non-neutropenic patients with candidemia should have a dilated ophthalmologic examination, preferably performed by an ophthalmologist, within the first week after diagnosis (AIII).

– Disseminated, chronic (hepatosplenic) infection	Initial therapy with lipid formulation AmB (5 mg/kg daily) OR an echinocandin (caspofungin 70 mg/m² IV loading dose on day 1 [max dose 70 mg], followed by 50 mg/m² IV [max dose 70 mg], on subsequent days OR micafungin 2 mg/kg/day q24h in children weighing <40 kg [max dose 100 mg]) for several weeks, followed by oral fluconazole in patients unlikely to have a fluconazole-resistant isolate (12 mg/kg/day q24h, after a load of 25 mg/kg/day) (AIII). Therapy should continue until lesions resolve on repeat imaging, which is usually several months. Premature discontinuation of antifungal therapy can lead to relapse (AIII).	If chemotherapy or hematopoietic cell transplantation is required, it should not be delayed because of the presence of chronic disseminated candidiasis, and antifungal therapy should be continued throughout the period of high risk to prevent relapse (AIII).

Preferred Therapy for Specific Fungal Pathogens

8

B. SYSTEMIC INFECTIONS (continued)

Infection	Therapy (evidence grade)	Comments
– Neonatal[52] (See Chapter 5.)	AmB-D (1 mg/kg/day) is recommended therapy (AII).[57] Fluconazole (12 mg/kg/day) is an alternative if patient has not been on fluconazole prophylaxis (AII).[58] For treatment of neonates and young infants (<120 days) on ECMO, fluconazole is loaded with 35 mg/kg on day 1, followed by 12 mg/kg/day q24h (BII). Lipid formulation AmB is an alternative but carries a theoretical risk of less urinary tract penetration compared with AmB-D (CIII). Duration of therapy for candidemia without obvious metastatic complications is for 2 wk after documented clearance and resolution of symptoms. Echinocandins should be used with caution and generally limited to salvage therapy or to situations in which resistance or toxicity preclude the use of AmB-D or fluconazole (CIII). Role of flucytosine in neonates with meningitis is questionable and not routinely recommended due to toxicity concerns. The addition of flucytosine (100 mg/kg/day div q6h) may be considered as salvage therapy in patients who have not had a clinical response to initial AmB therapy, but adverse effects are frequent (CIII).	In nurseries with high rates of candidiasis (>10%), IV or oral fluconazole prophylaxis (AI) (3–6 mg/kg twice weekly for 6 wk) in high-risk neonates (birth weight <1,000 g) is recommended. Oral nystatin, 100,000 units 3 times daily for 6 wk, is an alternative to fluconazole in neonates with birth weights <1,500 g in situations in which availability or resistance precludes the use of fluconazole (CII). Lumbar puncture and dilated retinal examination recommended in neonates with cultures positive for *Candida* spp from blood and/or urine (AIII). CT or ultrasound imaging of genitourinary tract, liver, and spleen should be performed if blood cultures are persistently positive (AIII). Meningoencephalitis in the neonate occurs at a higher rate than in older children/adults. Central venous catheter removal is strongly recommended. Infected CNS devices, including ventriculostomy drains and shunts, should be removed if possible.
– Oropharyngeal, esophageal[49]	Mild oropharyngeal disease: clotrimazole 10 mg troches PO 5 times daily OR nystatin 100,000 U/mL, 4–6 mL qid for 7–14 days. Alternatives also include miconazole mucoadhesive buccal 50-mg tablet to the mucosal surface over the canine fossa once daily for 7–14 days OR 1–2 nysta-	For fluconazole-refractory oropharyngeal or esophageal disease: itraconazole oral solution OR posaconazole OR AmB IV OR an echinocandin for up to 28 days (AII). Esophageal disease always requires systemic antifungal therapy. A diagnostic trial of antifungal therapy for esophageal candidiasis is appropriate before perform-

	Moderate–severe oropharyngeal disease: fluconazole 6 mg/kg qd PO for 7–14 days (AII). Esophageal candidiasis: oral fluconazole (6–12 mg/kg/day, after a loading dose of 25 mg/kg/day) for 14–21 days (AI). If cannot tolerate oral therapy, use fluconazole IV OR ABLC/L-AmB/AmB-D OR an echinocandin (AI).	Chronic suppressive therapy (3 times weekly) with fluconazole is recommended for recurrent infections (AI).
– Urinary tract infection	Cystitis: fluconazole 6 mg/kg qd IV or PO for 2 wk (AII). For fluconazole-resistant *C glabrata* or *C krusei*, AmB-D for 1–7 days (AIII). Pyelonephritis: fluconazole 12 mg/kg qd IV or PO for 2 wk (AIII) after a loading dose of 25 mg/kg/day. For fluconazole-resistant *C glabrata* or *C krusei*, AmB-D with or without flucytosine for 1–7 days (AIII).	Treatment is NOT recommended in asymptomatic candiduria unless neutropenic, low-birth weight neonate, or patient will undergo urologic manipulation (AIII). Removing Foley catheter, if present, may lead to a spontaneous cure in the normal host; check for additional upper urinary tract disease. AmB-D bladder irrigation is not generally recommended due to high relapse rate (an exception may be in fluconazole-resistant *Candida*) (CIII). For renal collecting system fungus balls, surgical debridement may be required in non-neonates (BIII). Echinocandins have poor urinary concentrations.
– Vulvovaginal[58]	Topical vaginal cream/tablets/suppositories (alphabetic order): butoconazole, clotrimazole, econazole, fenticonazole, miconazole, sertaconazole, terconazole, or tioconazole for 3–7 days (AI) OR fluconazole 10 mg/kg (max 150 mg) as a single dose (AI)	For uncomplicated vulvovaginal candidiasis, no topical agent is clearly superior. Avoid azoles during pregnancy. For recurring disease, consider 10–14 days of induction with topical agent or fluconazole, followed by fluconazole once weekly for 6 mo (AI).
Chromoblastomycosis (subcutaneous infection by dematiaceous fungi)[59–63]	Itraconazole oral solution 10 mg/kg/day div bid PO for 12–18 mo, in combination with surgical excision or repeated cryotherapy (AII)	Alternative: terbinafine plus surgery; heat and potassium iodide; posaconazole. Lesions are recalcitrant and difficult to treat.

8

Preferred Therapy for Specific Fungal Pathogens

8

B. SYSTEMIC INFECTIONS (continued)

Infection	Therapy (evidence grade)	Comments
Coccidioidomycosis[64–72]	For moderate infections: fluconazole 12 mg/kg PO q24h (AII) after loading dose of 25 mg/kg/day. For severe pulmonary disease: AmB-D 1 mg/kg/day IV q24h OR ABLC/L-AmB 5 mg/kg/day IV q24h (AIII) as initial therapy for several weeks until clear improvement, followed by an oral azole for total therapy of at least 12 mo, depending on genetic or immunocompromised risk factors. For meningitis: fluconazole 12 mg/kg/day IV q24h (AII) after loading dose of 25 mg/kg/day (AII). Itraconazole has also been effective (BII). If no response to azole, use intrathecal AmB-D (0.1–1.5 mg/dose) with or without fluconazole (AIII). Lifelong azole suppressive therapy required due to high relapse rate. Adjunctive corticosteroids in meningitis has resulted in less secondary cerebrovascular events.[73] For extrapulmonary (non-meningeal), particularly for osteomyelitis, an oral azole such as fluconazole or itraconazole solution 10 mg/kg/day div bid for at least 12 mo (AII), and AmB as an alternative for severe disease or if worsening.	Mild pulmonary disease does not require therapy in the normal host and only requires periodic reassessment. There is experience with posaconazole for disease in adults but little experience in children. Isavuconazole experience in adults is increasing. Treat until serum cocci complement fixation titers drop to 1:8 or 1:4, about 3–6 mo. Disease in immunocompromised hosts may need to be treated longer, including potentially lifelong azole secondary prophylaxis. Watch for relapse up to 1–2 y after therapy.
Cryptococcosis[74–78]	For mild–moderate pulmonary disease: fluconazole 12 mg/kg/day (max 400 mg) IV/PO q24h after loading dose of 25 mg/kg/day for 6–12 mo (AII). Itraconazole is alternative if cannot tolerate fluconazole.	Serum flucytosine concentrations should be obtained after 3–5 days to achieve a 2-h post-dose peak <100 µg/mL (ideally 30–80 µg/mL) to prevent neutropenia. For HIV-positive patients, continue maintenance therapy with fluconazole (6 mg/kg/day) indefinitely. Initiate HAART 2–10 wk after commencement of antifungal therapy to avoid immune reconstitution syndrome.

For meningitis or severe pulmonary disease: induction therapy with AmB-D 1 mg/kg/day IV q24h OR ABLC/L-AmB 5 mg/kg/day q24h; AND flucytosine 100 mg/kg/day PO div q6h for a minimum of 2 wk and a repeat CSF culture is negative, followed by consolidation therapy with fluconazole (12 mg/kg/day with max dose 400 mg after a loading dose of 25 mg/kg/day) for a minimum of 8 more wk (AI). Then use maintenance therapy with fluconazole (6 mg/kg/day) for 6–12 mo (AI).

Alternative induction therapies for meningitis or severe pulmonary disease (listed in order of preference): AmB product for 4–6 wk (AII); AmB product plus flucytosine for 2 wk, followed by fluconazole for 8 wk (BII); fluconazole plus flucytosine for 6 wk (BII).

In organ transplant recipients, continue maintenance fluconazole (6 mg/kg/day) for 6–12 mo after consolidation therapy with higher dose fluconazole.

For cryptococcal relapse, restart induction therapy (this time for 4–10 wk), repeat CSF analysis every 2 wk until sterile, and determine antifungal susceptibility of relapse isolate.

Successful use of voriconazole, posaconazole, and isavuconazole for cryptococcosis has been reported in adult patients.

Preferred Therapy for Specific Fungal Pathogens

B. SYSTEMIC INFECTIONS (continued)

Infection	Therapy (evidence grade)	Comments
Fusarium, Scedosporium prolificans, Pseudallescheria boydii (and its asexual form, *Scedosporium apiospermum*),[34,79-83] and other agents of **hyalohyphomycosis**	Voriconazole (AII) 18 mg/kg/day IV div q12h for a loading dose on the first day, then 16 mg/kg/day IV div q12h as a maintenance dose for children 2–12 y or 12–14 y and weighing <50 kg. In children ≥15 y or 12–14 y and weighing >50 kg, use adult dosing (load 12 mg/kg/day IV div q12h on the first day, then 8 mg/kg/day div q12h as a maintenance dose) (AII). When stable, may switch from voriconazole IV to voriconazole PO at a dose of 18 mg/kg/day div bid for children 2–12 y and at least 400 mg/day bid for children >12 y (AII). Dosing in children <2 y is less clear, but doses are generally higher (AIII). These are only initial dosing recommendations; continued dosing in all ages is guided by close monitoring of trough serum voriconazole concentrations in individual patients (AII). Unlike in adults, voriconazole PO bioavailability in children is only approximately 50%–60%, so trough levels are crucial at this stage.[29]	These can be highly resistant infections, so strongly recommend antifungal susceptibility testing against a wide range of agents to guide specific therapy and consultation with a pediatric infectious diseases expert. Optimal voriconazole trough serum concentrations (generally thought to be 2–5 µg/mL) are important for success. It is critical to monitor trough concentrations to guide therapy due to high inter-patient variability.[30] Low voriconazole concentrations are a leading cause of clinical failure. Younger children (especially <3 y) often have lower voriconazole levels and need much higher dosing. Often resistant to AmB in vitro. Alternatives: posaconazole (trough concentrations >0.7 µg/mL) can be active; echinocandins have been reportedly successful as salvage therapy in combination with azoles; while there are reports of promising in vitro combinations with terbinafine, terbinafine does not obtain good tissue concentrations for these disseminated infections; miltefosine (for leishmaniasis) use has been reported.
Histoplasmosis[84-86]	For severe acute pulmonary disease: ABLC/L-AmB 5 mg/kg/day q24h for 1–2 wk, followed by itraconazole 10 mg/kg/day div bid (max 400 mg daily) to complete a total of 12 wk (AIII). Add methylprednisolone (0.5–1.0 mg/kg/day) for first 1–2 wk in patients with hypoxia or significant respiratory distress.	Mild pulmonary disease may not require therapy and, in most cases, resolves in 1 mo. CNS histoplasmosis requires initial AmB therapy for 4–6 wk, followed by itraconazole for at least 12 mo and until CSF antigen resolution. Itraconazole oral solution provides greater and more reliable absorption than capsules and only the oral solution should be used (on an empty stomach);

8

	For mild–moderate acute pulmonary disease: if symptoms persist for >1 mo, itraconazole 10 mg/kg/day PO solution div bid for 6–12 wk (AIII). For progressive disseminated histoplasmosis: ABLC/L-AmB 5 mg/kg/day q24h for 4–6 wk; alternative treatment is lipid AmB for 1–2 wk followed by itraconazole 10 mg/kg/day div bid (max 400 mg daily) to complete a total of 12 wk (AIII). serum concentrations of itraconazole should be determined 2 wk after start of therapy to ensure adequate drug exposure. Maintain trough itraconazole concentrations at >1–2 µg/mL (values for both itraconazole and hydroxyl-itraconazole are added together). If only itraconazole capsules are available, use 20 mg/kg/day div q12h and take with cola product to increase gastric acidity and bioavailability. Potential lifelong suppressive itraconazole if cannot reverse immunosuppression. Corticosteroids recommended for 2 wk for pericarditis with hemodynamic compromise. Voriconazole and posaconazole use has been reported. Fluconazole is inferior to itraconazole.
Mucormycosis (previously known as zygomycosis)[28, 87–93]	Aggressive surgical debridement combined with induction antifungal therapy: L-AmB at 5–10 mg/kg/day q24h (AII) for 3 wk. Lipid formulations of AmB are preferred to AmB-D due to increased penetration and decreased toxicity. Some experts advocate induction or salvage combination therapy with L-AmB plus an echinocandin (although data are largely in diabetic patients with rhinocerebral disease) (CIII)[94] or combination of L-AmB plus posaconazole. For salvage therapy, isavuconazole (AII)[95] or posaconazole (AIII). Following successful induction antifungal therapy (for at least 3 wk), can continue consolidation therapy with posaconazole (or use intermittent L-AmB) (BII).	Following clinical response with AmB, long-term oral step-down therapy with posaconazole (trough concentrations ideally at >2 µg/mL) can be attempted for 2–6 mo. No pediatric dosing exists for isavuconazole. Voriconazole has NO activity against mucormycosis or other *Zygomycetes*. Return of immune function is paramount to treatment success; for children receiving corticosteroids, decreasing the corticosteroid dosage or changing to steroid-sparing protocols is also important.
Paracoccidioidomycosis[96–99]	Itraconazole 10 mg/kg/day (max 400 mg daily) PO solution div bid for 6 mo (AIII) OR voriconazole (dosing listed under Aspergillosis) (BI)	Alternatives: fluconazole; isavuconazole; sulfadiazine or TMP/SMX for 3–5 y. AmB is another alternative and may be combined with sulfa or azole antifungals.

Preferred Therapy for Specific Fungal Pathogens

Preferred Therapy for Specific Fungal Pathogens

B. SYSTEMIC INFECTIONS (continued)

Infection	Therapy (evidence grade)	Comments
Pneumocystis jiroveci (formerly *carinii*) pneumonia[100,101]	Severe disease; preferred regimen is TMP/SMX 15–20 mg TMP component/kg/day IV div q8h (AI) OR, for TMP/SMX intolerant or TMP/SMX treatment failure, pentamidine isethionate 4 mg base/kg/day IV daily (BII), for 3 wk. Mild–moderate disease: start with IV therapy, then after acute pneumonitis is resolved, TMP/SMX 20 mg TMP component/kg/day PO div qid for 3 wk total treatment course (AII).	Alternatives: TMP AND dapsone; OR primaquine AND clindamycin; OR atovaquone. Prophylaxis: preferred regimen is TMP/SMX (5 mg TMP component/kg/day) PO bid 3 times/wk on consecutive days; OR same dose, given qd, every day; OR atovaquone: 30 mg/kg/day for infants 1–3 mo; 45 mg/kg/day for infants/children 4–24 mo; and 30 mg/kg/day for children >24 mo; OR dapsone 2 mg/kg (max 100 mg) PO qd, OR dapsone 4 mg/kg (max 200 mg) PO once weekly. Use steroid therapy for more severe disease.
Sporotrichosis[102,103]	For cutaneous/lymphocutaneous: itraconazole 10 mg/kg/day div bid PO solution for 2–4 wk after all lesions gone (generally total of 3–6 mo) (AII) For serious pulmonary or disseminated infection or disseminated sporotrichosis: ABLC/L-AmB at 5 mg/kg/day q24h until favorable response, then step-down therapy with itraconazole PO for at least a total of 12 mo (AIII) For less severe disease, itraconazole for 12 mo	If no response for cutaneous disease, treat with higher itraconazole dose, terbinafine, or saturated solution of potassium iodide. Fluconazole is less effective. Obtain serum concentrations of itraconazole after 2 wk of therapy; want serum trough concentration >0.5 μg/mL. For meningeal disease, initial AmB should be 4–6 wk before change to itraconazole for at least 12 mo of therapy. Surgery may be necessary in osteoarticular or pulmonary disease.

C. LOCALIZED MUCOCUTANEOUS INFECTIONS

Infection	Therapy (evidence grade)	Comments
Dermatophytoses		
– Scalp (tinea capitis, including kerion)[104–109]	Griseofulvin ultramicrosize 10–15 mg/kg/day or microsize 20–25 mg/kg/day qd PO for 6–12 wk (All) (taken with milk or fatty foods to augment absorption). For kerion, treat concurrently with prednisone (1–2 mg/kg/day for 1–2 wk) (AIII). Terbinafine can be used for only 2–4 wk. Terbinafine dosing is 62.5 mg/day (<20 kg), 125 mg/day (20–40 kg), or 250 mg/day (>40 kg) (AII).	Griseofulvin is superior for *Microsporum* infections, but terbinafine is superior for *Trichophyton* infections. *Trichophyton tonsurans* predominates in United States. No need to routinely follow liver function tests in normal healthy children taking griseofulvin. Alternatives: itraconazole oral solution 5 mg/kg qd or fluconazole. 2.5% selenium sulfide shampoo, or 2% ketoconazole shampoo, 2–3 times/wk should be used concurrently to prevent recurrences.
– Tinea corporis (infection of trunk/limbs/face) – Tinea cruris (infection of the groin) – Tinea pedis (infection of the toes/feet)	Alphabetic order of topical agents: butenafine, ciclopirox, clotrimazole, econazole, haloprogin, ketoconazole, miconazole, naftifine, oxiconazole, sertaconazole, sulconazole, terbinafine, and tolnaftate (All); apply daily for 4 wk.	For unresponsive tinea lesions, use griseofulvin PO in dosages provided for scalp (tinea capitis, including kerion); fluconazole PO; itraconazole PO; OR terbinafine PO. For tinea pedis: terbinafine PO or itraconazole PO are preferred over other oral agents. Keep skin as clean and dry as possible, particularly for tinea cruris and tinea pedis.
– Tinea unguium (onychomycosis)[106,110,111]	Terbinafine 62.5 mg/day (<20 kg), 125 mg/day (20–40 kg), or 250 mg/day (>40 kg). Use for at least 6 wk (fingernails) or 12–16 wk (toenails) (AII).	Recurrence or partial response common. Alternative: itraconazole pulse therapy with 10 mg/kg/day div q12h for 1 wk per mo. Two pulses for fingernails and 3 pulses for toenails. Alternatives: fluconazole, griseofulvin.

Preferred Therapy for Specific Fungal Pathogens

C. LOCALIZED MUCOCUTANEOUS INFECTIONS (continued)

Infection	Therapy (evidence grade)	Comments
– Tinea versicolor (also pityriasis versicolor)[106,112,113]	Apply topically: selenium sulfide 2.5% lotion or 1% shampoo daily, leave on 30 min, then rinse; for 7 days, then monthly for 6 mo (AIII); OR ciclopirox 1% cream for 4 wk (BII); OR terbinafine 1% solution (BII); OR ketoconazole 2% shampoo daily for 5 days (BII) For small lesions, topical clotrimazole, econazole, haloprogin, ketoconazole, miconazole, or naftifine	For lesions that fail to clear with topical therapy or for extensive lesions: fluconazole PO or itraconazole PO are equally effective. Recurrence common.

9. Preferred Therapy for Specific Viral Pathogens

NOTE

- **Abbreviations:** AIDS, acquired immunodeficiency syndrome; ART, antiretroviral therapy; ARV, antiretroviral; bid, twice daily; BSA, body surface area; CDC, Centers for Disease Control and Prevention; CLD, chronic lung disease; CMV, cytomegalovirus; CrCl, creatinine clearance; div, divided; EBV, Epstein-Barr virus; FDA, US Food and Drug Administration; G-CSF, granulocyte-colony stimulating factor; HAART, highly active antiretroviral therapy; HBeAg, hepatitis B e antigen; HBV, hepatitis B virus; HCV, hepatitis C virus; HHS, US Department of Health and Human Services; HIV, human immunodeficiency virus; HSV, herpes simplex virus; IFN, interferon; IG, immune globulin; IM, intramuscular; IV, intravenous; NS5A, nonstructural protein 5A; PO, orally; postmenstrual age, weeks of gestation since last menstrual period PLUS weeks of chronologic age since birth; PTLD, posttransplant lymphoproliferative disorder; qd, once daily; qid, 4 times daily; RAV, resistance-associated variant; RSV, respiratory syncytial virus; SQ, subcutaneous; TAF, tenofovir alafenamide; tid, 3 times daily; WHO, World Health Organization.

Preferred Therapy for Specific Viral Pathogens

A. OVERVIEW OF NON-HIV VIRAL PATHOGENS AND USUAL PATTERN OF SUSCEPTIBILITY TO ANTIVIRALS

Virus	Interferon alfa-2b	Lamivudine	Acyclovir	Adefovir	Cidofovir	Daclatasvir Plus Sofosbuvir	Elbasvir/ Grazoprevir (Zepatier)	Entecavir	Famciclovir	Foscarnet	Ganciclovir
Cytomegalovirus					+					+	+
Hepatitis B virus[1]	+	+		+				+ +			
Hepatitis C virus[a]						+ + b,c	+ + d,e				
Herpes simplex virus	+ +		+ +						+ +	+	+
Influenza A and B											
Varicella-zoster virus	+ +		+ +						+ +	+	+

Virus	Ombitasvir/ Paritaprevir/Ritonavir Co-packaged With Dasabuvir (Viekira Pak)	Ombitasvir/ Paritaprevir/ Ritonavir Plus Ribavirin	Oseltamivir	Pegylated Interferon alfa-2a	Peramivir	Ribavirin
Cytomegalovirus						
Hepatitis B virus				+ +		
Hepatitis C virus[a]	+ + b	+ + e		+ + f		+ + f
Herpes simplex virus						
Influenza A and B			+ +		+	
Varicella-zoster virus						

9

Virus	Simeprevir Plus Sofosbuvir	Sofosbuvir/ Ledipasvir (Harvoni)	Sofosbuvir Plus Ribavirin	Sofosbuvir/ Velpatasvir (Epclusa)	Telbivudine	Tenofovir	Valacyclovir	Valganciclovir	Zanamivir
Cytomegalovirus								++	
Hepatitis B virus					+	++			
Hepatitis C virus[a]	++[b]	++[b,e,g]	++[c]	+[h]					
Herpes simplex virus							++	+	
Influenza A and B									+
Varicella-zoster virus							++		

NOTE: ++ = preferred therapy(ies); + = acceptable therapy.

[a] HCV treatment guidelines from the Infectious Diseases Society of America and the American Association for the Study of Liver Diseases available at www.hcvguidelines.org (accessed October 3, 2017).

[b] Treatment-naive patients with HCV genotype 1a and 1b infection who do not have cirrhosis.

[c] Treatment-naive patients with HCV genotype 2 and 3 infection who do not have cirrhosis.

[d] Treatment-naive patients with HCV genotype 1a and 1b infection in whom no baseline high fold-change NS5A RAVs for elbasvir are detected.

[e] Treatment-naive patients with HCV genotype 4 infection who do not have cirrhosis.

[f] Likely to be replaced in pediatric patients as studies of newer molecules are performed in children.

[g] Treatment-naive patients with HCV genotype 5 and 6 infection who do not have cirrhosis.

[h] Active against all genotypes of HCV.

Preferred Therapy for Specific Viral Pathogens

9

B. PREFERRED THERAPY FOR SPECIFIC VIRAL PATHOGENS

Infection	Therapy (evidence grade)	Comments
Adenovirus (pneumonia or disseminated infection in immunocompromised hosts)[2]	Cidofovir and ribavirin are active in vitro, but no prospective clinical data exist and both have significant toxicity. Two cidofovir dosing schedules have been employed in clinical settings: (1) 5 mg/kg/dose IV once weekly or (2) 1–1.5 mg/kg/dose IV 3 times/wk. If parenteral cidofovir is utilized, IV hydration and oral probenecid should be used to reduce renal toxicity.	Brincidofovir, the orally bioavailable lipophilic derivative of cidofovir also known as CMX001, is under investigation for the treatment of adenovirus in immunocompromised hosts. It is not yet commercially available.
Cytomegalovirus		
– Neonatal[3]	See Chapter 5.	
– Immunocompromised (HIV, chemotherapy, transplant-related)[4–16]	For induction: ganciclovir 10 mg/kg/day IV div q12h for 14–21 days (AII) (may be increased to 15 mg/kg/day IV div q12h). For maintenance: 5 mg/kg IV q24h for 5–7 days per week. Duration dependent on degree of immunosuppression (AII). CMV hyperimmune globulin may decrease morbidity in bone marrow transplant patients with CMV pneumonia (AII).	Use foscarnet or cidofovir for ganciclovir-resistant strains; for HIV-positive children on HAART, CMV may resolve without therapy. Also used for prevention of CMV disease posttransplant for 100–120 days. Data on valganciclovir dosing in young children for treatment of retinitis are unavailable, but consideration can be given to transitioning from IV ganciclovir to oral valganciclovir after improvement of retinitis is noted. Limited data on oral valganciclovir in infants[17,18] (32 mg/kg/day PO div bid) and children (dosing by BSA [dose (mg) = $7 \times BSA \times CrCl$]).[6]
– Prophylaxis of infection in immunocompromised hosts[5,19]	Ganciclovir 5 mg/kg IV daily (or 3 times/wk) (started at engraftment for stem cell transplant patients) (BII)	Neutropenia is a complication with ganciclovir prophylaxis and may be addressed with G-CSF. Prophylaxis and preemptive strategies are effective; neither has been shown clearly superior to the other.[10]

Valganciclovir at total dose in

milligrams = $7 \times$ BSA $\times$ CrCl (use maximum CrCl 150 mL/min/1.73 m^2) orally once daily with food for children 4 mo–16 y (max dose 900 mg/day) for primary prophylaxis in HIV patients[20] who are CMV antibody positive and have severe immunosuppression (CD4 count <50 cells/mm^3 in children ≥6 y; CD4 percentage <5% in children <6 y) (CIII)

Enterovirus	Supportive therapy; no antivirals currently FDA approved
	Pocapavir PO is currently under investigation for enterovirus (poliovirus).
	Pleconaril PO is currently under consideration for approval at FDA for treatment of neonatal enteroviral sepsis syndrome.[21]
Epstein-Barr virus	
– Mononucleosis, encephalitis[22-24]	Limited data suggest small clinical benefit of valacyclovir in adolescents for mononucleosis (3 g/day div tid for 14 days) (CIII).
	For EBV encephalitis: ganciclovir IV OR acyclovir IV (AIII).
	No prospective data on benefits of acyclovir IV or ganciclovir IV in EBV clinical infections of normal hosts.
	Patients suspected to have infectious mononucleosis should not be given ampicillin or amoxicillin, which cause nonallergic morbilliform rashes in a high proportion of patients with active EBV infection (AII).
	Therapy with short-course corticosteroids (prednisone 1 mg/kg per day PO [maximum 20 mg/day] for 7 days with subsequent tapering) may have a beneficial effect on acute symptoms in patients with marked tonsillar inflammation with impending airway obstruction, massive splenomegaly, myocarditis, hemolytic anemia, or hemophagocytic lymphohistiocytosis (BII).

Preferred Therapy for Specific Viral Pathogens

B. PREFERRED THERAPY FOR SPECIFIC VIRAL PATHOGENS (continued)

Infection	Therapy (evidence grade)	Comments
– Posttransplant lymphoproliferative disorder[25,26]	Ganciclovir (AIII)	Decrease immune suppression if possible, as this has the most effect on control of EBV, rituximab, methotrexate have been used but without controlled data. Preemptive treatment with ganciclovir may decrease PTLD in solid organ transplants.
Hepatitis B virus (chronic)[27-45]	IFN-alfa 3 million U/m² BSA SQ 3 times/wk for 1 wk, followed by dose escalation to 6 million U/m² BSA (max 10 million U/dose), to complete a 24-wk course for children 1–18 y; OR lamivudine 3 mg/kg/day (max 100 mg) PO q24h for 52 wk for children ≥2 y (children coinfected with HIV and HBV should use the approved dose for HIV) (AII); OR adefovir for children ≥12 y (10 mg PO q24h for a minimum of 12 mo; optimum duration of therapy unknown) (BII); OR entecavir for children ≥2 y (optimum duration of therapy unknown [BII]) No prior nucleoside therapy: ≥16 y: 0.5 mg qd 2–15 y: 10–11 kg: 0.15 mg oral solution qd >11–14 kg: 0.2 mg oral solution qd >14–17 kg: 0.25 mg oral solution qd >17–20 kg: 0.3 mg oral solution qd >20–23 kg: 0.35 mg oral solution qd >23–26 kg: 0.4 mg oral solution qd >26–30 kg: 0.45 mg oral solution qd >30 kg: 0.5 mg oral solution or tablet qd Prior nucleoside therapy: Double the dosage in each weight bracket	Indications for treatment of chronic HBV infection, with or without HIV coinfection, are (1) evidence of ongoing HBV viral replication, as indicated by serum HBV DNA (>20,000 without HBeAg positivity or >2,000 IU/mL with HBeAg positivity) for >6 mo and persistent elevation of serum transaminase levels for >6 mo, or (2) evidence of chronic hepatitis on liver biopsy (BII). Antiviral therapy is not warranted in children without necroinflammatory liver disease (BII). Treatment is not recommended for children with immunotolerant chronic HBV infection (ie, normal serum transaminase levels despite detectable HBV DNA) (BII). Standard IFN-alfa (IFN-2a or 2b) is recommended for treating chronic HBV infection with compensated liver disease in HIV-uninfected children aged ≥2 y who warrant treatment (AI). IFN-alfa therapy in combination with oral antiviral therapy cannot be recommended for pediatric HBV infection in HIV-uninfected children until more data are available (BII). In HIV/HBV-coinfected children who do not require ART for their HIV infection, IFN-alfa therapy is the preferred agent to treat chronic HBV (BIII), whereas adefovir can be considered in children ≥12 y (BIII). Treatment options for HIV/HBV-coinfected children who meet criteria for HBV therapy and who are already receiving lamivudine- or emtricitabine-containing HIV-suppressive ART include

9

the standard IFN-alfa therapy to the ARV regimen (BIII), or adefovir if the child can receive adult dosing (BIII), or use of tenofovir disoproxil fumarate in lamivudine- (or emtricitabine-) containing ARV regimen in children ≥2 y (BIII). HIV/HBV-coinfected children should not be given lamivudine (or emtricitabine) without additional anti-HIV drugs for treatment of chronic HBV (CIII).[20]

Alternatives

Tenofovir (adult and adolescent dose [≥12 y] 300 mg qd).

Telbivudine (adult dose 600 mg qd). There are not sufficient clinical data to identify the appropriate dose for use in children.

Lamivudine approved for children ≥2 y, but antiviral resistance develops on therapy in 30%.

Entecavir is superior to lamivudine in the treatment of chronic HBV infection and is the most potent anti-HBV agent available.

Preferred Therapy for Specific Viral Pathogens

9

B. PREFERRED THERAPY FOR SPECIFIC VIRAL PATHOGENS (continued)

Infection	Therapy (evidence grade)	Comments
Hepatitis C virus (chronic)[46-52]	Treatment of HCV infections in adults has been revolutionized in recent years with the licensure of numerous highly effective direct-acting antiviral drugs for use in adults. Studies of many of these drugs are underway in children, but their optimal use in children and adolescents has yet to be defined. Given the efficacy of these new treatment regimens in adults (AI),[53-68] strong consideration should be given to seeking out these studies if treatment is desired in children and adolescents. An alternative would be to not treat with the approved treatment regimen of IFN + ribavirin pending results of these pediatric studies. If treatment currently is desired and access to the studies of direct-acting antiviral agents is not available, the following treatment is the only one FDA approved for HCV infection in children 3–17 y: Pegylated IFN-alfa: 2a 180 μg/1.73 m² BSA SQ once per wk (maximum dose 180 μg) OR 2b 60 μg/m² BSA once per wk PLUS Ribavirin (oral) 7.5 mg/kg body weight bid (fixed dose by weight recommended) 25–36 kg: 200 mg in am and pm >36–49 kg: 200 mg in am and 400 mg in pm >49–61 kg: 400 mg in am and pm >61–75 kg: 400 mg in am and 600 mg in pm >75 kg: 600 mg in am and pm Treatment duration 24–48 wk (4m	None of the direct-acting antiviral HCV drugs currently have been approved for use in children <12 y. Sofosbuvir (Sovaldi) and sofosbuvir in a fixed dose combination tablet with ledipasvir (Harvoni) are now approved for patients ≥12 y. Treatment of children <3 y who have HCV infection usually is not recommended (BIII). HCV-infected, HIV-uninfected children ≥3 y should be individualized because HCV usually causes mild disease in this population and few data exist to identify risk factors differentiating those at greater risk for progression of liver disease. Those who are chosen for treatment should receive combination therapy with IFN-alfa and ribavirin for 48 wk for genotype 1 and 24 wk for genotypes 2 or 3 (AI) (see Therapy column). Treatment should be considered for all HIV/HCV-coinfected children aged >3 y who have no contraindications to treatment (BIII). A liver biopsy to stage disease is recommended before deciding whether to initiate therapy for chronic HCV genotype 1 infection (BIII). However, some specialists would treat children infected with HCV genotypes 2 or 3 without first obtaining a liver biopsy (BIII). IFN-alfa therapy is contraindicated for children with decompensated liver disease, substantial cytopenias, renal failure, severe cardiac or neuropsychiatric disorders, and non–HCV-related autoimmune disease (AII).[19]

Herpes simplex virus

– Third trimester maternal suppressive therapy[69,70]	Acyclovir or valacyclovir maternal suppressive therapy in pregnant women reduces HSV recurrences and viral shedding at the time of delivery but does not fully prevent neonatal HSV[70] (BIII).
– Neonatal	See Chapter 5.
– Mucocutaneous (normal host)	Acyclovir 80 mg/kg/day PO div qid (max dose 800 mg) for 5–7 days, or 15 mg/kg/day IV as 1–2 h infusion div q8h (AII) Suppressive therapy for frequent recurrence (no pediatric data): 20 mg/kg/dose given bid or tid (max dose 400 mg) for 6–12 mo, then reevaluate need (AIII) Valacyclovir 20 mg/kg/dose (max dose 1 g) PO bid[71] for 5–7 days (BII)	Foscarnet for acyclovir-resistant strains. Immunocompromised hosts may require 10–14 days of therapy. Topical acyclovir not efficacious and therefore is not recommended.
– Genital	Adult doses: acyclovir 400 mg PO tid for 7–10 days; OR valacyclovir 1 g PO bid for 10 days; OR famciclovir 250 mg PO tid for 7–10 days (AI)	All 3 drugs have been used as prophylaxis to prevent recurrence. Topical acyclovir not efficacious and therefore is not recommended.
– Encephalitis	Acyclovir 60 mg/kg/day IV as 1–2 h infusion div q8h; for 21 days for infants ≤4 mo. For older infants and children, 30–45 mg/kg/day IV as 1–2 h infusion div q8h (AIII).	Safety of high-dose acyclovir (60 mg/kg/day) not well defined beyond the neonatal period; can be used but monitor for neurotoxicity and nephrotoxicity.
– Keratoconjunctivitis	1% trifluridine or 0.15% ganciclovir ophthalmic gel (AII)	Treat in consultation with an ophthalmologist. Topical steroids may be helpful when used together with antiviral agents.

Preferred Therapy for Specific Viral Pathogens

9

B. PREFERRED THERAPY FOR SPECIFIC VIRAL PATHOGENS (continued)

Infection	Therapy (evidence grade)	Comments
Human herpesvirus 6		
– Immunocompromised children[72]	No prospective comparative data; ganciclovir 10 mg/kg/day IV div q12h used in case report (AIII)	May require high dose to control infection; safety and efficacy not defined at high doses.
Human immunodeficiency virus		
Current information on HIV treatment and opportunistic infections for children[73] is posted at http://aidsinfo.nih.gov/ContentFiles/PediatricGuidelines.pdf (accessed October 3, 2017); other information on HIV programs is available at www.cdc.gov/hiv/policies/index.html (accessed October 3, 2017). Consult with an HIV expert, if possible, for current recommendations, as treatment options are complicated and constantly evolving.		
– Therapy of HIV infection		
State-of-the-art therapy is rapidly evolving with introduction of new agents and combinations; currently there are 26 individual ARV agents approved for use by the FDA that have pediatric indications, as well as multiple combinations; guidelines for children and adolescents are continually updated on the AIDSinfo and CDC Web sites given previously.	Effective therapy (HAART) consists of ≥3 agents, including 2 nucleoside reverse transcriptase inhibitors, plus either a protease inhibitor, a non-nucleoside reverse transcriptase inhibitor, or an integrase inhibitor; many different combination regimens give similar treatment outcomes; choice of agents depends on the age of the child, viral load, consideration of potential viral resistance, and extent of immune depletion, in addition to judging the child's ability to adhere to the regimen.	Assess drug toxicity (based on the agents used) and virologic/immunologic response to therapy (quantitative plasma HIV and CD4 count) initially monthly and then every 3–6 mo during the maintenance phase.
– Children of any age	Any child with AIDS or significant HIV-related symptoms (clinical category C and most B conditions) should be treated (AI).	Adherence counseling and appropriate ARV formulations are critical for successful implementation.

Recent guidance from the WHO and HHS guidelines committees now recommends treatment for **all children** regardless of age, CD4 count, or clinical status, with situation-specific levels of urgency.

– First 3 y after birth	HAART with ≥3 drugs is now recommended for **all infants** ≤36 mo, regardless of clinical status or laboratory values (AI for <12 wk and for >1 y; AII for 12–52 wk).	Preferred therapy in the first year of life is zidovudine plus lamivudine (at any age) OR abacavir plus lamivudine (>3 mo) plus lopinavir/ritonavir (toxicity concerns preclude its use until a postmenstrual age of 42 wk and a postnatal age of at least 14 days is reached). Raltegravir is equally preferred with lopinavir/ritonavir for children between 2 and 3 y of age.
– HIV-infected children ≥3–<12 y	**Treat all** with special urgency for those with the following CD4 values: 1–<6 y with CD4 <1,000 or <25% (AII) 1–<6 y with CD4 ≥1,000 or ≥25% (BI) ≥6 y with CD4 <500 (AII) ≥6 y with CD4 ≥500 (BI)	Preferred regimens comprise zidovudine plus lamivudine (at any age) OR abacavir plus lamivudine (>3 mo) PLUS either lopinavir/ritonavir OR efavirenz OR atazanavir/ritonavir OR darunavir/ritonavir OR raltegravir.
– HIV-infected youth ≥12 y	**Treat all with evidence grades of AII–BI depending on CD4 count.**	Preferred regimens comprise tenofovir or TAF plus emtricitabine (adolescents/Tanner stage 4 or 5) OR abacavir plus lamivudine PLUS either atazanavir/ritonavir OR darunavir/ritonavir OR dolutegravir OR elvitegravir.
– Antiretroviral-experienced child	Consult with HIV specialist.	Consider treatment history and drug resistance testing and assess adherence.

Preferred Therapy for Specific Viral Pathogens

B. PREFERRED THERAPY FOR SPECIFIC VIRAL PATHOGENS (continued)

Infection	Therapy (evidence grade)	Comments
– HIV exposures, nonoccupational	Therapy recommendations for exposures available on the CDC Web site at www.cdc.gov/hiv/guidelines/preventing.html (accessed October 3, 2017)	Postexposure prophylaxis remains unproven but substantial evidence supports its use; consider individually regarding risk, time from exposure, and likelihood of adherence; prophylactic regimens administered for 4 wk.
– Negligible exposure risk (urine, nasal secretions, saliva, sweat, or tears—no visible blood in secretions) OR >72 h since exposure	Prophylaxis not recommended (BIII)	
– Significant exposure risk (blood, semen, vaginal, or rectal secretions from a known HIV-infected individual) AND <72 h since exposure	Prophylaxis recommended (BIII) Preferred regimens 4 wk–<2 y: zidovudine PLUS lamivudine PLUS either raltegravir or lopinavir/ritonavir 2–12 y: tenofovir PLUS emtricitabine PLUS raltegravir ≥13 y: tenofovir PLUS emtricitabine PLUS either raltegravir or dolutegravir	Consultation with a pediatric HIV specialist is advised.
– HIV exposure, occupational[74]	See guidelines on CDC Web site at www.cdc.gov/hiv/guidelines/preventing.html (accessed October 3, 2017).	

Influenza virus
Recommendations for the treatment of influenza can vary from season to season; access the American Academy of Pediatrics Web site (www.aap.org) and the CDC Web site (www.cdc.gov/flu/professionals/antivirals/summary-clinicians.htm; accessed October 3, 2017) for the most current, accurate information.

Influenza A and B

Infection	Therapy (evidence grade)	Comments
– Treatment[75–77]	Oseltamivir[75–77] Preterm, <38 wk postmenstrual age: 1 mg/kg/dose PO bid[75]	Oseltamivir currently is drug of choice for treatment of influenza infections.

Preterm, 38–40 wk postmenstrual age: 1.5 mg/kg/dose PO bid[75]
Preterm, >40 wk postmenstrual age: 3.0 mg/kg/dose PO bid
Term, birth–8 mo: 3.0 mg/kg/dose PO bid[76]
9–11 mo: 3.5 mg/kg/dose PO bid
12–23 mo: 30 mg/dose PO bid
2–12 y: ≤15 kg: 30 mg bid; 16–23 kg: 45 mg bid; 24–40 kg: 60 mg bid; >40 kg: 75 mg bid
≥13 y: 75 mg bid
OR
Zanamivir
≥7 y: 10 mg by inhalation bid for 5 days

For patients 12–23 mo, the original FDA-approved unit dose of 30 mg/dose may provide inadequate drug exposure; 3.5 mg/kg/dose PO bid has been studied,[76] but study population sizes were small.
Peramivir is a third neuraminidase inhibitor that was approved for use as a parenteral drug in adults in the United States in December 2014. Pediatric studies of parenteral peramivir are underway.
Studies of parenteral zanamivir have been completed in children.[78] This formulation of the drug is not yet approved in the United States, though.
The adamantanes, amantadine and rimantadine, currently are not effective for treatment due to near-universal resistance of influenza A.

– Chemoprophylaxis

Oseltamivir
3 mo–12 y: The mg dose given for prophylaxis is the same as for the treatment dose for all ages, but it is given qd for prophylaxis instead of bid for treatment.
Zanamivir
≥5 y: 10 mg by inhalation qd for as long as 28 days (community outbreaks) or 10 days (household setting)

Oseltamivir currently is drug of choice for chemoprophylaxis of influenza infection.
Unless the situation is judged critical, oseltamivir chemoprophylaxis not recommended for patients <3 mo because of limited safety and efficacy data in this age group.
The adamantanes, amantadine and rimantadine, currently are not effective for chemoprophylaxis due to near-universal resistance of influenza A.

Preferred Therapy for Specific Viral Pathogens

B. PREFERRED THERAPY FOR SPECIFIC VIRAL PATHOGENS (continued)

Infection	Therapy (evidence grade)	Comments
Measles[79]	No prospective data on antiviral therapy. Ribavirin is active against measles virus in vitro. Vitamin A is beneficial in children with measles and is recommended by WHO for all children with measles regardless of their country of residence (qd dosing for 2 days): for children ≥1 y: 200,000 IU; for infants 6–12 mo: 100,000 IU; for infants <6 mo: 50,000 IU (BII). Even in countries where measles is not usually severe, vitamin A should be given to all children with severe measles (eg, requiring hospitalization). Parenteral and oral formulations are available in the United States.	IG prophylaxis for exposed, susceptible children: 0.5 mL/kg (max 15 mL) IM
Respiratory syncytial virus[80,81]		
– Therapy (severe disease in compromised host)	Ribavirin (6-g vial to make 20 mg/mL solution in sterile water), aerosolized over 18–20 h daily for 3–5 days (BII)	Aerosol ribavirin provides a small benefit and should only be considered for use for life-threatening infection with RSV. Airway reactivity with inhalation precludes routine use.
– Prophylaxis (palivizumab, Synagis for high-risk infants) (BI)[80,81]	Prophylaxis: palivizumab (a monoclonal antibody) 15 mg/kg IM monthly (max 5 doses) for the following high-risk infants (AI): In first y after birth, palivizumab prophylaxis is recommended for infants born before 29 wk 0 days' gestation. Palivizumab prophylaxis is not recommended for otherwise healthy infants born at ≥29 wk 0 days' gestation.	Palivizumab does not provide benefit in the treatment of an active RSV infection. Palivizumab prophylaxis may be considered for children <24 mo who will be profoundly immunocompromised during the RSV season. Palivizumab prophylaxis is not recommended in the second year after birth except for children who required at least 28 days of supplemental oxygen after birth and who continue to require medical support (supplemental oxygen, chronic corticosteroid therapy, or diuretic therapy) during the 6-mo period before the start of the second RSV season.

9

	In first y after birth, palivizumab prophylaxis is recommended for preterm infants with CLD of prematurity, defined as birth at <32 wk 0 days' gestation and a requirement for >21% oxygen for at least 28 days after birth. Clinicians may administer palivizumab prophylaxis in the first y after birth to certain infants with hemodynamically significant heart disease.	Monthly prophylaxis should be discontinued in any child who experiences a breakthrough RSV hospitalization. Children with pulmonary abnormality or neuromuscular disease that impairs the ability to clear secretions from the upper airways may be considered for prophylaxis in the first year after birth. Insufficient data are available to recommend palivizumab prophylaxis for children with cystic fibrosis or Down syndrome. The burden of RSV disease and costs associated with transport from remote locations may result in a broader use of palivizumab for RSV prevention in Alaska Native populations and possibly in selected other American Indian populations. Palivizumab prophylaxis is not recommended for prevention of health care–associated RSV disease.
Varicella-zoster virus[82]		
– Infection in a normal host	Acyclovir 80 mg/kg/day as 1–2 h infusion 800 mg) PO div qid for 5 days (AI)	The sooner antiviral therapy can be started, the greater the clinical benefit.
– Severe primary chickenpox, disseminated infection (cutaneous, pneumonia, encephalitis, hepatitis); immunocompromised host with primary chickenpox or disseminated zoster	Acyclovir 30 mg/kg/day IV as 1–2 h infusion div q8h for 10 days (acyclovir doses of 45–60 mg/kg/day in 3 div doses IV should be used for disseminated or central nervous system infection). Dosing also can be provided as 1,500 mg/m²/day IV div q8h. Duration in immunocompromised children: 7–14 days, based on clinical response (AI).	Oral valacyclovir, famciclovir, foscarnet also active

10. Preferred Therapy for Specific Parasitic Pathogens

NOTES

- For some parasitic diseases, therapy may be available only from the Centers for Disease Control and Prevention (CDC), as noted. The CDC provides up-to-date information about parasitic diseases and current treatment recommendations at www.cdc.gov/parasites (accessed October 3, 2017). Consultation is available from the CDC for parasitic disease diagnostic services (www.cdc.gov/dpdx; accessed October 3, 2017); parasitic disease testing and experimental therapy at 404/639-3670; for malaria, 770/488-7788 or 855/856-4713 Monday through Friday, 9:00 am to 5:00 pm ET, and 770/488-7100 after hours, weekends, and holidays. Antiparasitic drugs available from the CDC can be reviewed and requested at www.cdc.gov/laboratory/drugservice/formulary.html (accessed October 3, 2017).

- Additional information about many of the organisms and diseases mentioned here, along with treatment recommendations, can be found in the appropriate sections in the American Academy of Pediatrics *Red Book*.

- **Abbreviations:** AmB, amphotericin B; A-P, atovaquone/proguanil; ASTMH, American Society of Tropical Medicine and Hygiene; bid, twice daily; BP, blood pressure; CDC, Centers for Disease Control and Prevention; CNS, central nervous system; CrCl, creatinine clearance; CSF, cerebrospinal fluid; DEC, diethylcarbamazine; div, divided; DS, double strength; ECG, electrocardiogram; FDA, US Food and Drug Administration; G6PD, glucose-6-phosphate dehydrogenase; GI, gastrointestinal; HIV, human immunodeficiency virus; IDSA, Infectious Diseases Society of America; IM, intramuscular; IV, intravenous; MRI, magnetic resonance imaging; PAIR, percutaneous aspiration, injection, re-aspiration; PHMB, polyhexamethylene biguanide; PO, orally; qd, once daily; qid, 4 times daily; qod, every other day; spp, species; tab, tablet; tid, 3 times daily; TMP/SMX, trimethoprim/sulfamethoxazole.

A. SELECTED COMMON PATGHOGENIC PARASITES AND SUGGESTED AGENTS FOR TREATMENT

	Albendazole/ Mebendazole	Metronidazole/ Tinidazole	Praziquantel	Ivermectin	Nitazoxanide	DEC	Pyrantel Pamoate	Paromomycin	TMP/SMX
Ascariasis	++			+	+		+		
Blastocystis spp		+			+			+	+
Cryptosporidiosis					+			+	
Cutaneous larva migrans	++			++					
Cyclosporiasis		-			+				++
Cystoisospora spp									++
Dientamoebiasis		++			+			+	
Liver fluke	+	+	++						
Lung fluke	-		++						
Giardia spp	+	++			++			+	
Hookworm	++			-			+		
Loiasis	+					++			
Mansonella ozzardi	-			+		-			
Mansonella perstans	++			-		-			
Onchocerciasis				++					
Pinworm	++						++		
Schistosomiasis			++						
Strongyloides spp	+			++					

Tapeworm		++		+
Toxocariasis	++		+	
Trichinellosis	++			
Trichomoniasis		++		
Trichuriasis	++			
Wuchereria bancrofti	+		++	

NOTE: + + = first-line agent or >90% effective; + = alternative or ≤90% effective; - = not likely to be effective.

Preferred Therapy for Specific Parasitic Pathogens

10

B. PREFERRED THERAPY FOR SPECIFIC PARASITIC PATHOGENS

Disease/Organism	Treatment (evidence grade)	Comments
Acanthamoeba	See MENINGOENCEPHALITIS.	
AMEBIASIS[1-5]		
Entamoeba histolytica		
– Asymptomatic intestinal colonization	Paromomycin 25–35 mg/kg/day PO div tid for 7 days; OR iodoquinol 30–40 mg/kg/day (max 650 mg/dose) PO tid for 20 days; OR diloxanide furoate (not commercially available in the United States) 20 mg/kg/day PO div tid (max 500 mg/dose) for 10 days (CII)	Follow-up stool examination to ensure eradication of carriage; screen/treat positive close contacts. *Entamoeba dispar* infections do not require treatment.
– Colitis	Metronidazole 35–50 mg/kg/day PO div tid for 10 days; OR tinidazole (age >3 y) 50 mg/kg/day PO (max 2 g) qd for 3 days FOLLOWED BY paromomycin or iodoquinol, as above, to eliminate cysts (BII)	Avoid antimotility drugs, steroids. Take tinidazole with food to decrease GI side effects; if unable to take tabs, pharmacists can crush tabs and mix with syrup. Avoid alcohol ingestion with metronidazole and tinidazole. Preliminary data support use of nitazoxanide to treat clinical infection, but it may not prevent parasitological failure: age ≥12 y, 500 mg bid for 3 days; ages 4–11 y, 200 mg bid for 3 days; ages 1–3 y, 100 mg bid for 3 days.
– Liver abscess, extraintestinal disease	Metronidazole 35–50 mg/kg/day IV q8h, switch to PO when tolerated, for 10 days; OR tinidazole (age >3 y) 50 mg/kg/day PO (max 2 g) qd for 5 days FOLLOWED BY paromomycin or iodoquinol, as above, to eliminate cysts (BII) Nitazoxanide 500 mg bid for 10 days (≥12 y)	Serologic assays >95% positive in extraintestinal amebiasis. Percutaneous or surgical drainage may be indicated for large liver abscesses or inadequate response to medical therapy. Avoid alcohol ingestion with metronidazole and tinidazole. Take tinidazole with food to decrease GI side effects; if unable to take tabs, pharmacists can crush tabs and mix with syrup.

AMEBIC MENINGOENCEPHALITIS[6-10]

Naegleria	AmB 1.5 mg/kg/day IV div 2 doses for 3 days, then 1 mg/kg/day qd for 11 days PLUS AmB intrathecally 1.5 mg qd for 2 days, then 1 mg/day qod for 8 days PLUS rifampin 10 mg/kg/day qd IV or PO (max 600 mg/day) for 28 days PLUS fluconazole 10 mg/kg/day IV or PO qd (max 600 mg/day) for 28 days PLUS miltefosine <45 kg 50 mg PO bid; ≥45 kg 50 mg PO tid for 28 days PLUS azithromycin 10 mg/kg/day IV or PO (max 500 mg/day) for 28 days; PLUS dexamethasone 0.6 mg/kg/day div qid for 4 days	Treatment recommendations based on regimens used for 5 known survivors; available at https://www.cdc.gov/parasites/naegleria/treatment-hcp.html (accessed October 3, 2017). Conventional amphotericin preferred; liposomal AmB is less effective in animal models. Treatment outcomes usually unsuccessful; early therapy (even before diagnostic confirmation if indicated) may improve survival.
Acanthamoeba	Combination regimens including miltefosine, fluconazole, and pentamidine favored by some experts; TMP/SMX, metronidazole, and a macrolide may be added. Other drugs that have been used alone or in combination include rifampin, azoles, pentamidine, sulfadiazine, flucytosine, and caspofungin. Keratitis: topical therapies include PHMB (0.02%) or biguanide chlorhexidine, combined with propamidine isethionate (0.1%) or hexamidine (0.1%) (topical therapies not approved in United States but available at compounding pharmacies).	Optimal treatment regimens uncertain; combination therapy favored. Keratitis should be evaluated by an ophthalmologist. Prolonged treatment often needed.
Balamuthia	Combination regimens preferred. Drugs that have been used alone or in combination include pentamidine, 5-flucytosine, fluconazole, macrolides, sulfadiazine, miltefosine, thioridazine, AmB, itraconazole, and albendazole.	Optimal treatment regimen uncertain; regimens based on case reports. Surgical resection of CNS lesions may be beneficial.
Ancylostoma braziliense	See CUTANEOUS LARVA MIGRANS.	
Ancylostoma caninum	See CUTANEOUS LARVA MIGRANS.	
Ancylostoma duodenale	See HOOKWORM.	

Preferred Therapy for Specific Parasitic Pathogens

Preferred Therapy for Specific Parasitic Pathogens

10

B. PREFERRED THERAPY FOR SPECIFIC PARASITIC PATHOGENS (continued)

Disease/Organism	Treatment (evidence grade)	Comments
ANGIOSTRONGYLIASIS[11–14]		
Angiostrongylus cantonensis (cerebral disease)	Supportive care	Most patients recover without antiparasitic therapy; treatment may provoke severe neurologic symptoms. Corticosteroids, analgesics, and repeat lumbar puncture may be of benefit. Prednisolone (1–2 mg/kg/day, up to 60 mg qd, in 2 div doses, for 2 wk) may shorten duration of headache and reduce need for repeat lumbar puncture. Ocular disease may require surgery or laser treatment.
Angiostrongylus costaricensis (eosinophilic enterocolitis)	Supportive care	Surgery may be pursued to exclude another diagnosis such as appendicitis or to remove inflamed intestine.
ASCARIASIS (Ascaris lumbricoides)[15]	First line: albendazole 400 mg PO once OR mebendazole 500 mg once or 100 mg tid for 3 days (BII) Pregnant women: pyrantel pamoate 11 mg/kg max 1 g once Alternatives: ivermectin 150–200 µg/kg PO once (CII); nitazoxanide 7.5 mg/kg once	Follow-up stool ova and parasite examination after therapy not essential. Take albendazole with food (bioavailability increases with food, especially fatty meals). Albendazole has theoretical risk of causing seizures in patients coinfected with cysticercosis.
BABESIOSIS (Babesia spp)[16–18]	Clindamycin 30 mg/kg/day IV or PO div tid (max 600 mg per dose), PLUS quinine 25 mg/kg/day PO (max 650 mg/dose) div tid for 7–10 days (BII) (preferred for severe disease); OR atovaquone 40 mg/kg/day (max 750 mg/dose) div bid, PLUS azithromycin 12 mg/kg/day (max 500 mg/dose) for 7–10 days (CII) (preferred for mild disease due to more favorable adverse event profile)	Daily monitoring of hematocrit and percentage of parasitized red blood cells (until <5%) should be done. Exchange blood transfusion may be of benefit for severe disease; Babesia divergens. Higher doses of medications and prolonged therapy may be needed for asplenic or immunocompromised individuals.
Balantidium coli[19]	Tetracycline (patients >7 y) 40 mg/kg/day PO div qid for 10 days (max 2 g/day) (CII); OR metronidazole 35–50 mg/kg/day PO div tid for 5 days; OR iodoquinol 30–40 mg/kg/day PO (max 2 g/day) div tid for 20 days	Repeated stool examination may be needed for diagnosis; prompt stool examination may increase detection of rapidly degenerating trophozoites. Follow-up stool examination if symptoms continue.

		None of these medications are approved for this indication. Nitazoxanide may also be effective.
Baylisascaris procyonis (raccoon roundworm)[20,21]	Albendazole 25–50 mg/kg/day PO div q12h for 10–20 days given as soon as possible after exposure (eg, ingestion of raccoon feces) might prevent clinical disease (CIII).	Therapy generally unsuccessful to prevent fatal outcome or severe neurologic sequelae once CNS disease present. Steroids may be of value in decreasing inflammation in CNS or ocular infection. Albendazole bioavailability increased with food, especially fatty meals.
Blastocystis spp[22,23]	Metronidazole 30 mg/kg/day (max 750 mg per dose) PO div tid for 5–10 days (BII); OR tinidazole 50 mg/kg (max 2 g) once (age >3 y) (BII)	Pathogenesis debated. Asymptomatic individuals do not need treatment; diligent search for other pathogenic parasites recommended for symptomatic individuals with *B hominis*. Paromomycin, nitazoxanide (200 mg PO bid for 3 days for age 4–11 y; 100 mg PO bid for 3 days for age 1–3 y), and TMP/SMX also may be effective. Metronidazole resistance may occur. Take tinidazole with food; tabs may be crushed and mixed with flavored syrup.
Brugia malayi, Brugia timori	See FILARIASIS.	
CHAGAS DISEASE (*Trypanosoma cruzi*)[24-26]	See TRYPANOSOMIASIS.	
Clonorchis sinensis	See FLUKES.	

Preferred Therapy for Specific Parasitic Pathogens

10

B. PREFERRED THERAPY FOR SPECIFIC PARASITIC PATHOGENS (continued)

Disease/Organism	Treatment (evidence grade)	Comments
CRYPTOSPORIDIOSIS (*Cryptosporidium parvum*)[27–30]	Nitazoxanide, age 12–47 mo, 5 mL (100 mg) bid for 3 days; age 4–11 y, 10 mL (200 mg) bid for 3 days; age ≥12 y, 500 mg (tab or suspension) PO bid for 3 days (BII). Paromomycin 30 mg/kg/day div bid–qid (CII); OR azithromycin 10 mg/kg/day for 5 days (CII); OR paromomycin AND azithromycin given as combination therapy may yield initial response but may not result in sustained cure in immunocompromised individuals.	Recovery depends largely on the immune status of the host; treatment not required in all immunocompetent individuals. Medical therapy may have limited efficacy in HIV-infected patients not receiving effective antiretroviral therapy. Longer courses (>2 wk) may be needed in solid organ transplant patients.
CUTANEOUS LARVA MIGRANS or **CREEPING ERUPTION**[31,32] (dog and cat hookworm) (*Ancylostoma caninum, Ancylostoma braziliense, Uncinaria stenocephala*)	Ivermectin 200 μg/kg PO for 1–2 days (CII); OR albendazole 15 mg/kg/day (max 400 mg) PO qd for 3 days (CII)	Albendazole bioavailability increased with food, especially fatty meals
Cyclospora spp[33,34] (cyanobacterium-like agent)	TMP/SMX 10 mg TMP/kg/day (max 1 DS tab bid) PO div bid for 7–10 days (BIII); nitazoxanide may be an alternative for TMP/SMX-allergic patients 500 mg bid for 7 days (adult dose).	HIV-infected patients may require higher doses/longer therapy. Ciprofloxacin 30 mg/kg/day div bid for 7 days may be an alternative; treatment failures have been reported.
CYSTICERCOSIS[35–38] (*Cysticercus cellulosae*; larva of *Taenia solium*)	Neurocysticercosis. Albendazole 15 mg/kg/day PO div bid (max 800 mg/day) (CII) plus steroids (prednisone 1.0 mg/kg/day or dexamethasone 0.1 mg/kg/day) for 5–10 days followed by rapid taper to reduce inflammation associated with dying organisms; OR praziquantel 50 mg/kg/day PO tid (CII) plus steroids (prednisone 1.0 mg/kg/day or dexamethasone 0.1 mg/kg/day) (AI) for 5–10 days followed by rapid taper.	Collaboration with a specialist with experience treating this condition is recommended. Management of seizures, edema, intracranial hypertension, or hydrocephalus, when present, is the focus of initial therapy.

	Combination therapy with albendazole plus praziquantel may be more effective than albendazole alone (CII). Optimal duration of therapy depends on form of disease (single enhancing lesions, 3–7 days; multiple viable parenchymal lesion, 10–14 days; subarachnoid disease, prolonged [≥28 days] therapy).	Treatment generally recommended for symptomatic patients with multiple live lesions; generally will not provide benefit when all lesions are calcified, although viable, live cysts may not be identified on MRI scans. Steroids may not be needed for single lesion disease, as there may be minimal CNS swelling with treatment, particularly if there are few viable parasites present at the time of treatment.[38] Intra-vesicular and intraocular cysts should be treated with surgical removal; antiparasitic therapy relatively contraindicated.
DIENTAMOEBIASIS[39,40] (*Dientamoeba fragilis*)	Metronidazole 35–50 mg/kg/day PO div tid for 10 days (max 500–750 mg/dose); OR paromomycin 25–35 mg/kg/day PO div tid for 7 days; OR iodoquinol 30–40 mg/kg/day (max 650 mg/dose) PO div tid for 20 days (BII)	Treatment indicated when no other cause except *Dientamoeba* found for abdominal pain or diarrhea lasting more than a week. Take paromomycin with meals and iodoquinol after meals. Tinidazole, nitazoxanide, tetracycline, and doxycycline also may be effective. Albendazole and mebendazole have no activity against *Dientamoeba*.
Diphyllobothrium latum	See TAPEWORMS.	
Dipylidium caninum	See TAPEWORMS.	
ECHINOCOCCOSIS[41,42]		
Echinococcus granulosus	Albendazole 15 mg/kg/day PO div bid (max 800 mg/day) for 1–6 mo alone (CIII) or as adjunctive therapy with surgery or percutaneous treatment; initiate 4–30 days before and continue for at least 1 mo after surgery.	Involvement with specialist with experience treating this condition recommended. Surgery is the treatment of choice for management of complicated cysts. PAIR technique effective for appropriate cysts. Praziquantel has proto-scolicidal activity but clinical efficacy variable; may be used in combination therapy with albendazole.

10

Preferred Therapy for Specific Parasitic Pathogens

10

B. PREFERRED THERAPY FOR SPECIFIC PARASITIC PATHOGENS (continued)

Disease/Organism	Treatment (evidence grade)	Comments
Echinococcus multilocularis	Surgical treatment generally the treatment of choice; postoperative albendazole 15 mg/kg/day PO div bid (max 800 mg/day) should be administered to reduce relapse; duration uncertain (at least 2 y with long-term monitoring for relapse). Benefit of preoperative albendazole unknown.	
Entamoeba histolytica	See AMEBIASIS.	
Enterobius vermicularis	See PINWORMS.	
Fasciola hepatica	See FLUKES.	
EOSINOPHILIC MENINGITIS.	See ANGIOSTRONGYLIASIS.	
FILARIASIS[43-45]		
– River blindness (*Onchocerca volvulus*)	Ivermectin 150 µg/kg PO once (AII); repeat q3–6mo until asymptomatic and no ongoing exposure; OR if no ongoing exposure, doxycycline 4 mg/kg/day PO (max 200 mg/day div bid) for 6 wk followed by a single dose of ivermectin; provide 1 dose of ivermectin for symptomatic relief 1 wk before beginning doxycycline.	Doxycycline targets *Wolbachia*, the endosymbiotic bacteria associated with *O volvulus*. Assess for *Loa loa* coinfection before using ivermectin if exposure occurred in settings where both *Onchocerca* and *L loa* are endemic.
– Tropical pulmonary eosinophilia[46]	DEC (from CDC) 6 mg/kg/day PO div tid for 12–21 days; antihistamines/corticosteroids for allergic reactions (CII)	
Loa loa	When no evidence of microfilaremia: DEC (from CDC) 8–10 mg/kg/day PO div tid for 21 days When microfilaremia present: day 1: 1 mg/kg (max 50 mg); day 2: 1 mg/kg (max 50 mg) div tid; day 3: 1–2 mg/kg (max 100 mg) div tid; days 4–21: 9 mg/kg/day PO div tid	Involvement with specialist with experience treating this condition recommended. Albendazole is an alternative agent.

Mansonella ozzardi	Ivermectin 200 µg/kg PO once may be effective.	DEC and albendazole not effective
Mansonella perstans	Albendazole 400 mg PO bid for 10 days or mebendazole 100 mg PO bid for 30 days	Relatively resistant to DEC and ivermectin; doxycycline 4 mg/kg/day PO (max 200 mg/day div bid) for 6 wk beneficial for clearing microfilaria in Mali
Wuchereria bancrofti, Brugia malayi, Brugia timori, Mansonella streptocerca	DEC (from CDC) 6 mg/kg/day div tid for 12 days OR 6 mg/kg/day PO as a single dose (AII). Consider adding doxycycline 4 mg/kg/day PO (max 200 mg/day div bid) for 4–6 wk.	Avoid DEC with Onchocerca and L loa coinfection; doxycycline (4 mg/kg/day PO, max 200 mg/day div bid, for 4–6 wk) may be used; albendazole is an alternative if doxycycline cannot be used.
FLUKES		
Liver flukes[47] (Clonorchis sinensis, Opisthorchis spp)	Praziquantel 75 mg/kg PO div tid for 2 days (BII); OR albendazole 10 mg/kg/day PO for 7 days (CIII) OR mebendazole 30 mg/kg for 20–30 days. Single 40 mg/kg dose praziquantel may be effective for Opisthorchis viverrini.[48]	Take praziquantel with liquids and food. Take albendazole with food (bioavailability increases with food, especially fatty meals).
Lung fluke[49,50] (Paragonimus westermani and other Paragonimus lung flukes)	Praziquantel 75 mg/kg PO div tid for 2–3 days (BII)	Triclabendazole (available from CDC) (10 mg/kg PO once or twice) may also be effective; triclabendazole should be taken with food to facilitate absorption.
Sheep liver fluke[51] (Fasciola hepatica)	Triclabendazole (from CDC) 10 mg/kg PO (take with food), age 12–47 mo, 100 mg/dose bid for 7 days; age 4–11 y, 200 mg/dose bid for 7 days; age ≥12 y, 1 tab (500 mg)/dose bid for 7 days (CII) OR nitazoxanide PO (BII)	Responds poorly to praziquantel; albendazole and mebendazole ineffective

10

Preferred Therapy for Specific Parasitic Pathogens

10

B. PREFERRED THERAPY FOR SPECIFIC PARASITIC PATHOGENS (continued)

Disease/Organism	Treatment (evidence grade)	Comments
GIARDIASIS (Giardia intestinalis [formerly lamblia])[52-54]	Metronidazole 15–30 mg/kg/day PO div tid for 5–7 days (BII); OR tinidazole 50 mg/kg/day (max 2 g) for 1 day (approved for age >3 years) (BII); OR nitazoxanide PO (take with food), age 1–3 y, 100 mg/dose bid for 3 days; age 4–11 y, 200 mg/dose bid for 3 days; age ≥12 y, 500 mg/dose bid for 3 days (BII)	Alternatives: albendazole 10–15 mg/kg/day (max 400 mg/dose) PO for 5 days (CII) OR mebendazole 200 mg PO tid for 5 days; OR paromomycin 30 mg/kg/day div tid for 5–10 days; furazolidone 6 mg/kg/day in 4 doses for 7–10 days (not available in United States). If therapy ineffective, may try a higher dose or longer course of the same agent, or an agent in a different class; combination therapy may be considered for refractory cases. Prolonged courses may be needed for immunocompromised patients (eg, hypogammaglobulinemia). Treatment of asymptomatic carriers not usually indicated.
HOOKWORM[55-57] Necator americanus, Ancylostoma duodenale	Albendazole 400 mg once (repeat dose may be necessary) (BII); OR mebendazole 100 mg PO for 3 days; OR pyrantel pamoate 11 mg/kg (max 1 g/day) (BII) PO qd for 3 days	
Hymenolepis nana	See TAPEWORMS.	
Cystoisospora belli (formerly Isospora belli)[19]	TMP/SMX 8–10 mg TMP/kg/day PO (or IV) div bid for 7–10 days (max 160 mg TMP/800 mg SMX bid); OR ciprofloxacin 500 mg PO bid for 7 days	Infection often self-limited in immunocompetent hosts; consider treatment if symptoms do not resolve by 5–7 days or are severe. Pyrimethamine plus leucovorin and nitazoxanide are alternatives. Immunocompromised patients should be treated; longer courses or suppressive therapy may be needed for severely immunocompromised patients.

LEISHMANIASIS[58-65]
(including kala-azar)
Leishmania spp

Visceral: liposomal AmB 3 mg/kg/day on days 1–5, day 14, and day 21 (AI); OR sodium stibogluconate (from CDC) 20 mg/kg/day IM or IV for 28 days (or longer) (BIII); OR miltefosine 2.5 mg/kg/day PO (max 150 mg/day) for 28 days (BII) (FDA-approved regimen: 50 mg PO bid for 28 days for weight 30–44 kg; 50 mg PO tid for 28 days for weight ≥45 kg); other AmB products available but not approved for this indication.

Cutaneous and mucosal disease: There is no generally accepted treatment of choice; treatment decisions should be individualized.

Uncomplicated cutaneous: combination of debridement of eschars, cryotherapy, thermotherapy, intralesional pentavalent antimony, and topical paromomycin (not available in United States).

Complicated cutaneous: oral or parenteral systemic therapy with miltefosine 2.5 mg/kg/day PO (max 150 mg/day) for 28 days (FDA-approved regimen: 50 mg PO bid for 28 days for weight 30–44 kg; 50 mg PO tid for 28 days for weight ≥45 kg) (BII); OR sodium stibogluconate 20 mg/kg/day IM or IV for 20 days (BIII); OR pentamidine isethionate 2–4 mg/kg/day IV or IM qod for 4–7 doses; OR amphotericin (various regimens); OR azoles (fluconazole 200–600 mg PO qd for 6 wk; or ketoconazole or itraconazole); also intralesional and topical alternatives.

Mucosal: sodium stibogluconate 20 mg/kg/day IM or IV for 28 days; OR amphotericin B (Fungizone) 0.5–1 mg/kg/day IV qd or qod for cumulative total of ~20–45 mg/kg; OR AmB ~3 mg/kg/day IV qd for cumulative total of ~20–60 mg/kg; OR miltefosine 2.5 mg/kg/day PO (max 150 mg/day) for 28 days (FDA-approved regimen: 50 mg PO bid for 28 days for weight 30–44 kg; 50 mg PO tid for 28 days for weight ≥45 kg); OR pentamidine isethionate 2–4 mg/kg/day IV or IM qod or 3 times per week for 15 or more doses (considered a lesser alternative).

Consultation with a specialist familiar with management of leishmaniasis is advised strongly, especially when treating patients with HIV coinfection. See IDSA/ASTMH guidelines.[58]

Region where infection acquired, spp of *Leishmania*, skill of practitioner with some local therapies, and drugs available in the United States affect therapeutic choices.

For immunocompromised patients with visceral disease, FDA-approved dosing of liposomal amphotericin is 4 mg/kg on days 1–5, 10, 17, 24, 31, and 38, with further therapy on an individual basis.

Preferred Therapy for Specific Parasitic Pathogens

10

B. PREFERRED THERAPY FOR SPECIFIC PARASITIC PATHOGENS (continued)

Disease/Organism	Treatment (evidence grade)	Comments
LICE *Pediculosis capitis or humanus, Phthirus pubis*[66,67]	Follow manufacturer's instructions for topical use: permethrin 1% (≥2 mo) OR pyrethrin (children aged ≥2 y) (BII); OR 0.5% ivermectin lotion (≥6 mo) (BII); OR spinosad 0.9% topical suspension (≥6 mo) (BII); OR benzyl alcohol lotion 5% (≥6 mo) (BIII); OR malathion 0.5% (children aged ≥2 y) (BIII); OR topical or oral ivermectin 200 μg/kg PO once (400 μg/kg for ≥15 kg): repeat 7–10 days later.	Launder bedding and clothing; for eyelash infestation, use petrolatum; for head lice, remove nits with comb designed for that purpose. Benzyl alcohol can be irritating to skin; parasite resistance unlikely to develop. Consult health care professional before re-treatment with ivermectin lotion; re-treatment with spinosad topical suspension usually not needed unless live lice seen 1 wk after treatment. Administration of 3 doses of ivermectin (1 dose/wk separately by weekly intervals) may be needed to eradicate heavy infection.
MALARIA[68–72] *Plasmodium falciparum, Plasmodium vivax, Plasmodium ovale, Plasmodium malariae*	CDC Malaria Hotline 770/488-7788 or 855/856-4713 toll-free (Monday–Friday, 9:00 am–5:00 pm ET) or emergency consultation after hours 770/488-7100; online information at www.cdc.gov/malaria (accessed October 3, 2017). Consult infectious diseases or tropical medicine specialist if unfamiliar with malaria.	Consultation with a specialist familiar with management of malaria is advised, especially for severe malaria. No antimalarial drug provides absolute protection against malaria; fever after return from an endemic area should prompt an immediate evaluation. Emphasize personal protective measures (insecticides, bed nets, clothing, and avoidance of dusk–dawn mosquito exposures).
Prophylaxis		See https://wwwnc.cdc.gov/travel/yellowbook/2018/infectious-diseases-related-to-travel/malaria#5217 (accessed October 3, 2017).
For areas with chloroquine-resistant *P falciparum* or *P vivax*	A-P: 5–8 kg, ½ pediatric tab/day; ≥9–10 kg, ¾ pediatric tab/day; ≥11–20 kg, 1 pediatric tab (62.5 mg atovaquone/25 mg proguanil); ≥21–30 kg, 2 pediatric tabs; ≥31–40 kg, 3 pediatric tabs; ≥40 kg, 1 adult	Avoid mefloquine for persons with a history of seizures or psychosis, active depression, or cardiac conduction abnormalities; see black box warning. Avoid A-P in severe renal impairment (CrCl <30).

tab (250 mg atovaquone/100 mg proguanil) PO qd starting 1–2 days before travel and continuing 7 days after last exposure; for children <5 kg, data on A-P limited (BII); OR mefloquine: for children <5 kg, 5 mg/kg; ≥5–9 kg, 1/8 tab; ≥10–19 kg, ¼ tab; ≥20–30 kg, ½ tab; ≥31–45 kg, ¾ tab; ≥45 kg (adult dose), 1 tab PO once weekly starting the wk before arrival in area and continuing for 4 wk after leaving area (BII); OR doxycycline (patients >7 y): 2 mg/kg (max 100 mg) PO qd starting 1–2 days before arrival in area and continuing for 4 wk after leaving area (BII); OR primaquine (check for G6PD deficiency before administering): 0.5 mg/kg base qd starting 1 day before travel and continuing for 5 days after last exposure (BII)

P falciparum resistance to mefloquine exists along the borders between Thailand and Myanmar and Thailand and Cambodia, Myanmar and China, and Myanmar and Laos; isolated resistance has been reported in southern Vietnam.

Take doxycycline with adequate fluids to avoid esophageal irritation and food to avoid GI side effects; use sunscreen and avoid excessive sun exposure.

| For areas without chloroquine-resistant *P falciparum* or *P vivax* | Chloroquine phosphate 5 mg base/kg (max 300 mg base) PO once weekly, beginning the wk before arrival in area and continuing for 4 wk after leaving area (available in suspension outside the United States and Canada and at compounding pharmacies) (AII). For heavy or prolonged (months) exposure to mosquitoes: consider treatment with primaquine (check for G6PD deficiency before administering) 0.5 mg base/kg PO qd with final 2 wk of chloroquine for prevention of relapse with *P ovale* or *P vivax*. | |

Preferred Therapy for Specific Parasitic Pathogens

10

B. PREFERRED THERAPY FOR SPECIFIC PARASITIC PATHOGENS (continued)

Disease/Organism	Treatment (evidence grade)	Comments
Treatment of disease		See https://www.cdc.gov/malaria/resources/pdf/treatmenttable.pdf (accessed October 3, 2017).
– Chloroquine-resistant P falciparum or P vivax	Oral therapy: artemether/lumefantrine 6 doses over 3 days at 0, 8, 24, 36, 48, and 60 h; <15 kg, 1 tab/dose; ≥15–25 kg, 2 tabs/dose; ≥25–35 kg, 3 tabs/dose; ≥35 kg, 4 tabs/dose (BII); A-P: for children <5 kg, data limited; ≥5–8 kg, 2 pediatric tabs (62.5 mg atovaquone/25 mg proguanil) PO qd for 3 days; ≥9–10 kg, 3 pediatric tabs qd for 3 days; ≥11–20 kg, 1 adult tab (250 mg atovaquone/100 mg proguanil) qd for 3 days; >20–30 kg, 2 adult tabs qd for 3 days; >30–40 kg, 3 adult tabs qd for 3 days; >40 kg, 4 adult tabs qd for 3 days (BII); OR quinine 30 mg/kg/day (max 2 g/day) PO div tid for 3–7 days AND doxycycline (age >7 y) 4 mg/kg/day div bid for 7 days OR clindamycin 30 mg/kg/day div tid (max 900 mg tid) for 7 days. Parenteral therapy (check with CDC): quinidine gluconate salt 10 mg/kg (max 600 mg) IV (1 h infusion in physiologic [normal] saline solution) followed by continuous infusion of 0.02 mg/kg/min until oral therapy can be given (BII); alternative: artesunate 2.4 mg/kg/dose IV for 3 days at 0, 12, 24, 48, and 72 h (from CDC) (BI) AND a second oral agent (A-P, clindamycin, or doxycycline for aged ≥7 y). For prevention of relapse with P vivax, P ovale: primaquine (check for G6PD deficiency before administering) 0.5 mg base/kg/day PO for 14 days.	Mild disease may be treated with oral antimalarial drugs; severe disease (impaired level of consciousness, convulsion, hypotension, or parasitemia >5%) should be treated parenterally. Avoid mefloquine for treatment of malaria, if possible, given higher dose and increased incidence of adverse events. Take clindamycin and doxycycline with plenty of liquids. Do not use primaquine during pregnancy. For relapses of primaquine-resistant P vivax or P ovale, consider retreating with primaquine 30 mg (base) for 28 days. Continuously monitor ECG, BP, and glucose in patients receiving quinidine. Avoid artemether/lumefantrine and mefloquine in patients with cardiac arrhythmias, and avoid concomitant use of drugs that prolong QT interval. Take A-P and artemether/lumefantrine with food or milk. Use artesunate for quinidine intolerance, lack of quinidine availability, or treatment failure; www.cdc.gov/malaria/resources/pdf/treatmenttable.pdf (accessed October 3, 2017); artemisinin should be used in combination with other drugs to avoid resistance.

– Chloroquine-susceptible P falciparum, chloroquine-susceptible P vivax, P ovale, P malariae	Oral therapy: chloroquine 10 mg/kg base (max 600 mg base) PO then 5 mg/kg 6, 24, and 48 h after initial dose. Parenteral therapy: quinidine, as above. See above in Chloroquine-resistant P falciparum or P vivax for prevention of relapse due to P vivax and P ovale. Alternative if chloroquine not available: hydroxychloroquine 10 mg base/kg PO immediately, followed by 5 mg base/kg PO at 6, 24, and 48 h.
Mansonella ozzardi, Mansonella perstans, Mansonella streptocerca	See FILARIASIS.
Naegleria	See MENINGOENCEPHALITIS.
Necator americanus	See HOOKWORM.
Onchocerca volvulus	See FILARIASIS.
Opisthorchis spp	See FLUKES.
Paragonimus westermani	See FLUKES.
PINWORMS (Enterobius vermicularis)	Mebendazole 100 mg once, repeat in 2 wk; OR albendazole <20 kg, 200 mg PO once; ≥20 kg, 400 mg PO once; repeat in 2 wk (BII); OR pyrantel pamoate 11 mg/kg (max 1 g) PO once (BII); repeat in 2 wk.	Treat entire household (and if this fails, consider close child care/school contacts); re-treatment of contacts after 2 wk may be needed to prevent reinfection.
Plasmodium spp	See MALARIA.
PNEUMOCYSTIS	See Chapter 8, Table 8B, Pneumocystis jiroveci (formerly carinii) pneumonia.
SCABIES (Sarcoptes scabiei)[73]	Permethrin 5% cream applied to entire body (including scalp in infants), left on for 8–14 h then bathe, repeat in 1 wk (BII); OR ivermectin 200 µg/kg PO once weekly for 2 doses (BII); OR crotamiton 10% applied topically overnight on days 1, 2, 3, and 8, bathe in am (BII).	Launder bedding and clothing. Reserve lindane for patients who do not respond to other therapy. Crotamiton treatment failure has been observed. Ivermectin safety not well established in children <15 kg and pregnant women. Itching may continue for weeks after successful treatment; can be managed with antihistamines.

10

Preferred Therapy for Specific Parasitic Pathogens

Preferred Therapy for Specific Parasitic Pathogens

10

B. PREFERRED THERAPY FOR SPECIFIC PARASITIC PATHOGENS (continued)

Disease/Organism	Treatment (evidence grade)	Comments
SCHISTOSOMIASIS (*Schistosoma haematobium, Schistosoma japonicum, Schistosoma mansoni, Schistosoma mekongi, Schistosoma intercalatum*)[74–76]	Praziquantel 40 (for *S haematobium, S mansoni*, and *S intercalatum*) or 60 (for *S japonicum* and *S mekongi* mg/kg/day PO bid (if 40 mg/day) or tid (if 60 mg/day) for 1 day (AI)	Take praziquantel with food and liquids. Oxamniquine (not available in United States) 20 mg/kg PO div bid for 1 day (Brazil) or 40–60 mg/kg/day for 2–3 days (most of Africa) (BII).
STRONGYLOIDIASIS (*Strongyloides stercoralis*)[77,78]	Ivermectin 200 μg/kg PO qd for 1–2 days (BI); OR albendazole 400 mg PO bid for 7 days (or longer for disseminated disease) (BII)	Albendazole is less effective but may be adequate if longer courses used. For immunocompromised patients (especially with hyperinfection syndrome), parenteral veterinary formulations may be lifesaving. Ivermectin safety not well established in children <15 kg and pregnant women.
TAPEWORMS – *Taenia saginata, Taenia solium, Hymenolepis nana, Diphyllobothrium latum, Dipylidium caninum*	Praziquantel 5–10 mg/kg PO once (25 mg/kg once; for *H nana*) (BII); OR niclosamide 50 mg/kg (max 2 g) PO once, chewed thoroughly (not available in United States)	Nitazoxanide may be effective (published clinical data limited) 500 mg PO bid for 3 days for age >11 y; 200 mg PO bid for 3 days for age 4–11 y; 100 mg PO bid for 3 days for age 1–3 y.
TOXOCARIASIS[79] (*Toxocara canis* [dog roundworm] and *Toxocara cati* [cat roundworm])	Visceral larval migrans: albendazole 400 mg PO bid for 5 days (BII) Ocular larva migrants: albendazole 400 mg PO, 15 mg/kg/day div bid, max 800 mg/day (800 mg div bid for adults) for 2–4 wk with prednisone (0.5–1 mg/kg/day with slow taper)	Mild disease often resolves without treatment. Corticosteroids may be used for severe symptoms in visceral larval migrans. Mebendazole (100–200 mg/day PO bid for 5 days) and DEC (available only from CDC) are alternatives.

TOXOPLASMOSIS (*Toxoplasma gondii*)[80–82]	Pyrimethamine 2 mg/kg/day PO div bid for 2 days (max 100 mg) then 1 mg/kg/day (max 25 mg/day) PO qd AND sulfadiazine 120 mg/kg/day PO qid (max 6 g/day); with supplemental folinic acid and leucovorin 10–25 mg with each dose of pyrimethamine (AI) for 3–6 wk. See Chapter 5 for congenital infection. For treatment in pregnancy, spiramycin 50–100 mg/kg/day PO div qid (available as investigational therapy through the FDA at 301/796-0563) (CII).	Experienced ophthalmologic consultation encouraged for treatment of ocular disease. Treatment continued for 2 wk after resolution of illness (approximately 3–6 wk); concurrent corticosteroids given for ocular or CNS infection. Prolonged therapy if HIV positive. Take pyrimethamine with food to decrease GI adverse effects; sulfadiazine should be taken on an empty stomach with water. Clindamycin, azithromycin, or atovaquone plus pyrimethamine may be effective for patients intolerant of sulfa-containing drugs. Consult expert advice for treatment during pregnancy and management of congenital infection.
TRAVELERS' DIARRHEA[83–86]	Azithromycin 10 mg/kg qd for 1–3 days (AII); OR rifaximin 200 mg PO tid for 3 days (ages ≥12 y) (BIII); OR ciprofloxacin (BIII); OR rifaximin 200 mg tid for 3 days for ages ≥12 y (BII).	Azithromycin preferable to ciprofloxacin for travelers to Southeast Asia and India given high prevalence of fluoroquinolone-resistant *Campylobacter*. Do not use rifaximin for *Campylobacter*, *Salmonella*, *Shigella* and other causes of invasive diarrhea. Antibiotic regimens may be combined with loperamide (≥2 y).
TRICHINELLOSIS (*Trichinella spiralis*)[87]	Albendazole 400 mg PO bid for 8–14 days (BII) OR mebendazole 200–400 mg PO tid for 3 days, then 400–500 mg PO tid for 10 days	Therapy ineffective for larvae already in muscles. Anti-inflammatory drugs, steroids for CNS or cardiac involvement or severe symptoms.
TRICHOMONIASIS (*Trichomonas vaginalis*)[88]	Tinidazole 50 mg/kg (max 2 g) PO for 1 dose (BII) OR metronidazole 2 gm PO for 1 dose OR metronidazole 500 mg PO bid for 7 days (BII)	Treat sex partners simultaneously. Metronidazole resistance occurs and may be treated with higher-dose metronidazole or tinidazole.
Trichuris trichiura	See WHIPWORM (TRICHURIASIS).	

10

Preferred Therapy for Specific Parasitic Pathogens

Preferred Therapy for Specific Parasitic Pathogens

10

B. PREFERRED THERAPY FOR SPECIFIC PARASITIC PATHOGENS (continued)

Disease/Organism	Treatment (evidence grade)	Comments
TRYPANOSOMIASIS		
– Chagas disease[24-26] (*Trypanosoma cruzi*)	Benznidazole PO (from CDC): age <12 y, 5–7.5 mg/kg/day div bid for 60 days; ≥12 y, 5–7 mg/kg/day div bid for 60 days (BIII); OR nifurtimox PO (from CDC): age 1–10 y, 15–20 mg/kg/day div tid or qid for 90 days; 11–16 y, 12.5–15 mg/kg/day div tid or qid for 90 days; ≥17 y, 8–10 mg/kg/day div tid–qid for 90–120 days (BIII)	Therapy recommended for acute and congenital infection, reactivated infection, and chronic infection in children aged <18 y; consider in those up to age 50 with chronic infection without advanced cardiomyopathy. Side effects fairly common. Both drugs contraindicated in pregnancy.
Sleeping sickness[89-92] – Acute (hemolymphatic) stage (*Trypanosoma brucei gambiense* [West African]; *T brucei rhodesiense* [East African])	*Tb gambiense:* pentamidine isethionate 4 mg/kg/day (max 300 mg) IM or IV for 7–10 days (BII) *Tb rhodesiense:* suramin (from CDC) 100–200 mg test dose IV, then 20 mg/kg (max 1 g) IV on days 1, 3, 7, 14, and 21 (BII)	CSF examination required for all patients to assess CNS involvement. Consult with infectious diseases or tropical medicine specialist if unfamiliar with trypanosomiasis. Examination of the buffy coat of peripheral blood may be helpful. *Tb gambiense* may be found in lymph node aspirates.
– Late (CNS) stage (*Trypanosoma brucei gambiense* [West African]; *T brucei rhodesiense* [East African])	*Tb gambiense:* eflornithine (from CDC) 400 mg/kg/day IV div bid for 7 days PLUS nifurtimox 5 mg/kg PO tid for 10 days (BIII); OR eflornithine 400 mg/kg/day IV div qid for 14 days; OR melarsoprol (from CDC) 2.2 mg/kg/day (max 180 mg) in 10 daily injections (BIII). *Tb rhodesiense:* melarsoprol, 2–3.6 mg/kg/day IV for 3 days; after 7 days, 3.6 mg/kg/day for 3 days; after 7 days, 3.6 mg/kg/day for 3 days; corticosteroids often given with melarsoprol to decrease risk of CNS toxicity.	CSF examination needed for management (double-centrifuge technique recommended); perform repeat CSF examinations every 6 mo for 2 y to detect relapse.
Uncinaria stenocephala	See CUTANEOUS LARVA MIGRANS.	

WHIPWORM (TRICHURIASIS)		
Trichuris trichiura	Mebendazole 100 mg PO bid for 3 days; OR albenda-zole 400 mg PO for 3 days; OR ivermectin 200 µg/kg/day PO qd for 3 days (BII)	Treatment can be given for 5–7 days for heavy infestation.
Wuchereria bancrofti	See FILARIASIS.	
YAWS	Azithromycin 30 mg/kg max 2 g once (also treats bejel and pinta)	Alternative regimens include IM benzathine penicillin and second-line agents doxycycline, tetracycline, and erythromycin.

11. Alphabetic Listing of Antimicrobials

NOTES

- Higher dosages in a dose range are generally indicated for more serious infections. For pathogens with higher minimal inhibitory concentrations against beta-lactam antibiotics, a more prolonged infusion of the antibiotic will allow increased antibacterial effect (see Chapter 3).

- Maximum dosages for adult-sized children (eg, ≥40 kg) are based on US Food and Drug Administration (FDA)-approved product labeling or post-marketing data.

- Antiretroviral medications are not listed in this chapter. See Chapter 9.

- Drugs with FDA-approved dosage, or dosages based on randomized clinical trials, are given a Level of Evidence I. Dosages for which data are collected from noncomparative trials or small comparative trials are given a Level of Evidence II. Dosages based on expert or consensus opinion or case reports are given a Level of Evidence III.

- If no oral liquid form is available, round the child's dose to a combination of available solid dosage forms. Consult a pediatric pharmacist for recommendations on mixing with food (crushing tablets, emptying capsule contents) and the availability of extemporaneously compounded liquid formulations.

- Cost estimates are in US dollars per course, or per month for continual regimens. Estimates are based on costs at the editor's institution. These may differ from that of the reader due to contractual differences, regional market forces, and supply fluctuations. Legend: $ = <$100, $$ = $100–$400, $$$ = $401–$1,000, $$$$ = >$1,000, $$$$$ = >$10,000.

- There are some agents that we do not recommend even though they may be available. We believe they are significantly inferior to those we do recommend (see chapters 5–10) and could possibly lead to poor outcomes if used. Such agents are not listed.

- **Abbreviations:** 3TC, lamivudine; AOM, acute otitis media; AUC:MIC, area under the curve–minimum inhibitory concentration; bid, twice daily; BSA, body surface area; CABP, community-acquired bacterial pneumonia; CA-MRSA, community-associated methicillin-resistant *Staphylococcus aureus;* cap, capsule or caplet; CDC, Centers for Disease Control and Prevention; CF, cystic fibrosis; CMV, cytomegalovirus; CNS, central nervous system; CrCl, creatinine clearance; div, divided; DR, delayed release; EC, enteric coated; ER, extended release; FDA, US Food and Drug Administration; HCV, hepatitis C virus; hs, bedtime; HSV, herpes simplex virus; IBW, ideal body weight; IM, intramuscular; IV, intravenous; IVPB, intravenous piggyback (premixed bag); LD, loading dose; MAC, *Mycobacterium avium* complex; MRSA, methicillin-resistant *S aureus;* NS, normal saline (physiologic saline solution); oint, ointment; OPC, oropharyngeal candidiasis; ophth, ophthalmic; PCP, *Pneumocystis* pneumonia; PEG, pegylated; PIP, piperacillin; PMA, post-menstrual age; PO, oral; pwd, powder;

qd, once daily; qhs, every bedtime; qid, 4 times daily; RSV, respiratory syncytial virus; RTI, respiratory tract infection; SIADH, syndrome of inappropriate antidiuretic hormone; SMX, sulfamethoxazole; soln, solution; SPAG-2, small particle aerosol generator model-2; SQ, subcutaneous; SSSI, skin and skin structure infection; STI, sexually transmitted infection; susp, suspension; tab, tablet; TB, tuberculosis; TBW, total body weight; tid, 3 times daily; TMP, trimethoprim; top, topical; UTI, urinary tract infection; vag, vaginal; VZV, varicella-zoster virus.

A. SYSTEMIC ANTIMICROBIALS WITH DOSAGE FORMS AND USUAL DOSAGES

Generic and Trade Names	Dosage Form (cost estimate)	Route	Dose (evidence level)	Interval
Acyclovir,[a] Zovirax (See Valacyclovir as another oral formulation to achieve therapeutic acyclovir serum concentrations.)	50-mg/mL in 10- and 20-mL vial ($)	IV	15–45 mg/kg/day (I) (See chapters 5 and 9.) Max 1,500 mg/m²/day (II) (See Chapter 12.)	q8h
	200-mg/5-mL susp ($$) 200-mg cap ($) 400-, 800-mg tab ($)	PO	900 mg/m²/day (I) 60–80 mg/kg/day, max 4 g/day (I) (See chapters 5 and 9.)	q8h q6–8h
Albendazole, Albenza	200-mg tab ($$$$)	PO	15 mg/kg/day, max 800 mg/day (I) (See Chapter 10 for other dosages.)	q12h
Amikacin,[a] Amikin	250-mg/mL in 2- or 4-mL vials ($–$$)	IV, IM	15–22.5 mg/kg/day[b] (I) (See Chapter 1.) 30–35 mg/kg/day[b] for CF (II)	q8–24h q24h
		Intravesical	50–100 mL of 0.5 mg/mL in NS (III)	q12h
Amoxicillin,[a] Amoxil	125-, 200-, 250-, 400-mg/5-mL susp ($) 125-, 250-mg chew tab ($) 250-, 500-mg cap ($) 500-, 875-mg tab ($)	PO	Standard dose: 40–45 mg/kg/day (I) High dose: 80–90 mg/kg/day (I) 150 mg/kg/day for penicillin-resistant *Streptococcus pneumoniae* otitis media (III) Max 4 g/day (III)	q8–12h q12h q8h
Amoxicillin extended release,[a] Moxatag	775-mg tab ($$)	PO	≥12 y and adults 775 mg/day	q24h

11

Alphabetic Listing of Antimicrobials

A. SYSTEMIC ANTIMICROBIALS WITH DOSAGE FORMS AND USUAL DOSAGES (continued)

Generic and Trade Names	Dosage Form (cost estimate)	Route	Dose (evidence level)	Interval
Amoxicillin/clavulanate,[a] Augmentin	16:1 Augmentin XR: 1,000/62.5-mg tab ($$)	PO	16:1 formulation: ≥40 kg and adults 4,000-mg amoxicillin/day (not per kg) (I)	q12h
	14:1 Augmentin ES: 600/42.9-mg/5-mL susp ($)	PO	14:1 formulation: 90-mg amoxicillin component/kg/day (I), max 4,000 mg/day (III)	q12h
	7:1 Augmentin ($): 875/125-mg tab 200/28.5-, 400/57-mg chew tab 200/28.5-, 400/57-mg/5-mL susp	PO	7:1 formulation: 25- or 45-mg amoxicillin component/kg/day, max 1,750 mg/day (I)	q12h
	4:1 Augmentin: 500/125-mg tab ($) 125/31.25-mg/5-mL susp ($$$) 250/62.5-mg/5-mL susp ($)	PO	20- or 40-mg amoxicillin component/kg/day (max 1,500 mg/day) (I)	q8h
	2:1 Augmentin: 250 mg/125-mg tab	PO	2:1 formulation: ≥40 kg and adults 750-mg amoxicillin/day (not per kg) (I)	q8h
Amphotericin B deoxycholate,[a] Fungizone	50-mg vial ($$)	IV	1–1.5 mg/kg pediatric and adults (I), no max 0.5 mg/kg for Candida esophagitis or cystitis (II)	q24h
		Intravesical	50–100 µg/mL in sterile water × 50–100 mL (III)	q8h
Amphotericin B, lipid complex, Abelcet	100-mg/20-mL vial ($$$$)	IV	5 mg/kg pediatric and adult dose (I) No max	q24h
Amphotericin B, liposomal, AmBisome	50-mg vial ($$$$)	IV	5 mg/kg pediatric and adult dose (I) No max	q24h
Ampicillin sodium[a]	125-, 250-, 500-mg vial ($) 1-, 2-, 10-g vial ($)	IV, IM	50–200 mg/kg/day, max 8 g/day (I) 300–400 mg/kg/day, max 12 g/day endocarditis/meningitis (III)	q6h q4–6h

11

Drug	Formulation	Route	Dosage	Frequency
Ampicillin trihydrate[a]	500-mg cap ($)	PO	50–100 mg/kg/day if <20 kg (I) ≥20 kg and adults 1–2 g/day (I)	q6h
Ampicillin/sulbactam,[a] Unasyn	1/0.5-, 2/1-, 10/5-g vial ($)	IV, IM	200-mg ampicillin component/kg/day (I) ≥40 kg and adults 4–max 8 g/day (I)	q6h
Anidulafungin, Eraxis	50-, 100-mg vial ($$)	IV	1.5–3 mg/kg LD, then 0.75–1.5 mg/kg (II) Max 200-mg LD, then 100 mg (I)	q24h
Atovaquone,[a] Mepron	750-mg/5-mL susp ($$$)	PO	30 mg/kg/day if 1–3 mo or >24 mo (I) 45 mg/kg/day if >3–24 mo (I) Max 1,500 mg/day (I)	q12h q24h for prophylaxis
Atovaquone and proguanil,[a] Malarone	62.5/25-mg pediatric tab ($-$$) 250/100-mg adult tab ($$)	PO	Prophylaxis for malaria: 11–20 kg: 1 pediatric tab, 21–30 kg: 2 pediatric tabs, 31–40 kg: 3 pediatric tabs, >40 kg: 1 adult tab (I) Treatment: 5–8 kg: 2 pediatric tabs, 9–10 kg: 3 pediatric tabs, 11–20 kg: 1 adult tab, 21–30 kg: 2 adult tabs, 31–40 kg: 3 adult tabs, >40 kg: 4 adult tabs (I)	q24h

Alphabetic Listing of Antimicrobials

A. SYSTEMIC ANTIMICROBIALS WITH DOSAGE FORMS AND USUAL DOSAGES (continued)

Generic and Trade Names	Dosage Form (cost estimate)	Route	Dose (evidence level)	Interval
Azithromycin,[a] Zithromax	250-, 500-, 600-mg tab (S) 100-, 200-mg/5-mL susp (S) 1-g packet for susp (S) 2-g/60-mL ER susp (Zmax) ($$)	PO	Otitis: 10 mg/kg/day for 1 day, then 5 mg/kg for 4 days; or 10 mg/kg/day for 3 days; or 30 mg/kg once (I). Pharyngitis: 12 mg/kg/day for 5 days, max 2,500-mg total dose (I). Sinusitis: 10 mg/kg/day for 3 days, max 1.5-g total dose (I). CABP: 10 mg/kg/day for 1 day, then 5 mg/kg/day for 4 days (max 1.5-g total dose), or 60 mg/kg once of ER (Zmax) susp, max 2 g (I). MAC prophylaxis: 5 mg/kg/day, max 250 mg (I), or 20 mg/kg, max 1.2 g weekly. Adult dosing for RTI: 500 mg day 1, then 250 mg daily for 4 days or 500 mg for 3 days. Adult dosing for STI: Non-gonorrhea: 1 g once Gonorrhea: 2 g once See other indications in Chapter 6.	q24h
Aztreonam,[a] Azactam	500-mg vial[a] (S)	IV	10 mg/kg, max 500 mg (II)	q24h
	1-, 2-g vial ($$–$$$)	IV, IM	90–120 mg/kg/day, max 8 g/day (I)	q6–8h
Bezlotoxumab, Zinplava	1,000-mg/40-mL vial ($$$$)	IV	Adults: 10 mg/kg	One time
Capreomycin, Capastat	1-g vial ($$$$)	IV, IM	15–30 mg/kg (III), max 1 g (I)	q24h
Caspofungin, Cancidas	50-, 70-mg vial ($$$$)	IV	Load with 70 mg/m² once, then 50 mg/m², max 70 mg (I)	q24h
Cefaclor,[a] Ceclor	125-, 250-, 375-mg/5-mL susp ($$) 250-, 500-mg cap (S) 500-mg ER tab ($$)	PO	20–40 mg/kg/day, max 1 g/day (I)	q12h

Cefadroxil,[a] Duricef	250-, 500-mg/5-mL susp ($) 500-mg cap ($) 1-g tab ($)	PO	30 mg/kg/day, max 2 g/day (I)	q12–24h
Cefazolin,[a] Ancef	0.5-, 1-, 10-, 20-g vial ($)	IV, IM	25–100 mg/kg/day (I) 100–150 mg/kg/day for serious infections (III), max 12 g/day	q8h q6h
Cefdinir,[a] Omnicef	125-, 250-mg/5-mL susp ($) 300-mg cap ($)	PO	14 mg/kg/day, max 600 mg/day (I)	q24h
Cefepime,[a] Maxipime	1-, 2-g vial ($) 1-, 2-g IVPB ($$$)	IV, IM	100 mg/kg/day, max 4 g/day (I) 150 mg/kg/day empiric therapy of fever with neutropenia, max 6 g/day (I)	q12h q8h
Cefixime, Suprax	100-, 200-mg/5-mL susp[a] ($$) 100-, 200-mg chew tab ($$) 400-mg cap ($$)	PO	8 mg/kg/day, max 400 mg/day (I) For convalescent oral therapy of serious infections, up to 20 mg/kg/day (III)	q24h q12h
Cefotaxime,[a] Claforan	0.5-, 1-, 2-, 10-g vial ($)	IV, IM	150–180 mg/kg/day, max 8 g/day (I) 200–225 mg/kg/day for meningitis, max 12 g/day (I)	q8h q6h
Cefotetan,[a] Cefotan	1-, 2-g vial ($$) 1-, 2-g IVPB ($$)	IV, IM	60–100 mg/kg/day, max 6 g/day (I)	q12h
Cefoxitin,[a] Mefoxin	1-, 2-, 10-g vial ($) 1-, 2-g IVPB ($$)	IV, IM	80–160 mg/kg/day, max 12 g/day (I)	q6–8h
Cefpodoxime,[a] Vantin	100-mg/5-mL susp ($–$$) 100-, 200-mg tab ($)	PO	10 mg/kg/day, max 400 mg/day (I)	q12h
Cefprozil,[a] Cefzil	125-, 250-mg/5-mL susp ($) 250-, 500-mg tab ($)	PO	15–30 mg/kg/day, max 1 g/d (I)	q12h

11

Alphabetic Listing of Antimicrobials

Alphabetic Listing of Antimicrobials

11

A. SYSTEMIC ANTIMICROBIALS WITH DOSAGE FORMS AND USUAL DOSAGES (continued)

Generic and Trade Names	Dosage Form (cost estimate)	Route	Dose (evidence level)	Interval
Ceftaroline, Teflaro	400-, 600-mg vial ($$$$)	IV	For skin or CABP (I): ≥2 mo–<2 y: 24 mg/kg/day ≥2 y: 36 mg/kg/day, max 1.2 g/day For complicated pneumonia (see Chapter 6) (II): ≥2–<6 mo: 30 mg/kg/day ≥6 mo: 45 mg/kg/day, max 1.8 g/day	q8h
Ceftazidime,[a] Tazicef, Fortaz	0.5-, 1-, 2-, 6-g vial ($$)	IV, IM	90–150 mg/kg/day, max 6 g/day (I)	q8h
	1-, 2-g IVPB ($$)	IV	200–300 mg/kg/day for serious *Pseudomonas* infection, max 12 g/day (II)	q8h
Ceftazidime/avibactam, Avycaz	2-g/0.5-g vial ($$$$)	IV	Adults 7.5 g (6 g/1.5 g)/day (I)	q8h
Ceftolozane/tazobactam, Zerbaxa	1.5-g (1-g/0.5-g) vial ($$$$)	IV	Adults 4.5 g (3 g/1.5 g)/day (I)	q8h
Ceftriaxone,[a] Rocephin	0.25-, 0.5-, 1-, 2-, 10-g vial ($)	IV, IM	50–75 mg/kg/day, max 2 g/day (I)	q24h
	1-, 2-g IVPB ($)		Meningitis: 100 mg/kg/day, max 4 g/day (I) 50 mg/kg, max 1 g, 1–3 doses q24h for AOM (II)	q12h
Cefuroxime, Ceftin (PO), Zinacef (IV)	125-, 250-mg/5-mL susp ($$) 250-, 500-mg tab[a] ($)	PO	20–30 mg/kg/day, max 1 g/day (I) For bone and joint infections, up to 100 mg/kg/day, max 3 g/day (III)	q12h q8h
	0.75-, 1.5-, 7.5-g vial[a] ($)	IV, IM	100–150 mg/kg/day, max 6 g/day (I)	q8h
Cephalexin,[a] Keflex	125-, 250-mg/5-mL susp ($) 250-, 500-mg cap, tab ($) 333-, 750-mg cap ($$)	PO	25–50 mg/kg/day (I) 75–100 mg/kg/day for bone and joint, or severe infections (II), max 4 g/day (I)	q12h q6–8h

2018 Nelson's Pediatric Antimicrobial Therapy — 207

Chloroquine phosphate,[a] Aralen	250-, 500-mg (150-, 300-mg base) tabs ($$)	PO	See Chapter 10.
Cidofovir,[a] Vistide	375-mg/5-mL vial ($$$)	IV	5 mg/kg (III); see Chapter 9.	Weekly
Ciprofloxacin, Cipro	250-, 500-mg/5-mL susp ($$) 250-, 500-, 750-mg tab[a] ($)	PO	20–40 mg/kg/day, max 1.5 g/day (I)	q12h
	100-mg tab[a] ($)		Adult females 200 mg/day for 3 days (I)	
	200-, 400-mg vial, IVPB[a] ($)	IV	20–30 mg/kg/day, max 1.2 g/day (I)	q12h
Ciprofloxacin extended release,[a] Cipro XR	500-, 1,000-mg ER tab ($)	PO	Adults 500–1,000 mg (I)	q24h
Clarithromycin,[a] Biaxin	125-, 250-mg/5-mL susp ($-$$) 250-, 500-mg tab ($)	PO	15 mg/kg/day, max 1 g/day (I)	q12h
Clarithromycin extended release,[a] Biaxin XL	500-mg ER tab ($)	PO	Adults 1 g (I)	q24h
Clindamycin,[a] Cleocin	75 mg/5-mL soln ($-$$) 75-, 150-, 300-mg cap ($)	PO	10–25 mg/kg/day, max 1.8 g/day (I) 30–40 mg/kg/day for CA-MRSA, intra-abdominal infection, or AOM (III)	q8h
	0.3-, 0.6-, 0.9- 9-g vial ($) 0.3-, 0.6-, 0.9-g IVPB ($)	IV, IM	20–40 mg/kg/day, max 2.7 g/day (I)	q8h
Clotrimazole,[a] Mycelex	10-mg lozenge ($)	PO	≥3 y and adults, dissolve lozenge in mouth (I).	5 times daily
Colistimethate,[a] Coly-Mycin M	150-mg (colistin base) vial ($$) 1-mg base = 2.7-mg colistimethate	IV, IM	2.5- to 5-mg base/kg/day based on IBW (I) Up to 5- to 7-mg base/kg/day (III)	q8h
Cycloserine, Seromycin	250-mg cap ($$$$)	PO	10–20 mg/kg/day (III) Adults max 1 g/day (I)	q12h
Daclatasvir, Daklinza	30-, 60-, 90-mg tab ($$$$$)	PO	Adults 30–90 mg + sofosbuvir (I)	q24h

Alphabetic Listing of Antimicrobials

A. SYSTEMIC ANTIMICROBIALS WITH DOSAGE FORMS AND USUAL DOSAGES (continued)

Generic and Trade Names	Dosage Form (cost estimate)	Route	Dose (evidence level)	Interval
Dalbavancin, Dalvance	500-mg vial ($$$$)	IV	Adults 1 g one time then 500 mg in 1 wk	Once weekly
Dapsone[a]	25-, 100-mg tab ($)	PO	2 mg/kg, max 100 mg (I)	q24h
			4 mg/kg, max 200 mg (I)	Once weekly
Daptomycin,[a] Cubicin	500-mg vial ($$$)	IV	For SSSI: Concern for toxicity in infants <1 y 1–2 y: 10 mg/kg (I) 2–6 y: 9 mg/kg (I) 7–11 y: 7 mg/kg (I) ≥12 y: 5 mg/kg (I) For other indications, see Chapter 6. Adults: 4–6 mg/kg TBW (I)	q24h
Dasabuvir co-packaged with ombitasvir, paritaprevir, ritonavir (Viekira Pak)	Ombitasvir/paritaprevir/ritonavir (12.5-/75-/50-mg) tab + dasabuvir 250-mg tab ($$$$$)	PO	Adults 2 ombitasvir, paritaprevir, ritonavir tabs PLUS 1 dasabuvir 250-mg tab	qam q12h
Delafloxacin, Baxdela	450-mg tab ($$$$) 300-mg vial ($$$$)	PO IV	Adults 450 mg PO or 300 mg IV	q12h
Demeclocycline,[a] Declomycin	150-, 300-mg tab ($$)	PO	≥8 y: 7–13 mg/kg/day, max 600 mg/day (I). Dosage differs for SIADH.	q6h
Dicloxacillin,[a] Dynapen	250-, 500-mg cap ($)	PO	12–25 mg/kg/day (adults 0.5–1 g/day) (I) For bone and joint infections, up to 100 mg/kg/day, max 2 g/day (III)	q6h
Doxycycline, Vibramycin	25-mg/5-mL susp[a] ($) 50-mg/5-mL syrup ($$) 20-, 50-, 75-, 100-mg tab/cap[a] ($)	PO	≥8 y: 4 mg/kg/day loading dose on day 1, then 2–4 mg/kg/day, max 200 mg/day (I)	q12h 12–24h
	100-mg vial[a] ($$)	IV		

Drug	Forms (cost)	Route	Adults/Pediatric dose	Interval
Elbasvir/Grazoprevir, Zepatier	50-mg/100-mg tab ($$$$$)	PO	Adults 1 tab	q24h
Entecavir, Baraclude See Chapter 9, Hepatitis B virus.	0.05-mg/mL soln ($$$) 0.5-, 1-mg tab ($$$$)	PO	2–<16 y (II): use PO soln for doses <0.5 mg 10–11 kg: 0.15 mg >11–14 kg: 0.2 mg >14–17 kg: 0.25 mg >17–20 kg: 0.3 mg >20–23 kg: 0.35 mg >23–26 kg: 0.4 mg >26–30 kg: 0.45 mg >30 kg: 0.5 mg ≥16 y: 0.5 mg (I) Double dose if 3TC exposed (I)	q24h
Ertapenem, Invanz	1-g vial ($$$)	IV, IM	30 mg/kg/day, max 1 g/day (I) ≥13 y and adults: 1 g/day (I)	q12h q24h
Erythromycin base	250-, 500-mg tab 250-mg EC cap[a] 333-, 500-mg EC particle tab (PCE) 250-, 333-, 500-mg DR tab (Ery-Tab) All forms ($$-$$$)	PO	50 mg/kg/day, max 4 g/day (I)	q6–8h
Erythromycin ethylsuccinate, EES, EryPed	200-, 400-mg/5-mL susp ($$) 400-mg tab ($$)	PO	50 mg/kg/day, max 4 g/day (I)	q6–8h
Erythromycin lactobionate, Erythrocin	0.5-g vial ($$$)	IV	20 mg/kg/day, max 4 g/day (I)	q6h
Erythromycin stearate	250-mg tab ($$)	PO	50 mg/kg/day, max 4 g/day (I)	q6–8h
Ethambutol,[a] Myambutol	100-, 400-mg tab ($)	PO	15–25 mg/kg, max 2.5 g (I)	q24h
Ethionamide, Trecator	250-mg tab ($$)	PO	15–20 mg/kg/day, max 1 g/day (I)	q12–24h

Alphabetic Listing of Antimicrobials

11

A. SYSTEMIC ANTIMICROBIALS WITH DOSAGE FORMS AND USUAL DOSAGES (continued)

Generic and Trade Names	Dosage Form (cost estimate)	Route	Dose (evidence level)	Interval
Famciclovir,[a] Famvir	125-, 250-, 500-mg tab ($)	PO	Adults 0.5–2 g/day (I)	q8–12h
Fluconazole,[a] Diflucan	50-, 100-, 150-, 200-mg tab ($) 50-, 200-mg/5-mL susp ($)	PO	6–12 mg/kg/day, max 800 mg/day (I). 800–1,000 mg/day may be used for some CNS fungal infections. See Chapter 8.	q24h
	100-, 200-, 400-mg IVPB ($)	IV		
Flucytosine,[a] Ancobon	250-, 500-mg cap ($$$$)	PO	100 mg/kg/day (I)[c]	q6h
Foscarnet, Foscavir	6-g vial ($$$$)	IV	CMV/VZV: 180 mg/kg/day (I)	q8–12h
			CMV suppression: 90–120 mg/kg (I)	q24h
			HSV: 120 mg/kg/day (I)	q8–12h
Ganciclovir,[a] Cytovene	500-mg vial ($$–$$$)	IV	CMV treatment: 10 mg/kg/day (I)	q12h
			CMV suppression: 5 mg/kg (I)	q24h
			VZV: 10 mg/kg/day (III)	q12h
Gentamicin[a,c]	20-mg/2-mL ($) 40-mg/mL in 2-mL and 20-mL ($)	IV, IM	3–7.5 mg/kg/day, CF 7–10 mg/kg/day See Chapter 1 for q24h dosing.	q8–24h
		Intravesical	0.5 mg/mL in NS x 50–100 mL (III)	
Griseofulvin microsize,[a] Grifulvin V	125-mg/5-mL susp ($) 500-mg tab ($$)	PO	20–25 mg/kg (II), max 1 g (I)	q24h
Griseofulvin ultramicrosize,[a] Gris-PEG	250-mg tab ($$)	PO	10–15 mg/kg (II), max 750 mg (I)	q24h
Imipenem/cilastatin,[a] Primaxin	250/250-, 500/500-mg vial ($$)	IV, IM	60–100 mg/kg/day, max 4 g/day (I) IM form not approved for <12 y	q6h

Interferon-PEG Alfa-2a, Pegasys Alfa-2b, PegIntron Sylatron	All ($$$$) Vials, prefilled syringes: 180-µg 50-µg 200-, 300-, 600-µg	SQ	See Chapter 9, Hepatitis C virus. Weekly
Isavuconazonium (isavuconazole), Cresemba	186-mg cap (100-mg base) ($$$$) 372-mg vial (200-mg base) ($$$$)	PO IV	Adults 200 mg base per dose PO/IV (base = isavuconazole) q8h x 6 doses, then q24h
Isoniazid,[a] Nydrazid	50-mg/5-mL syrup ($$) 100-, 300-mg tab ($) 1,000-mg vial ($$)	PO IV, IM	10–15 mg/kg/day, max 300 mg/day (I) q12–24h With directly observed biweekly therapy, dosage is 20–30 mg/kg, max 900 mg/dose (I). Twice weekly
Itraconazole, Sporanox	50-mg/5-mL soln ($$$) 100-mg cap[a] ($$)	PO	10 mg/kg/day (III), max 200 mg/day q12h 5 mg/kg/day for chronic mucocutaneous Candida (III) q24h
Ivermectin,[a] Stromectol	3-mg tab ($)	PO	0.15–0.2 mg/kg, no max (I) 1 dose
Ketoconazole,[a] Nizoral	200-mg tab ($)	PO	≥2 y: 3.3–6.6 mg/kg, max 400 mg (I) q24h
Levofloxacin,[a] Levaquin	125-mg/5-mL soln ($) 250-, 500-, 750-mg tab ($) 500-, 750-mg vial ($) 250-, 500-, 750-mg IVPB ($)	PO, IV	For postexposure anthrax prophylaxis (I): <50 kg: 16 mg/kg/day, max 500 mg/day q12h ≥50 kg: 500 mg q24h For respiratory infections: <5 y: 20 mg/kg/day (II) q12h ≥5 y: 10 mg/kg/day, max 500 mg/day (II) q24h

Alphabetic Listing of Antimicrobials

A. SYSTEMIC ANTIMICROBIALS WITH DOSAGE FORMS AND USUAL DOSAGES (continued)

Generic and Trade Names	Dosage Form (cost estimate)	Route	Dose (evidence level)	Interval
Linezolid,[a] Zyvox	100-mg/5-mL susp ($$$) 600-mg tab ($) 200-, 600-mg IVPB ($$)	PO, IV	Pneumonia, complicated SSSI: (I) Birth–11 y: 30 mg/kg/day >11 y: 1.2 g/day Uncomplicated SSSI: (I) Birth–<5 y: 30 mg/kg/day 5–11 y: 20 mg/kg/day >11–18 y: 1.2 g/day	q8h q12h q8h q12h q12h
Mebendazole See Chapter 10.	100-mg chew tab, Emverm ($$$$)	PO	≥2y: 100 mg (not per kg) (I)	q12h for 3 days 1 dose for pinworm
	500-mg chew tab, Vermox		≥1 y: 500 mg	1 dose
Mefloquine,[a] Lariam	250-mg tab ($)	PO	See Chapter 10, Malaria.	
Meropenem,[a] Merrem	0.5-, 1-g vial ($$)	IV	60 mg/kg/day, max 3 g/day (I) 120 mg/kg/day meningitis, max 6 g/day (I)	q8h q8h
Methenamine hippurate,[a] Hiprex	1-g tab ($)	PO	6–12 y: 1–2 g/day (I) >12 y: 2 g/day (I)	q12h
Methenamine mandelate[a]	0.5-, 1-g tab ($)	PO	<6 y: 75 mg/kg/day (I) 6–12 y: 2 g/day (I) >12 y: 4 g/day (I)	q6h
Metronidazole,[a] Flagyl	250-, 500-mg tab ($) 250-mg/5-mL susp ($) 375-mg cap ($$)	PO	30–50 mg/kg/day, max 2,250 mg/day (I)	q8h
	500-mg IVPB ($)	IV	22.5–40 mg/kg/day (II), max 4 g/day (I)	q6–8h
Micafungin, Mycamine	50-, 100-mg vial ($$$)	IV	2–4 mg/kg, max 150 mg (I)	q24h

Miltefosine, Impavido[a]	50-mg cap Available from CDC	PO	2.5 mg/kg/day (II). See Chapter 10. ≥12 y (I): 30–44 kg: 100 mg/day ≥45 kg: 150 mg/day	bid bid tid
Minocycline, Minocin	50-, 75-, 100-mg cap[a] ($) 50-, 75-, 100-mg tab[a] ($) 100-mg vial ($$$$)	PO, IV	≥8 y: 4 mg/kg/day, max 200 mg/day (I)	q12h
Minocycline, Solodyn, Minolira	55-, 65-, 80-, 105-, 115-, 135-mg ER tabs ($$$)	PO	≥12 y: 1 mg/kg/day for acne	q24h
Moxifloxacin,[a] Avelox	400-mg tab ($), IVPB ($$)	PO, IV	Adults 400 mg/day (I)	q24h
Nafcillin,[a] Nallpen	1-, 2-, 10-g vial ($)	IV, IM	150–200 mg/kg/day (II) Max 12 g/day div q4h (I)	q6h
Neomycin sulfate[a]	500-mg tab ($)	PO	50–100 mg/kg/day (II), max 12 g/day (I)	q6–8h
Nitazoxanide, Alinia	100-mg/5-mL susp ($$$) 500-mg tab ($$$)	PO	1–3 y: 200 mg/day (I) 4–11 y: 400 mg/day (I) ≥12 y: 1 g/day (I)	q12h
Nitrofurantoin,[a] Furadantin	25-mg/5-mL susp ($$$)	PO	5–7 mg/kg/day, max 400 mg/day (I)	q6h
			1–2 mg/kg for UTI prophylaxis (I)	q24h
Nitrofurantoin macrocrystals,[a] Macrodantin	50-, 100-mg cap ($) 25-mg cap ($$)	PO	Same as susp	
Nitrofurantoin monohydrate and macrocrystalline,[a] Macrobid	100-mg cap ($)	PO	>12 y: 200 mg/day (I)	q12h
Nystatin,[a] Mycostatin	500,000-U/5-mL susp ($) 500,000-U tabs ($)	PO	Infants 2 mL/dose, children 4–6 mL/dose, to coat oral mucosa Tabs: 3–6 tabs/day	q6h tid–qid

Alphabetic Listing of Antimicrobials

11

Alphabetic Listing of Antimicrobials

11

A. SYSTEMIC ANTIMICROBIALS WITH DOSAGE FORMS AND USUAL DOSAGES (continued)

Generic and Trade Names	Dosage Form (cost estimate)	Route	Dose (evidence level)	Interval
Obiltoxaximab, Anthim	600-mg/6-mL vial	IV	≤15 kg: 32 mg/kg (I) >15–40 kg: 24 mg/kg (I) >40 kg and adults: 16 mg/kg (I)	One time
Oritavancin, Orbactiv	400-mg vial ($$$$)	IV	Adults 1.2 g/day (I)	One time
Oseltamivir, Tamiflu (See chapters 5 and 9, Influenza.)	30-mg/5-mL susp ($$) 30-, 45-, 75-mg cap[a] ($$)	PO	Preterm, <38 wk PMA (II): 2 mg/kg/day Preterm, 38–40 wk PMA (II): 3 mg/kg/day Preterm, >40 wk PMA (II), and term, birth–8 mo (I): 6 mg/kg/day 9–11 mo (II): 7 mg/kg/day ≥12 mo (I): ≤15 kg: 60 mg/day >15–23 kg: 90 mg/day >23–40 kg: 120 mg/day >40 kg: 150 mg/day	q12h
			Prophylaxis: Give half the daily dose q24h. Not recommended for infants <3 mo.	q24h
Oxacillin,[a] Bactocill	1-, 2-, 10-g vial ($$)	IV, IM	100 mg/kg/day, max 12 g/day (I) 150–200 mg/kg/day for meningitis (III)	q4–6h
Palivizumab, Synagis	50-, 100-mg vial ($$$$)	IM	15 mg/kg (I)	Monthly during RSV season, maximum of 5 doses
Paromomycin,[a] Humatin	250-mg cap ($–$$)	PO	25–35 mg/kg/day, max 4 g/day (I)	q8h

Penicillin G intramuscular

– Penicillin G benzathine, Bicillin L-A	600,000 U/mL in 1-, 2-, 4-mL prefilled syringes ($$)	IM	50,000 U/kg for newborns and infants, children <60 lb: 300,000–600,000 U, children ≥60 lb: 900,000 U (I) (FDA approved in 1952 for dosing by pounds) Adults 1.2–2.4 million U	1 dose
– Penicillin G benzathine/procaine, Bicillin C-R	1,200,000 IU per 2 mL prefilled syringe as 600,000 IU benzathine + 600,000 IU procaine per mL ($)	IM	<30 lb: 600,000 U; 30–60 lb: 900,000–1,200,000 U; >60 lb: 2,400,000 U (I)	1 dose (may need repeat injections q2–3d)

Penicillin G intravenous

– Penicillin G K,[a] Pfizerpen	5-, 20-million U vial ($)	IV, IM	100,000–300,000 U/kg/day (I). Max daily dose is 24 million U.	q4–6h
– Penicillin G sodium[a]	5-million U vial ($$)	IV, IM	100,000–300,000 U/kg/day (I). Max daily dose is 24 million U.	q4–6h

Penicillin V oral

– Penicillin V K[a]	125-, 250-mg/5-mL soln ($); 250-, 500-mg tab ($)	PO	25–50 mg/kg/day, max 2 g/day (I)	q6h
Pentamidine Pentam, Nebupent	300-mg vial ($$$)	IV, IM	4 mg/kg/day (I), max 300 mg	q24h
	300-mg vial ($)	Inhaled	300 mg monthly for prophylaxis (I)	Monthly
Peramivir, Rapivab	200-mg vial ($$–$$$)	IV	10 mg/kg (II), max 600 mg (I)	One time
Piperacillin/tazobactam,[a] Zosyn	2/0.25-, 3/0.375-, 4/0.5-, 12/1.5-, 36/4.5-g vial ($)	IV	≤40 kg: 240–300 mg PIP/kg/day, max 16 g PIP/day (I)	q8h
Polymyxin B[a]	500,000 U vial ($); 1 mg = 10,000 U	IV	2.5 mg/kg/day (I) Adults 2 mg/kg LD, then 2.5–3 mg/kg/day, dose based on TBW, no max (II)	q12h

Alphabetic Listing of Antimicrobials

11

A. SYSTEMIC ANTIMICROBIALS WITH DOSAGE FORMS AND USUAL DOSAGES (continued)

Generic and Trade Names	Dosage Form (cost estimate)	Route	Dose (evidence level)	Interval
Posaconazole, Noxafil (See Chapter 8.)	200-mg/5-mL susp ($$$$)	PO	<13 y: under investigation, 18 mg/kg/day with serum trough monitoring	q8h
			≥13 y and adults (I):	
			Candida or Aspergillus prophylaxis: 600 mg/day	q8h
			OPC treatment: 100 mg q12h for 1 day, then 100 mg/day	q24h
			Refractory OPC: 800 mg/day	q12h
	100-mg DR tab ($$$$) 300-mg/16.7-mL vial ($$$$)	PO, IV	≥13 y and adults (I): Candida or Aspergillus prophylaxis: 300 mg q12h for 1 day, then 300 mg/day	q24h
Praziquantel, Biltricide	600-mg tri-scored tab ($$)	PO	20–25 mg/kg, no max (I)	q4–6h for 3 doses
Primaquine phosphate[a]	15-mg base tab ($) (26.3-mg primaquine phosphate)	PO	0.3 mg base/kg, max 30 mg (III) (See Chapter 10.)	q24h
Pyrantel pamoate[a]	250-mg base/5-mL susp ($)	PO	11 mg (base)/kg, max 1 g (I) (144-mg pyrantel pamoate = 50-mg base)	Once
Pyrazinamide[a]	500-mg tab ($)	PO	30 mg/kg/day, max 2 g/day (I)	q24h
			Directly observed biweekly therapy, 50 mg/kg (I) use IBW, no max.	Twice weekly
Quinupristin/dalfopristin, Synercid	150/350-mg vial (500-mg total) ($$$$)	IV	22.5 mg/kg/day (II) Adults 15–22.5 mg/kg/day, no max (I)	q8h q8–12h

Raxibacumab	1,700-mg/35-mL vial Available from CDC	IV	≤15 kg: 80 mg/kg >15–50 kg: 60 mg/kg >50 kg: 40 mg/kg (I)	Once
Ribavirin, Rebetol	200-mg/5-mL soln ($) 200-mg cap/tab[a] ($) 400-, 600-mg tab ($$$$) 600-, 800-, 1,000-, 1,200-mg dose paks ($$$$)	PO	15 mg/kg/day (I) Given as combination therapy with other agents for HCV; see Chapter 9.	q12h
Ribavirin, Virazole	6-g vial ($$$$$)	Inhaled	1 vial by SPAG-2; see Chapter 9, Respiratory syncytial virus.	q24h
Rifabutin,[a] Mycobutin	150-mg cap ($$$)	PO	5 mg/kg for MAC prophylaxis (II) 10–20 mg/kg for MAC or TB treatment (I) Max 300 mg/day	q24h
Rifampin,[a] Rifadin	150-, 300-mg cap ($) 600-mg vial ($$–$$$)	PO, IV	10–20 mg/kg, max 600 mg for TB (I)	q24h
			With directly observed biweekly therapy, dosage is still 10–20 mg/kg/dose (max 600 mg).	Twice weekly
			20 mg/kg/day for 2 days for meningococcus prophylaxis, max 1.2 g/day (I)	q12h
Rifampin/isoniazid/pyrazinamide, Rifater	120-/50-/300-mg tab ($$$)	PO	≥15 y and adults: ≤44 kg: 4 tab 45–54 kg: 5 tab ≥55 kg: 6 tab	q24h
Rifapentine, Priftin	150-mg tab ($$)	PO	≥12 y and adults: 600 mg/dose (I)	Twice weekly
Rifaximin, Xifaxan	200-mg tab ($$$)	PO	≥12 y and adults: 600 mg/day (I) 20–30 mg/kg/day, max 1.6 g/day (III)	q8h
Simeprevir, Olysio	150-mg cap ($$$$$)	PO	Adults: 150 mg (I)	q24h
Sofosbuvir, Sovaldi	400-mg tab ($$$$$)	PO	≥12 y and adults: 400 mg (I)	q24h

11

Alphabetic Listing of Antimicrobials

A. SYSTEMIC ANTIMICROBIALS WITH DOSAGE FORMS AND USUAL DOSAGES (continued)

Generic and Trade Names	Dosage Form (cost estimate)	Route	Dose (evidence level)	Interval
Sofosbuvir/Ledipasvir, Harvoni	400-/90-mg tab ($$$$$)	PO	≥12 y and adults: 1 tab (I)	q24h
Sofosbuvir/Velpatasvir, Epclusa	400-/100-mg tab ($$$$$)	PO	Adults 1 tab (I)	q24h
Streptomycin[a]	1-g vial ($$)	IM, IV	20–40 mg/kg/day, max 1 g/day[c] (I)	q12–24h
Sulfadiazine[a]	500-mg tab ($$)	PO	120–150 mg/kg/day, max 4–6 g/day (I) See Chapter 10.	q6h
			Rheumatic fever secondary prophylaxis 500 mg qd if ≤27 kg, 1,000 mg qd if >27 kg (II)	q24h
Tedizolid, Sivextro	200-mg tab ($$$$) 200-mg vial ($$$$)	PO, IV	Adults 200 mg (I)	q24h
Telavancin, Vibativ	250-, 750-mg vial ($$$$)	IV	Adults 10 mg/kg	q24h
Telbivudine, Tyzeka	600-mg tab ($$$$)	PO	≥16 y and adults: 600 mg/day (I)	q24h
Terbinafine, Lamisil	125-, 187.5-mg granules ($$$) 250-mg tab[a] ($)	PO	>4 y: <25 kg: 125 mg/day 25–35 kg: 187.5 mg/day >35 kg: 250 mg/day (I)	q24h
Tetracycline[a]	250-, 500-mg cap ($$)	PO	≥8 y: 25–50 mg/kg/day (I)	q6h
Tinidazole,[a] Tindamax	250-, 500-mg tab ($)	PO	50 mg/kg, max 2 g (I) See Chapter 10.	q24h
Tobramycin,[a] Nebcin	20-mg/2-mL vial ($) 40-mg/mL 2-, 30-, 50-mL vial ($) 1.2-g vial ($)	IV, IM	3–7.5 mg/kg/day (CF 7–10);[c] see Chapter 1 regarding q24h dosing.	q8–24h
Tobramycin inhalation,[a] Tobi	300-mg ampule ($$$$)	Inhaled	≥6 y: 600 mg/day (I)	q12h

Tobi Podhaler	28-mg cap for inhalation ($$$$)	Inhaled	≥6 y: 224 mg/day via Podhaler device (I)	q12h
Trimethoprim/ sulfamethoxazole,[a] Bactrim, Septra	80-mg TMP/400-mg SMX tab (single strength) ($)	PO, IV	8–10 mg TMP/kg/day (I)	q12h
	160-mg TMP/800-mg SMX tab (double strength) ($)		2 mg TMP/kg/day for UTI prophylaxis (I)	q24h
	40-mg TMP/200-mg SMX per 5-mL oral susp ($)		15–20 mg TMP/kg/day for PCP treatment (I), no max	q6–8h
	16-mg TMP/80-mg SMX per mL injection soln in 5-, 10-, 30-mL vial ($$)		150 mg TMP/m²/day, OR 5 mg TMP/kg/day for PCP prophylaxis (I), max 160 mg TMP/day	q12h 3 times a wk OR q24h
Valacyclovir,[a] Valtrex (provides therapeutic acyclovir serum concentrations)	500-mg, 1-g tab ($)	PO	VZV: ≥3 mo: 60 mg/kg/day (I, II) HSV: ≥3 mo: 40 mg/kg/day (II) Max single dose 1 g (I)	q8h q12h
Valganciclovir,[a] Valcyte (provides therapeutic ganciclovir serum concentrations)	250-mg/5-mL soln ($$$$) 450-mg tab ($$$$)	PO	Congenital CMV treatment: 32 mg/kg/day (II). See Chapter 5. CMV prophylaxis (mg): 7 × BSA × CrCl (using the modified Schwartz formula for CrCl), max 900 mg (I). See Chapter 9.	q12h q24h
Vancomycin,[a] Vancocin	125-, 250-mg/5-mL susp ($) 125-, 250-mg cap ($$–$$$)	PO	40 mg/kg/day (I), max 500 mg/day (III)	q6h
	0.5-, 0.75-, 1-, 5-, 10-g vial ($)	IV	30–40 mg/kg/day[c] (I) For life-threatening invasive MRSA infection, 60–70 mg/kg/day adjusted to achieve an AUC:MIC of >400 mg/L × h (II)	q6–8h

Alphabetic Listing of Antimicrobials

A. SYSTEMIC ANTIMICROBIALS WITH DOSAGE FORMS AND USUAL DOSAGES (continued)

Generic and Trade Names	Dosage Form (cost estimate)	Route	Dose (evidence level)	Interval
Voriconazole,[a,c] Vfend (See Chapter 8.)	200-mg/5-mL susp ($$$$) 50-, 200-mg tab ($$)	PO	≥2 y and <50 kg: 18 mg/kg/day, max 700 mg/day (I) ≥50 kg: 400–600 mg/day (I)	q12h
	200-mg vial ($$$)	IV	≥2 y and <50 kg: 18 mg/kg/day LD for 1 day, then 16 mg/kg/day (I) ≥50 kg: 12 mg/kg/day LD for 1 day, then 8 mg/kg/day (I)	q12h
Zanamivir, Relenza	5-mg blister cap for inhalation ($)	Inhaled	Prophylaxis: ≥5 y: 10 mg/day (I)	q24h
			Treatment: ≥7 y: 20 mg/day (I)	q12h

[a] Available in a generic formulation.
[b] Given as a cocktail with ribavirin ± interferon-PEG.
[c] Monitor serum concentrations.

11

B. TOPICAL ANTIMICROBIALS (SKIN, EYE, EAR)

Generic and Trade Names	Dosage Form	Route	Dose	Interval
Acyclovir, Sitavig	50-mg tab	Buccal	Adults 50 mg, for herpes labialis	One time
Azithromycin, AzaSite	1% ophth soln	Ophth	1 drop	bid for 2 days then qd for 5 days
Bacitracin[a]	Ophth oint	Ophth	Apply to affected eye.	q3–4h
	Oint[b]	Top	Apply to affected area.	bid–qid
Benzyl alcohol, Ulesfia	5% lotion	Top	Apply to scalp and hair.	Once; repeat in 7 days.
Besifloxacin, Besivance	0.6% ophth susp	Ophth	≥1 y: 1 drop to affected eye	tid
Butenafine, Mentax, Lotrimin-Ultra	1% cream	Top	≥12 y: apply to affected area.	qd
Butoconazole, Gynazole-1	2% prefilled cream	Vag	Adults 1 applicatorful	One time
Ciclopirox,[a] Loprox, Penlac	0.77% cream, gel, lotion	Top	≥10 y: apply to affected area.	bid
	1% shampoo		≥16 y: apply to scalp.	Twice weekly
	8% nail lacquer		≥12 y: apply to infected nail.	qd
Ciprofloxacin,[a] Cetraxal	0.2% otic soln	Otic	≥1 y: apply 3 drops to affected ear.	bid for 7 days
Ciprofloxacin, Ciloxan	0.3% ophth soln[a]	Ophth	Apply to affected eye.	q2h for 2 days then q4h for 5 days
	0.3% ophth oint			q8h for 2 days then q12h for 5 days
Ciprofloxacin, Otiprio	6% otic susp	Otic	≥6 mo: 0.1 mL each ear intratympanic	One time

Alphabetic Listing of Antimicrobials

B. TOPICAL ANTIMICROBIALS (SKIN, EYE, EAR) (continued)

Generic and Trade Names	Dosage Form	Route	Dose	Interval
Ciprofloxacin + dexamethasone, Ciprodex	0.3% + 0.1% otic soln	Otic	≥6 mo: apply 4 drops to affected ear.	bid for 7 days
Ciprofloxacin + fluocinolone, Otovel	0.3% + 0.025% otic soln	Otic	≥6 mo: instill 0.25 mL to affected ear.	bid for 7 days
Ciprofloxacin + hydrocortisone, Cipro HC	0.2% + 1% otic soln	Otic	≥1 y: apply 3 drops to affected ear.	bid for 7 days
Clindamycin				
Cleocin	100-mg ovule	Vag	1 ovule	qhs for 3 days
	2% vaginal cream[a]		1 applicatorful	qhs for 3–7 days
Cleocin-T[a]	1% soln, gel, lotion	Top	Apply to affected area.	qd–bid
Clindesse	2% cream	Vag	Adolescents and adults 1 applicatorful	One time
Evoclin[a]	1% foam			qd
Clindamycin + benzoyl peroxide, BenzaClin	1% gel[a]	Top	≥12 y: apply to affected area.	bid
Acanya	1.2% gel	Top	Apply small amount to face.	q24h
Clindamycin + tretinoin, Ziana, Veltin	1.2% gel	Top	Apply small amount to face.	hs
Clotrimazole,[a,b] Lotrimin	1% cream, lotion, soln	Top	Apply to affected area.	bid
Gyne-Lotrimin-3[a,b]	2% cream	Vag	≥12 y: 1 applicatorful	qhs for 7–14 days
Gyne-Lotrimin-7[a,b]	1% cream			qhs for 3 days
Clotrimazole + betamethasone,[a] Lotrisone	1% + 0.05% cream, lotion	Top	≥12 y: apply to affected area.	bid

Drug	Formulation	Route	Application	Frequency
Colistin + neomycin + hydrocortisone, Coly-Mycin S, Cortisporin TC otic	0.3% otic susp	Otic	Apply 3–4 drops to affected ear canal; may use with wick.	q6–8h
Cortisporin; bacitracin + neomycin + polymyxin B + hydrocortisone	Oint	Top	Apply to affected area.	bid–qid
Cortisporin; neomycin + polymyxin B + hydrocortisone	Otic soln[a]	Otic	3 drops to affected ear	bid–qid
	Cream	Top	Apply to affected area.	bid–qid
Dapsone, Aczone	5% gel	Top	≥12 y: Apply to affected area.	bid
	7.5% gel			qd
Econazole,[a] Spectazole	1% cream	Top	Apply to affected area.	qd–bid
Efinaconazole, Jublia	10% soln	Top	Apply to toenail.	qd for 48 wk
Erythromycin[a]	0.5% ophth oint	Ophth	Apply to affected eye.	q4h
Akne-Mycin	2% oint	Top	Apply to affected area.	bid
Ery Pads	2% pledgets[a]			
Eryderm,[a] Erygel[a]	2% soln, gel			
Erythromycin + benzoyl peroxide,[a] Benzamycin	3% gel	Top	≥12 y: apply to affected area.	qd–bid
Ganciclovir, Zirgan	0.15% ophth gel	Ophth	≥2 y: 1 drop in affected eye	q3h while awake (5 times/day) until healed then tid for 7 days
Gatifloxacin,[a] Zymaxid	0.5% ophth soln	Ophth	Apply to affected eye.	q2h for 1 day then q6h
Gentamicin,[a] Garamycin	0.1% cream, oint	Top	Apply to affected area.	tid–qid
	0.3% ophth soln, oint	Ophth	Apply to affected eye.	q1–4h (soln) q4–8h (oint)

Alphabetic Listing of Antimicrobials

B. TOPICAL ANTIMICROBIALS (SKIN, EYE, EAR) (continued)

Generic and Trade Names	Dosage Form	Route	Dose	Interval
Gentamicin + prednisolone, Pred-G	0.3% ophth soln, oint	Ophth	Adults: apply to affected eye.	q1–4h (soln)
				qd–tid (oint)
Imiquimod,[a] Aldara	5% cream	Top	≥12y: to perianal or external genital warts	3 times per week
Ivermectin, Sklice	0.5% lotion	Top	≥6 mo: thoroughly coat hair and scalp, rinse after 10 minutes.	Once
Ivermectin, Soolantra	1% cream	Top	Adults: apply to face.	qd
Ketoconazole,[a] Nizoral	2% shampoo	Top	≥12 y: apply to affected area.	qd
	2% cream			qd–bid
Extina, Xolegel	2% foam, gel			bid
Nizoral A-D	1% shampoo			bid
Levofloxacin,[a] Quixin	0.5% ophth soln	Ophth	Apply to affected eye.	q1–4h
Luliconazole, Luzu	1% cream	Top	Adults: apply to affected area.	q24h for 1–2 wk
Mafenide, Sulfamylon	8.5% cream	Top	Apply to burn.	qd–bid
	5-g pwd for reconstitution		To keep burn dressing wet	q4–8h as needed
Malathion,[a] Ovide	0.5% soln	Top	≥6 y: apply to hair and scalp.	Once
Maxitrol[a]; neomycin + polymyxin + dexamethasone	Susp, oint	Ophth	Apply to affected eye.	q4h (oint)
				q1–4h (susp)
Metronidazole[a]	0.75% cream, gel, lotion	Top	Adults: apply to affected area.	bid
	0.75% vag gel	Vag	Adults 1 applicatorful	qd–bid
	1% gel	Top	Adults: apply to affected area.	qd

Noritate	1% cream	Top	Adults: apply to affected area.	qd
Miconazole				
Fungoid[a,b]	2% tincture	Top	Apply to affected area.	bid
Micatin[a,b] and others	2% cream, pwd, oint, spray, lotion, gel	Top	Apply to affected area.	qd–bid
Monistat-1[a,b]	1.2-g ovule + 2% cream	Vag	≥12 y: insert one ovule (plus cream to external vulva bid as needed).	Once
Monistat-3[a,b]	200-mg ovule, 4% cream			qhs for 3 days
Monistat-7[a,b]	100-mg ovule, 2% cream			qhs for 7 days
Vusion	0.25% oint	Top	To diaper dermatitis	Each diaper change for 7 days
Moxifloxacin, Vigamox	0.5% ophth soln	Ophth	Apply to affected eye.	tid
Mupirocin, Bactroban	2% oint,[a] cream,[a] nasal oint	Top	Apply to infected skin or nasal mucosa.	tid
Naftifine, Naftin	1%, 2% cream[a] 2% gel	Top	Apply to affected area.	qd
Natamycin, Natacyn	5% ophth soln	Ophth	Adults: apply to affected eye.	q1–4h
Neosporin[a]				
bacitracin + neomycin + polymyxin B	Ophth oint	Ophth	Apply to affected eye.	q4h
	Oint[a,b]	Top	Apply to affected area.	bid–qid
gramicidin + neomycin + polymyxin B	Ophth soln	Ophth	Apply to affected eye.	q4h
Nystatin,[a] Mycostatin	100,000 U/g cream, oint, pwd	Top	Apply to affected area.	bid–qid
Nystatin + triamcinolone,[a] Mycolog II	100,000 U/g + 0.1% cream, oint	Top	Apply to affected area.	bid

Alphabetic Listing of Antimicrobials

11

Alphabetic Listing of Antimicrobials

B. TOPICAL ANTIMICROBIALS (SKIN, EYE, EAR) (continued)

Generic and Trade Names	Dosage Form	Route	Dose	Interval
Ofloxacin,[a] Floxin Otic, Ocuflox	0.3% otic soln	Otic	5–10 drops to affected ear	qd–bid
	0.3% ophth soln	Ophth	Apply to affected eye.	q1–6h
Oxiconazole, Oxistat	1% cream,[a] lotion	Top	Apply to affected area.	qd–bid
Permethrin, Nix[a,b]	1% cream	Top	Apply to hair/scalp.	Once for 10 min
Elimite[a]	5% cream		Apply to all skin surfaces.	Once for 8–14 h
Piperonyl butoxide + pyrethrins,[a,b] Rid	4% + 0.3% shampoo, gel	Top	Apply to affected area.	Once for 10 min
Polysporin,[a] polymyxin B + bacitracin	Ophth oint	Ophth	Apply to affected eye.	qd–tid
	Oint[b]	Top	Apply to affected area.	qd–tid
Polytrim,[a] polymyxin B + trimethoprim	Ophth soln	Ophth	Apply to affected eye.	q3–4h
Retapamulin, Altabax	1% oint	Top	Apply thin layer to affected area.	bid for 5 days
Selenium sulfide,[a] Selsun	2.5% lotion 2.25% shampoo	Top	Lather into scalp or affected area.	Twice weekly then every 1–2 wk
Selsun Blue[a,b]	1% shampoo			qd
Sertaconazole, Ertaczo	2% cream	Top	≥12 y: apply to affected area.	bid
Silver sulfadiazine,[a] Silvadene	1% cream	Top	Apply to affected area.	qd–bid
Spinosad,[a] Natroba	0.9% susp	Top	Apply to scalp and hair.	Once; may repeat in 7 days.
Sulconazole, Exelderm	1% soln, cream	Top	Adults: apply to affected area.	qd–bid
Sulfacetamide sodium[a]	10% soln	Ophth	Apply to affected eye.	q1–3h
	10% ophth oint			q4–6h
	10% lotion, wash, cream	Top	≥12 y: apply to affected area.	bid–qid

Drug	Formulation	Route	Directions	Frequency
Sulfacetamide sodium + prednisolone,[a] Blephamide	10% ophth oint, soln	Ophth	Apply to affected eye.	tid–qid
Tavaborole, Kerydin	5% soln	Top	Adults: apply to toenail.	qd for 48 wk
Terbinafine,[b] Lamisil-AT	1% cream,[a] spray, gel	Top	Apply to affected area.	qd–bid
Terconazole,[a] Terazol	0.4% cream	Vag	Adults 1 applicatorful or 1 suppository	qhs for 7 days
	0.8% cream 80-mg suppository			qhs for 3 days
Tioconazole[a,b]	6.5% ointment	Vag	≥12 y: 1 applicatorful	One time
Tobramycin, Tobrex	0.3% soln,[a] oint	Ophth	Apply to affected eye.	q1–4h (soln) q4–8h (oint)
Tobramycin + dexamethasone, Tobradex	0.3% soln,[a] oint	Ophth	Apply to affected eye.	q2–6h (soln) q6–8h (oint)
Tobramycin + loteprednol, Zylet	0.3% + 0.5% ophth susp	Ophth	Adults: apply to affected eye.	q4–6h
Tolnaftate,[a,b] Tinactin	1% cream, soln, pwd, spray	Top	Apply to affected area.	bid
Trifluridine,[a] Viroptic	1% ophth soln	Ophth	1 drop (max 9 drops/day)	q2h

[a] Generic available.
[b] Over the counter.

11

Alphabetic Listing of Antimicrobials

12. Antibiotic Therapy for Children Who Are Obese

When prescribing an antimicrobial for a child who is obese, selecting a dose based on milligrams per kilograms of total body weight (TBW) may expose the child to supratherapeutic plasma concentrations if the drug doesn't freely distribute into fat tissue. The aminoglycosides are an example of such potentially problematic antibiotics; they are hydrophilic molecules with distribution volumes that correlate with extracellular fluid. This likely explains why their weight-adjusted distribution volumes are lower in obese compared with nonobese children.

For **aminoglycosides** in obese adults and children, a 40% adjustment in dosing weight has been recommended. When performing this empiric dosing strategy with aminoglycosides in children who are obese, we recommend closely following serum concentrations.

Vancomycin is traditionally dosed based on TBW in obese adults due to increases in kidney size and glomerular filtration rate. In children who are obese, weight-adjusted distribution volume and clearance area are lower, and TBW-based dosing may result in supratherapeutic concentrations. Dosing adjustments using body surface area may be more appropriate. We recommend closely following serum concentrations.

In the setting of **cephalosporins** for surgical prophylaxis (see Chapter 14), adult studies of obese patients have generally found that distribution to the subcutaneous fat tissue target is subtherapeutic when standard doses are used. Given the wide safety margin of these agents in the short-term setting of surgical prophylaxis, maximum single doses are recommended in obese adults (eg, cefazolin 2–3 g instead of the standard 1 g) with re-dosing at 4-hour intervals for longer cases. Based on the adult data, we recommend dosing cephalosporins for surgical prophylaxis based on TBW up to the adult maximum.

In critically ill obese adults, extended infusion times have been shown to increase the likelihood of achieving therapeutic serum concentrations with **carbapenems** and **piperacillin/tazobactam**.

Monitor creatine kinase when using **daptomycin** in a child who is obese.

Listed in the Table are the major classes of antimicrobials and our suggestion on how to calculate the most appropriate dose. The levels of evidence to support these recommendations are Level II–III (pharmacokinetic studies in children, extrapolations from adult studies, and expert opinion). Whenever a dose is used that is greater than one prospectively investigated for efficacy and safety, the clinician must weigh the benefits with potential risks. Data are not available on all agents.

DRUG CLASS	DOSING RECOMMENDATIONS		
	BY EBW[a]	INTERMEDIATE DOSING	BY TBW[b]
ANTIBACTERIALS			
Beta-lactams		EBW 1 0.5 (TBW-EBW)	
Penicillins		X	
Cephalosporins		X	X (surgical prophylaxis)
Carbapenems		X	
Macrolides			
Erythromycin	X		
Azithromycin	X (for gastrointestinal infections)		X
Clarithromycin	X		
Lincosamides			
Clindamycin			X
Glycopeptides			
Vancomycin		1,500–2,000 mg/m²/d	X
Aminoglycosides		EBW + 0.4 (TBW-EBW)	
Gentamicin		X	
Tobramycin		X	
Amikacin		X	
Fluoroquinolones		EBW + 0.45 (TBW-EBW)	
Ciprofloxacin		X	
Levofloxacin		X	
Rifamycins			
Rifampin	X		
Miscellaneous			
TMP/SMX			X
Metronidazole	X		
Linezolid	X		
Daptomycin			X

DRUG CLASS	DOSING RECOMMENDATIONS		
	BY EBW[a]	INTERMEDIATE DOSING	BY TBW[b]
ANTIFUNGALS			
Polyenes			
Amphotericin B (conventional and lipid formulations)			X
Azoles			
Fluconazole			X (max 1,200 mg/day)
Posaconazole	X		
Voriconazole	X		
Pyrimidine Analogues			
Flucytosine	X		
Echinocandins			
Anidulafungin	X		
Caspofungin			X (max 150 mg/day)
Micafungin			
ANTIVIRALS (NON-HIV)			
Nucleoside analogues (acyclovir, ganciclovir)	X		
Oseltamivir	X		
ANTIMYCOBACTERIALS			
Isoniazid	X		
Rifampin			X (max 1,200 mg/day)
Pyrazinamide			X (max 2,000 mg/day)
Ethambutol			X (max 1,600 mg/day)

Abbreviations: BMI, body mass index; EBW, expected body weight; HIV, human immunodeficiency virus; TBW, total body weight; TMP/SMX, trimethoprim/sulfamethoxazole.

[a] EBW (kg) = BMI 50th percentile for age × actual height (m)^2; from Le Grange D, et al. *Pediatrics.* 2012;129(2): e438–e446.

[b] Actual measured body weight.

Bibliography

Camaione L, et al. *Pharmacotherapy.* 2013;33(12):1278–1287

Hall RG. *Curr Pharm Des.* 2015;21(32):4748–4751

Harskamp-van Ginkel MW, et al. *JAMA Pediatr.* 2015;169(7):678–685

Heble DE Jr, et al. *Pharmacotherapy.* 2013;33(12):1273–1277

Le J, et al. *Clin Ther.* 2015;37(6):1340–1351

Pai MP, et al. *Antimicrob Agents Chemother.* 2011;55(12):5640–5645

Payne KD, et al. *Expert Rev Anti Infect Ther.* 2014;12(7):829–854

Payne KD, et al. *Expert Rev Anti Infect Ther.* 2016;14(2):257–267

Sampson M, et al. *GaBI J.* 2013;2(2):76–81

Smith M, et al. *E-PAS.* 2015:4194.689

13. Sequential Parenteral-Oral Antibiotic Therapy (Oral Step-down Therapy) for Serious Infections

The concept of oral step-down therapy is not new; evidence-based recommendations from Nelson and colleagues appeared 40 years ago in the *Journal of Pediatrics*.[1,2] Bone and joint infections,[3–5] complicated bacterial pneumonia with empyema,[6] deep-tissue abscesses, and appendicitis,[7,8] as well as cellulitis or pyelonephritis,[9] may require initial parenteral therapy to control the growth and spread of pathogens and minimize injury to tissues. For abscesses in soft tissues, joints, bones, and empyema, most organisms are removed by surgical drainage and, presumably, killed by the initial parenteral therapy. When the signs and symptoms of infection begin to resolve, often within 2 to 4 days, continuing intravenous (IV) therapy may not be required, as a normal host neutrophil response begins to assist in clearing the infection.[10] In addition to following the clinical response prior to oral switch, following objective laboratory markers, such as C-reactive protein (CRP) or procalcitonin (PCT), during the hospitalization may also help the clinician better assess the response to antibacterial therapy, particularly in the infant or child who is difficult to examine.[11,12]

For the beta-lactam class of antibiotics, absorption of orally administered antibiotics in *standard* dosages provides peak serum concentrations that are routinely only 5% to 20% of those achieved with IV or intramuscular administration. However, *high-dose* oral beta-lactam therapy provides the tissue antibiotic exposure thought to be required to eradicate the remaining pathogens at the infection site as the tissue perfusion improves. For beta-lactams, begin with a dosage 2 to 3 times the normal dosage (eg, 75–100 mg/kg/day of amoxicillin or 100 mg/kg/day of cephalexin). High-dose oral beta-lactam antibiotic therapy of osteoarticular infections has been associated with treatment success since 1978.[3] It is reassuring that high-quality retrospective cohort data have recently confirmed similar outcomes achieved in those treated with oral step-down therapy compared with those treated with IV.[10,13] High-dose prolonged oral beta-lactam therapy may be associated with reversible neutropenia; checking for hematologic toxicity every few weeks during therapy is recommended.[14]

Clindamycin and many antibiotics of the fluoroquinolone class (ciprofloxacin, levofloxacin)[15] and oxazolidinone class (linezolid, tedizolid) have excellent absorption of their oral formulations and provide virtually the same tissue antibiotic exposure at a particular mg/kg dose, compared with that dose given intravenously. Trimethoprim/sulfamethoxazole and metronidazole are also very well absorbed.

One must also assume that the parent and child are compliant with the administration of each antibiotic dose, that the oral antibiotic will be absorbed from the gastrointestinal tract into the systemic circulation (no vomiting or diarrhea), and that the parents will seek medical care if the clinical course does not continue to improve for their child.

Monitor the child clinically for a continued response on oral therapy; follow CRP or PCT after the switch to oral therapy, if there are concerns about continued response, to make sure the antibiotic and dosage you selected are appropriate and the family is compliant. From some of the first published cases of oral step-down therapy, failures caused by noncompliance have occurred.[16]

14. Antimicrobial Prophylaxis/Prevention of Symptomatic Infection

This chapter provides a summary of recommendations for prophylaxis of infections, defined as providing therapy prior to the onset of clinical signs or symptoms of infection. Prophylaxis can be considered in several clinical scenarios.

A. Postexposure Antimicrobial Prophylaxis to Prevent Infection

Given for a relatively short, specified period after exposure to specific pathogens/organisms, where the risks of acquiring the infection are felt to justify antimicrobial treatment to eradicate the pathogen or prevent symptomatic infection in situations in which the child (healthy or with increased susceptibility to infection) is likely to have been inoculated/exposed (eg, asymptomatic child closely exposed to meningococcus; a neonate born to a mother with active genital herpes simplex virus).

B. Long-term Antimicrobial Prophylaxis to Prevent Symptomatic New Infection

Given to a particular, defined population of children who are of relatively high risk of acquiring a severe infection from a single or multiple exposures (eg, a child postsplenectomy; a child with documented rheumatic heart disease to prevent subsequent streptococcal infection), with prophylaxis provided during the period of risk, potentially months or years.

C. Prophylaxis of Symptomatic Disease in Children Who Have Asymptomatic Infection/Latent Infection

Where a child has a documented but asymptomatic infection and targeted antimicrobials are given to prevent the development of symptomatic disease (eg, latent tuberculosis infection or therapy of a stem cell transplant patient with documented cytomegalovirus viremia but no symptoms of infection or rejection, to prevent reactivation of herpes simplex virus). Treatment period is usually defined, particularly in situations in which the latent infection can be cured (tuberculosis), but other circumstances, such as reactivation of a latent virus, may require months or years of prophylaxis.

D. Surgical/Procedure Prophylaxis

A child receives a surgical/invasive catheter procedure, planned or unplanned, in which the risk of infection postoperatively or post-procedure may justify prophylaxis to prevent an infection from occurring (eg, prophylaxis to prevent infection following spinal rod placement). Treatment is usually short-term, beginning just prior to the procedure and ending at the conclusion of the procedure, or within 24 to 48 hours.

E. Travel-Related Exposure Prophylaxis

Not discussed in this chapter; please refer to information on specific disease entities (eg, traveler's diarrhea, Chapter 6) or pathogens (eg, malaria, Chapter 10). Constantly updated, current information for travelers about prophylaxis and current worldwide infection risks can be found on the Centers for Disease Control and Prevention Web site at www.cdc.gov/travel (accessed October 4, 2017).

NOTE

- Abbreviations: AHA, American Heart Association; ALT, alanine aminotransferase; amox/clav, amoxicillin/clavulanate; ARF, acute rheumatic fever; bid, twice daily; CDC, Centers for Disease Control and Prevention; CSF, cerebrospinal fluid; div, divided; DOT, directly observed therapy; GI, gastrointestinal; HSV, herpes simplex virus; IGRA, interferon-gamma release assay; IM, intramuscular; INH, isoniazid; IV, intravenous; MRSA, methicillin-resistant *Staphylococcus aureus*; N/A, not applicable; PCR, polymerase chain reaction; PO, orally; PPD, purified protein derivative; qd, once daily; qid, 4 times daily; spp, species; TB, tuberculosis; tid, 3 times daily; TIG, tetanus immune globulin; TMP/SMX, trimethoprim/sulfamethoxazole; UTI, urinary tract infection.

A. POSTEXPOSURE ANTIMICROBIAL PROPHYLAXIS TO PREVENT INFECTION

Prophylaxis Category	Therapy (evidence grade)	Comments
Bacterial		
Bites, animal and human[1-5] (*Pasteurella multocida* [animal], *Eikenella corrodens* [human], *Staphylococcus* spp, and *Streptococcus* spp)	Amox/clav 45 mg/kg/day PO div tid (amox/clav 7:1; see Chapter 1 for amox/clav description) for 3–5 days (AII) OR ampicillin and clindamycin (BII). For penicillin allergy, consider ciprofloxacin (for *Pasteurella*) plus clindamycin (BIII).	Recommended for children who are (1) immunocompromised; (2) asplenic; (3) have moderate to severe injuries, especially to the hand or face; or (4) have injuries that may have penetrated the periosteum or joint capsule (AII).[3] Consider rabies prophylaxis for at-risk animal bites (AII)[6]; consider tetanus prophylaxis.[7] Human bites have a very high rate of infection (do not close open wounds routinely). Cat bites have a higher rate of infection than dog bites. *Staphylococcus aureus* coverage is only fair with amox/clav and provides no coverage for MRSA.

Endocarditis prophylaxis[8,9]. Given that (1) endocarditis is rarely caused by dental/GI procedures and (2) prophylaxis for procedures prevents an exceedingly small number of cases, the risks of antibiotics most often outweigh benefits. However, some "highest risk" conditions are currently recommended for prophylaxis: (1) prosthetic heart valve (or prosthetic material used to repair a valve); (2) previous endocarditis; (3) cyanotic congenital heart disease that is unrepaired (or palliatively repaired with shunts and conduits); (4) congenital heart disease that is repaired but with defects at the site of repair adjacent to prosthetic material; (5) completely repaired congenital heart disease using prosthetic material, for the first 6 months after repair; or (6) cardiac transplant patients with valvulopathy. Routine prophylaxis no longer is recommended for children with native valve abnormalities. Follow-up data in children suggest that following these new guidelines, no increase in endocarditis has been detected,[10] but in adults in the United States[11] and in the United Kingdom,[12] some concern for increase in the number of cases of endocarditis has been documented since widespread prophylaxis was stopped. More recent data from California and New York do not support an increase in infective endocarditis with the current approach to prophylaxis.[13]

14

A. POSTEXPOSURE ANTIMICROBIAL PROPHYLAXIS TO PREVENT INFECTION (continued)

Prophylaxis Category	Therapy (evidence grade)	Comments
Bacterial (continued)		
– In highest-risk patients: dental procedures that involve manipulation of the gingival or periodontal region of teeth	Amoxicillin 50 mg/kg PO 1 h before procedure OR ampicillin or ceftriaxone or cefazolin, all at 50 mg/kg IM/IV 30–60 min before procedure	If penicillin allergy: clindamycin 20 mg/kg PO (60 min before) or IV (30 min before) OR azithromycin 15 mg/kg or clarithromycin 15 mg/kg (1 h before)
– Genitourinary and gastrointestinal procedures	None	No longer recommended
Lyme disease (*Borrelia burgdorferi*)[14]	Doxycycline 4 mg/kg (up to 200 mg max), once. Dental staining should not occur with a single dose of doxycycline. Amoxicillin prophylaxis is not well studied, and experts recommend a full 14-day course if amoxicillin is used.	ONLY (1) for those in highly Lyme-endemic areas AND (2) the tick has been attached for >36 h (and is engorged) AND (3) prophylaxis started within 72 h of tick removal.
Meningococcus (*Neisseria meningitidis*)[15]	For prophylaxis of close contacts, including household members, child care center contacts, and anyone directly exposed to the patient's oral secretions (eg, through kissing, mouth-to-mouth resuscitation, endotracheal intubation, endotracheal tube management) in the 7 days before symptom onset Rifampin Infants <1 mo: 5 mg/kg PO q12h for 4 doses Children ≥1 mo: 10 mg/kg PO q12h for 4 doses (max 600 mg/dose) OR Ceftriaxone Children <15 y: 125 mg IM once Children ≥16 y: 250 mg IM once OR Ciprofloxacin 500 mg PO once (adolescents and adults)	A single dose of ciprofloxacin should not present a significant risk of cartilage damage, but no prospective data exist in children for prophylaxis of meningococcal disease. For a child, an equivalent exposure for ciprofloxacin to that in adults would be 15–20 mg/kg as a single dose (max 500 mg). A few ciprofloxacin-resistant strains have now been reported. Insufficient data to recommend azithromycin at this time. Meningococcal vaccines may also be recommended in case of an outbreak.

Pertussis[16,17]

Same regimen as for treatment of pertussis: azithromycin 10 mg/kg/day qd for 5 days OR clarithromycin (for infants >1 mo) 15 mg/kg/day div bid for 7 days OR erythromycin (estolate preferable) 40 mg/kg/day PO div qid for 14 days (AII) Alternative: TMP/SMX 8 mg/kg/day div bid for 14 days (BIII)

Prophylaxis to family members; contacts defined by CDC: persons within 21 days of exposure to an infectious pertussis case, who are at high risk of severe illness or who will have close contact with a person at high risk of severe illness (including infants, pregnant women in their third trimester, immunocompromised persons, contacts who have close contact with infants <12 mo). Close contact can be considered as face-to-face exposure within 3 feet of a symptomatic person; direct contact with respiratory, nasal, or oral secretions; or sharing the same confined space in close proximity to an infected person for ≥1 h.

Community-wide prophylaxis is not currently recommended.

Azithromycin and clarithromycin are better tolerated than erythromycin (see Chapter 5); azithromycin is preferred in exposed very young infants to reduce pyloric stenosis risk.

Tetanus
(*Clostridium tetani*)[7,18,19]

NEED FOR TETANUS VACCINE OR TIG[a]

Number of past tetanus vaccine doses	Clean Wound		Contaminated Wound	
	Need for tetanus vaccine	Need for TIG 500 U IM[a]	Need for tetanus vaccine	Need for TIG 500 U IM[a]
<3 doses	Yes	No	Yes	Yes
≥3 doses	No (if <10 y[b]) Yes (if ≥10 y[b])	No	No (if <5 y[b]) Yes (if ≥5 y[b])	No

[a] IV immune globulin should be used when TIG is not available.
[b] Years since last tetanus-containing vaccine dose.

For deep, contaminated wounds, wound debridement is essential. For wounds that cannot be fully debrided, consider metronidazole 30 mg/kg/day PO div q8h until wound healing is underway and anaerobic conditions no longer exist, as short as 3–5 days (BIII).

14

Antimicrobial Prophylaxis/Prevention of Symptomatic Infection

A. POSTEXPOSURE ANTIMICROBIAL PROPHYLAXIS TO PREVENT INFECTION (continued)

Prophylaxis Category	Therapy (evidence grade)	Comments
Bacterial (continued)		
Tuberculosis (*Mycobacterium tuberculosis*) Exposed children <4 y, or immunocompromised patient (high risk of dissemination)[20,21] For treatment of latent TB infection, see Table 14C.	Scenario 1: Previously uninfected child becomes exposed to a person with active disease. Exposed children <4 y, or immunocompromised patient (high risk of dissemination): INH 10–15 mg/kg PO qd for at least 2–3 mo (AIII) at which time the PPD/IGRA may be assessed. Older children may also begin prophylaxis postexposure, but if exposure is questionable, can wait 2–3 mo after exposure to assess for infection; if PPD/IGRA at 2–3 mo is positive and child remains asymptomatic at that time, start INH for 9–12 mo.	If PPD or IGRA remains negative at 2–3 mo and child remains well, consider stopping empiric therapy. However, tests at 2–3 mo may not be reliable in immunocompromised patients. This regimen is to prevent infection in a compromised host after exposure, rather than to treat latent asymptomatic infection.
	Scenario 2: Asymptomatic child is found to have a positive skin test/IGRA test for TB, documenting latent TB infection. INH 10–15 mg/kg PO qd for 9 mo (≥12 mo for an immunocompromised child) OR INH 20–30 mg/kg PO directly observed therapy twice weekly for 9 mo	Other options For INH intolerance or INH resistance if a direct contact can be tested: rifampin 10 mg/kg PO qd for 4 mo For children ≥12 y, can use once-weekly DOT with INH AND rifapentine for 12 wk; much less data for children 2–12 y[22]
Viral		
Herpes simplex virus		
During pregnancy	For women with recurrent genital herpes: acyclovir 400 mg PO bid; valacyclovir 500 mg PO qd OR 1-g PO qd from 36-wk gestation until delivery (CII)[23]	Development of neonatal HSV disease after maternal suppression has been documented.[24]

Neonatal: Primary or nonprimary maternal infection, neonate exposed at delivery[25]	Asymptomatic, exposed neonate: at 24 h of life, culture mucosal sites (see Comments), obtain CSF and whole-blood PCR for HSV DNA, obtain ALT, and start preemptive therapeutic acyclovir IV (60 mg/kg/day div q8h) for 10 days (AII). Some experts would evaluate at birth for exposure following presumed maternal primary infection and start preemptive therapy rather than wait 24 h.	Reference 21 provides a management algorithm that determines the type of maternal infection and, thus, the appropriate evaluation and preemptive therapy of the neonate. Mucosal sites for culture: conjunctivae, mouth, nasopharynx, rectum. Any symptomatic baby, at any time, requires a full evaluation for invasive infection and IV acyclovir therapy for 14–21 days, depending on extent of disease.
Neonatal: Recurrent maternal infection, neonate exposed at delivery[25]	Asymptomatic, exposed neonate: at 24 h of life, culture mucosal sites, obtain whole-blood PCR for HSV DNA. Hold on therapy unless cultures or PCR are positive, at which time the diagnostic evaluation should be completed (CSF PCR for HSV DNA, serum ALT) and preemptive therapeutic IV acyclovir (60 mg/kg/day div q8h) should be administered for 10 days (AIII).	Reference 21 provides a management algorithm that determines the type of maternal infection and, thus, the appropriate evaluation and preemptive therapy of the neonate. Mucosal sites for culture: conjunctivae, mouth, nasopharynx, rectum. Any symptomatic baby, at any time, requires a full evaluation for invasive infection and IV acyclovir therapy for 14–21 days, depending on extent of disease.
Neonatal: Following symptomatic disease, to prevent recurrence during first year of life[25] See page 245 in Table 14C.		
Keratitis (ocular) in otherwise healthy children See page 245 in Table 14C.		

Antimicrobial Prophylaxis/Prevention of Symptomatic Infection

Antimicrobial Prophylaxis/Prevention of Symptomatic Infection

A. POSTEXPOSURE ANTIMICROBIAL PROPHYLAXIS TO PREVENT INFECTION (continued)

Prophylaxis Category	Therapy (evidence grade)	Comments
Viral (continued)		
Influenza virus (A or B)[26]	Oseltamivir prophylaxis (AI) 3–≤8 mo: 3.0 mg/kg/dose qd for 10 days 9–11 mo: 3.5 mg/kg/dose PO qd for 10 days[27] Based on body weight for children ≥12 mo ≤15 kg: 30 mg qd for 10 days >15–23 kg: 45 mg qd for 10 days >23–40 kg: 60 mg qd for 10 days >40 kg: 75 mg qd for 10 days Zanamivir prophylaxis (AI) Children ≥5 y: 10 mg (two 5-mg inhalations) qd for as long as 28 days (community outbreaks) or 10 days (household settings)	Not recommended for infants 0 to ≤3 mo unless situation judged critical because of limited data on use and variability of drug exposure in this age group.
Rabies virus[28]	Rabies immune globulin, 20 IU/kg, infiltrate around wound, with remaining volume injected IM (AII) PLUS Rabies immunization (AII)	For dog, cat, or ferret bite from symptomatic animal, immediate rabies immune globulin and immunization; otherwise, can wait 10 days for observation of animal, if possible, prior to rabies immune globulin or vaccine. Bites of squirrels, hamsters, guinea pigs, gerbils, chipmunks, rats, mice and other rodents, rabbits, hares, and pikas almost never require antirabies prophylaxis. For bites of bats, skunks, raccoons, foxes, most other carnivores, and woodchucks, immediate rabies immune globulin and immunization (regard as rabid unless geographic area is known to be free of rabies or until animal proven negative by laboratory tests).

14

Fungal

Pneumocystis jiroveci (previously *Pneumocystis carinii*)[29,30]	TMP/SMX as 5 mg TMP/kg/day PO, div 2 doses, q12h, either qd or 3 times/wk on consecutive days (AI); OR TMP/SMX 5 mg TMP/kg/day PO as a *single dose*, qd, given 3 times/wk on consecutive days (AI) (once-weekly regimens have also been successful); OR dapsone 2 mg/kg (max 100 mg) PO qd, or 4 mg/kg (max 200 mg) once weekly; OR atovaquone 30 mg/kg/day for infants 1–3 mo; 45 mg/kg/day for infants/children 4–24 mo; and 30 mg/kg/day for children >24 mo until no longer immunocompromised, based on oncology or transplant treatment regimen	Prophylaxis in specific populations based on degree of immunosuppression

Antimicrobial Prophylaxis/Prevention of Symptomatic Infection

14

B. LONG-TERM ANTIMICROBIAL PROPHYLAXIS TO PREVENT SYMPTOMATIC NEW INFECTION

Prophylaxis Category	Therapy (evidence grade)	Comments
Bacterial otitis media[31,32]	Amoxicillin or other antibiotics can be used in half the therapeutic dose qd or bid to prevent infections if the benefits outweigh the risks of (1) development of resistant organisms for that child and (2) the risk of antibiotic side effects.	To prevent recurrent infections, also consider the risks and benefits of placing tympanostomy tubes to improve middle ear ventilation as an alternative to antibiotic prophylaxis. Studies have demonstrated that amoxicillin, sulfisoxazole, and TMP/SMX are effective. However, antimicrobial prophylaxis may alter the nasopharyngeal flora and foster colonization with resistant organisms, compromising long-term efficacy of the prophylactic drug. Continuous PO-administered antimicrobial prophylaxis should be reserved for control of recurrent acute otitis media, only when defined as ≥3 distinct and well-documented antimicrobial prophylaxis during a period of 6 mo or ≥4 episodes during a period of 12 mo. Although prophylactic administration of an antimicrobial agent limited to a period when a person is at high risk of otitis media has been suggested (eg, during acute viral respiratory tract infection), this method has not been evaluated critically.
Acute rheumatic fever	For >27.3 kg (>60 lb): 1.2 million U penicillin G benzathine, q4wk (q3wk for high-risk children) For <27.3 kg: 600,000 U penicillin G benzathine, q4wk (q3wk for high-risk children) OR Penicillin V (phenoxymethyl) oral, 250 mg PO bid	AHA policy statement at http://circ.ahajournals.org/content/119/11/1541.full.pdf (accessed October 4, 2017). Doses studied many years ago, with no new data; ARF is an uncommon disease currently in the United States. Alternatives to penicillin include sulfisoxazole or macrolides, including erythromycin, azithromycin, and clarithromycin.
Urinary tract infection, recurrent[33–36]	TMP/SMX 3 mg/kg/dose TMP PO QD OR nitrofurantoin 1–2 mg/kg PO qd at bedtime; more rapid resistance may develop using beta-lactams (BII).	Only for those with grade III–V reflux or with recurrent febrile UTI: prophylaxis no longer recommended for patients with grade I–II (some also exclude grade III) reflux and no evidence of renal damage. Prophylaxis prevents infection but may not prevent scarring. Early treatment of new infections is recommended for these children. Resistance eventually develops to every antibiotic; follow resistance patterns for each patient.

C. PROPHYLAXIS OF SYMPTOMATIC DISEASE IN CHILDREN WHO HAVE ASYMPTOMATIC INFECTION/LATENT INFECTION

Prophylaxis Category	Therapy (evidence grade)	Comments
Herpes simplex virus		
Neonatal: Following symptomatic disease, to prevent recurrence during first year after birth[25]	300 mg/m²/dose PO tid for 6 mo following cessation of IV acyclovir treatment of acute disease (AI)	Follow absolute neutrophil counts at 2 and 4 wk, then monthly during prophylactic/suppressive therapy.
Keratitis (ocular) in otherwise healthy children	Suppressive therapy for frequent recurrence (no pediatric data): 20 mg/kg/dose bid (up to 400 mg) for ≥1 y (AIII)	Based on data from adults. Anecdotally, some children may require tid dosing to prevent recurrences. Check for acyclovir resistance for those who relapse while on appropriate therapy. Suppression oftentimes required for many years. Watch for severe recurrence at conclusion of suppression.
Tuberculosis[20,21] (latent TB infection [asymptomatic infection], defined by a positive skin test or IGRA, with no clinical or x-ray evidence of active disease)	INH 10–15 mg/kg/day (max 300 mg) PO qd for 9 mo (12 mo for immunocompromised patients) (AII); treatment with INH at 20–30 mg twice weekly for 9 mo is also effective (AIII).	Single drug therapy if no clinical or radiographic evidence of active disease. For exposure to known INH-resistant but rifampin-susceptible strains, use rifampin 10 mg/kg PO qd for 6 mo (AIII). For children ≥12 y, can use once weekly DOT with INH AND rifapentine for 12 wk; much less data for children 2–12 y.[22] For exposure to multidrug-resistant strains, consult with TB specialist.

Antimicrobial Prophylaxis/Prevention of Symptomatic Infection

14

D. SURGICAL/PROCEDURE PROPHYLAXIS[37–45]

The CDC National Healthcare Safety Network uses a classification of surgical procedure-related wound infections based on an estimation of the load of bacterial contamination: Class I, clean; Class II, clean-contaminated; Class III, contaminated; Class IV, dirty/infected.[38,41] Other major factors creating risk for postoperative surgical site infection include the duration of surgery (a longer-duration operation, defined as one that exceeded the 75th percentile for a given procedure) and the medical comorbidities of the patient, as determined by an American Society of Anesthesiologists score of III, IV, or V (presence of severe systemic disease that results in functional limitations, is life-threatening, or is expected to preclude survival from the operation). The virulence/pathogenicity of bacteria inoculated and the presence of foreign debris/devitalized tissue/surgical material in the wound are also considered risk factors for infection.

For all categories of surgical prophylaxis, dosing recommendations are derived from (1) choosing agents based on the organisms likely to be responsible for inoculation of the surgical site; (2) giving the agents shortly before starting the operation to achieve appropriate serum and tissue exposures at the time of incision through the end of the procedure; (3) providing additional doses during the procedure at times based on the standard dosing guideline for that agent; and (4) stopping the agents at the end of the procedure but no longer than 24–48 h after the procedure.[39–42,44,45]

Procedure/Operation	Recommended Agents	Preoperative Dose	Re-dosing Interval (h) for Prolonged Surgery
Cardiovascular			
Cardiac	Cefazolin, OR	30 mg/kg	4
Staphylococcus epidermidis, Staphylococcus aureus, Corynebacterium spp	Vancomycin, if MRSA likely[42]	15 mg/kg	8
	Ampicillin/sulbactam if enteric Gram-negative bacilli a concern	50 mg/kg of ampicillin	3
Vascular	Cefazolin, OR	30 mg/kg	4
S epidermidis, S aureus, Corynebacterium spp, Gram-negative enteric bacilli, particularly for procedures in the groin	Vancomycin, if MRSA likely[42]	15 mg/kg	8

Thoracic (noncardiac)

Indication	Agent	Dose	Interval (h)
Lobectomy, video-assisted thoracoscopic surgery, thoracotomy (but no prophylaxis needed for simple chest tube placement for pneumothorax)	Cefazolin, OR	30 mg/kg	4
	Ampicillin/sulbactam if enteric Gram-negative bacilli a concern	50 mg/kg of ampicillin	3
	Vancomycin or clindamycin if drug allergy or MRSA likely[42]	15 mg/kg vancomycin	8
		10 mg/kg clindamycin	6

Gastrointestinal

Indication	Agent	Dose	Interval (h)
Gastroduodenal Enteric Gram-negative bacilli, respiratory tract Gram-positive cocci	Cefazolin	30 mg/kg	4
Biliary procedure, open Enteric Gram-negative bacilli, enterococci, *Clostridia*	Cefazolin, OR	30 mg/kg	4
	Cefoxitin	40 mg/kg	2
Appendectomy, non-perforated	Cefoxitin, OR	40 mg/kg	2
	Cefazolin and metronidazole	30 mg/kg cefazolin and 10 mg/kg metronidazole	4 for cefazolin 8 for metronidazole
Complicated appendicitis or other ruptured colorectal viscus Enteric Gram-negative bacilli, anaerobes. For complicated appendicitis, antibiotics provided to treat ongoing infection, rather than prophylaxis.	Cefazolin and metronidazole, OR	30 mg/kg cefazolin and 10 mg/kg metronidazole	4 for cefazolin 8 for metronidazole
	Cefoxitin, OR	40 mg/kg	2
	Ceftriaxone and metronidazole, OR	50 mg/kg ceftriaxone and 10 mg/kg metronidazole	12 for ceftriaxone 8 for metronidazole
	Ertapenem, OR	30 mg/kg	8
	Meropenem, OR	20 mg/kg	4
	Imipenem	20 mg/kg	4

D. SURGICAL/PROCEDURE PROPHYLAXIS[37-45] (continued)

Procedure/Operation	Recommended Agents	Preoperative Dose	Re-dosing Interval (h) for Prolonged Surgery
Genitourinary			
Cystoscopy (only requires prophylaxis for children with suspected active UTI or those having foreign material placed)	Cefazolin, OR	30 mg/kg	4
	TMP/SMX (if low local resistance), OR	4–5 mg/kg	N/A
Enteric Gram-negative bacilli, enterococci	Select a 3rd-generation cephalosporin (cefotaxime) or fluoroquinolone (ciprofloxacin) if the child is colonized with cefazolin-resistant, TMP/SMX-resistant strains.		
Open or laparoscopic surgery Enteric Gram-negative bacilli, enterococci	Cefazolin	30 mg/kg	4
Head and Neck Surgery			
Assuming incision through respiratory tract mucosa	Clindamycin, OR	10 mg/kg	6
Anaerobes, enteric Gram-negative bacilli, S aureus	Cefazolin and metronidazole	30 mg/kg cefazolin and 10 mg/kg metronidazole	4 for cefazolin 8 for metronidazole
	Ampicillin/sulbactam if enteric Gram-negative bacilli a concern	50 mg/kg of ampicillin	3
Neurosurgery			
Craniotomy, ventricular shunt placement	Cefazolin, OR	30 mg/kg	4
S epidermidis, S aureus	Vancomycin, if MRSA likely	15 mg/kg	8

Orthopedic			
Internal fixation of fractures, spinal rod placement,[43] prosthetic joints S epidermidis, S aureus	Cefazolin, OR	30 mg/kg	4
	Vancomycin, if MRSA likely[42]	15 mg/kg	8
Trauma			
Exceptionally varied; no prospective, comparative data in children; agents should focus on skin flora (S epidermidis, S aureus) as well as the flora inoculated into the wound, that may include enteric Gram-negative bacilli, anaerobes (including Clostridia spp), and fungi. Cultures at time of wound exploration are critical to focus therapy.	Cefazolin (for skin), OR	30 mg/kg	4
	Vancomycin (for skin), if MRSA likely, OR	15 mg/kg	8
	Meropenem OR imipenem (for anaerobes, including Clostridia spp, and non-fermenting Gram-negative bacilli), OR	20 mg/kg for either	4
	Gentamicin and metronidazole (for anaerobes, including Clostridia spp. and non-fermenting Gram-negative bacilli), OR	2.5 mg/kg gentamicin and 10 mg/kg metronidazole	6 for gentamicin 8 for metronidazole
	Piperacillin/tazobactam	100 mg/kg piperacillin component	2

Antimicrobial Prophylaxis/Prevention of Symptomatic Infection

14

15. Adverse Reactions to Antimicrobial Agents

A good rule of clinical practice is to be suspicious of an adverse drug reaction when a patient's clinical course deviates from the expected. This section focuses on reactions that may require close observation or laboratory monitoring because of their frequency or severity. For more detailed listings of reactions, review the US Food and Drug Administration (FDA)-approved package labels available at the National Library of Medicine (NLM) (http://dailymed.nlm.nih.gov, accessed October 3, 2017), with the more recently approved agents actually having adverse events listed for the new agent and the comparator agent from the phase 3 prospective clinical trials. This allows one to assign drug-attributable side effects for specific drugs, such as oseltamivir, used for influenza, when influenza and the antiviral may both cause nausea. The NLM also provides an online drug information service for patients (MedlinePlus) at www.nlm.nih.gov/medlineplus/druginformation.html (accessed October 3, 2017).

Antibacterial Drugs

Aminoglycosides. Any of the aminoglycosides can cause serious nephrotoxicity and ototoxicity. Monitor all patients receiving aminoglycoside therapy for more than a few days for renal function with periodic determinations of blood urea nitrogen and creatinine to assess potential problems of drug accumulation with deteriorating renal function. Common practice has been to measure the peak serum concentration 0.5 to 1 hour after a dose to make sure one is in a therapeutic range and to measure a trough serum concentration immediately preceding a dose to assess for drug accumulation and pending toxicity. Monitoring is especially important in patients with any degree of renal insufficiency. Elevated trough concentrations (>2 mg/mL for gentamicin and tobramycin; >10 mg/mL for amikacin) suggest drug accumulation and should be a warning to decrease the dose, even if the peak is not yet elevated. Renal toxicity may be related to the total exposure of the kidney to the aminoglycoside over time. With once-daily administration regimens, peak values are 2 to 3 times greater, and trough values are usually very low. Nephrotoxicity is less common in adults with once-daily (as opposed to 3 times daily) dosing regimens, but data are generally lacking in children.[1-3] In patients with cystic fibrosis with pulmonary exacerbations, once-daily aminoglycosides appear less toxic and equally effective.[4]

The "loop" diuretics (furosemide and bumetanide) and other nephrotoxic drugs may potentiate the ototoxicity of the aminoglycosides. Aminoglycosides potentiate botulinum toxin neuromuscular junction dysfunction and are to be avoided in young infants with infant botulism.

Minor side effects, such as allergies, rashes, and drug fever, are rare.

Beta-lactam Antibiotics. The most feared reaction to penicillins, anaphylactic shock, is extremely rare, and no absolutely reliable means of predicting its occurrence exists. For most infections, alternative therapy to penicillin or beta-lactams exists. However, in certain situations, the benefits of penicillin or a beta-lactam may outweigh the risk of anaphylaxis, requiring that skin testing and desensitization be performed in a medically supervised environment. The commercially available skin testing material, benzylpenicilloyl polylysine (Pre-Pen, AllerQuest), contains the major determinants thought to be primarily responsible for urticarial reactions but does not contain the minor determinants that are more often associated with anaphylaxis. No commercially available minor determinant mixture is available. For adults, the Centers for Disease Control and Prevention (CDC) suggests using a dilute solution of freshly prepared benzyl penicillin G as the skin test material in place of a standardized mixture of minor determinants.[5] Testing should be performed on children with a credible history of a possible reaction to a penicillin before these drugs are used in oral or parenteral formulations. Anaphylaxis has been reported in adults receiving penicillin skin testing. Recent reviews provide more in-depth discussion,[6,7] with additional information on desensitization available in the CDC "Sexually Transmitted Diseases Treatment Guidelines, 2015."[5] Cross-reactions between classes of beta-lactam antibiotics (penicillins, cephalosporins, carbapenems, and monobactams) occur at a rate of less than 5% to 20%, with the rate of reaction to cephalosporins in patients with a *history* of penicillin allergy of about 0.1%.[8] No commercially available skin-testing reagent has been developed for beta-lactam antibiotics other than penicillin.

Amoxicillin and other aminopenicillins are associated with minor adverse effects. Diarrhea, oral or diaper-area candidiasis, morbilliform, and blotchy rashes are not uncommon. The kinds of non-urticarial rashes that may occur while a child is receiving amoxicillin are not known to predispose to anaphylaxis and may not actually be caused by amoxicillin itself; they do not represent a routine contraindication to subsequent use of amoxicillin or any other penicillins. Rarely, beta-lactams cause serious, life-threatening pseudomembranous enterocolitis due to suppression of normal bowel flora and overgrowth of toxin-producing strains of *Clostridium difficile*. Drug-related fever may occur; serum sickness is uncommon. Reversible neutropenia and thrombocytopenia may occur with any of the beta-lactams and seem to be related to dose and duration of therapy, but the neutropenia does not appear to carry the same risk of bacterial superinfection that is present with neutropenia in oncology patients.

The cephalosporins have been a remarkably safe series of antibiotics. Third-generation cephalosporins cause profound alteration of normal flora on mucosal surfaces, and all have caused pseudomembranous colitis on occasion. Ceftriaxone commonly causes loose stools, but it is rarely severe enough to require stopping therapy. Ceftriaxone in high dosages may cause fine "sand" (a calcium complex of ceftriaxone) to develop in the gallbladder. In adults, and rarely in children, these deposits may cause biliary tract symptoms; these are not gallstones, and the deposits are reversible after stopping the drug. In neonates receiving calcium-containing hyperalimentation concurrent with intravenous (IV) ceftriaxone, precipitation of ceftriaxone-calcium in the bloodstream resulting in death has been reported,[9] leading to an FDA warning against the concurrent use of ceftriaxone and parenteral calcium in neonates younger than 28 days. As ceftriaxone may also displace bilirubin from albumin-binding sites and increase free bilirubin in serum, the antibiotic is not routinely used in neonatal infections until the normal physiologic jaundice is resolving after the first few weeks of life. Cefotaxime is the preferred IV third-generation cephalosporin for neonates.

Imipenem/cilastatin, meropenem, and ertapenem have rates of adverse effects on hematopoietic, hepatic, and renal systems that are similar to other beta-lactams. However, children treated with imipenem for bacterial meningitis were noted to have an increase in probable drug-related seizures not seen with meropenem therapy in controlled studies.[10] For children requiring carbapenem therapy, meropenem is preferred for those with any underlying central nervous system inflammatory condition.

Fluoroquinolones (FQs). All quinolone antibiotics (nalidixic acid, ciprofloxacin, levofloxacin, gatifloxacin, and moxifloxacin) cause cartilage damage to weight-bearing joints in toxicity studies in various immature animals; however, no conclusive data indicate similar toxicity in young children.[11] Studies to evaluate cartilage toxicity and failure to achieve predicted growth have not consistently found statistically significant differences between those children treated with FQs and controls, although in an FDA-requested, blinded, prospective study of complicated urinary tract infections (2004), the number of muscular/joint/tendon events was greater in the ciprofloxacin-treated group than in the comparator (www.fda.gov/downloads/Drugs/DevelopmentApprovalProcess/DevelopmentResources/UCM162536.pdf, accessed October 3, 2017). This continues to be an area of active investigation by the pediatric infectious disease community as well as the FDA. Fluoroquinolone toxicities in adults, which vary in incidence considerably between individual agents, include cardiac dysrhythmias, hepatotoxicity, and photodermatitis; other reported side effects include gastrointestinal symptoms, dizziness, headaches, tremors, confusion, seizures, and alterations of glucose metabolism producing hyperglycemia and hypoglycemia. The American Academy of Pediatrics published a clinical report and a 2016 update on the use of fluoroquinolones and, based on the best available evidence, concluded that IV fluoroquinolones should be used when safer IV antibiotic alternatives were not available and that oral fluoroquinolones should be used if no other safe and effective *oral* therapy existed, even if effective alternative IV therapy existed.[12]

Lincosamides. Clindamycin can cause nausea, vomiting, and diarrhea. Pseudomembranous colitis due to suppression of normal flora and overgrowth of *C difficile* is uncommon, especially in children, but potentially serious. Urticaria, glossitis, pruritus, and skin rashes occur occasionally. Serum sickness, anaphylaxis, and photosensitivity are rare, as are hematologic and hepatic abnormalities. Extensive use of clindamycin since 2000 for treatment of community-associated methicillin-resistant *Staphylococcus aureus* infections has not been accompanied by reports of substantially increasing rates of *C difficile*–mediated colitis in children, although rates of colitis are being watched carefully.

Macrolides. Erythromycin is one of the safest antimicrobial agents but has largely been replaced by azithromycin because of substantially decreased epigastric distress and nausea. Intravenous erythromycin lactobionate causes phlebitis and should be administered slowly (1–2 hours); the gastrointestinal side effects seen with oral administration also accompany IV use. However, IV azithromycin is better tolerated than IV erythromycin and has been evaluated for pharmacokinetics in limited numbers of children.[13]

Erythromycin therapy has been associated with pyloric stenosis in newborns and young infants; due to this toxicity and with limited data on safety of azithromycin in the first months of life (with a few reports of pyloric stenosis), azithromycin is now the preferred macrolide for treatment of pertussis in neonates and young infants.[14]

Oxazolidinones. Linezolid represents the first oxazolidinone antibiotic approved for all children, including neonates, by the FDA. Toxicity is primarily hematologic, with thrombocytopenia and neutropenia that is dependent on dosage and duration of therapy, occurring most often with treatment courses of 2 weeks or longer. Routine monitoring for bone marrow toxicity every 1 to 2 weeks is recommended for children on long-term therapy. Peripheral neuropathy and optic neuritis may also occur with long-term therapy.[15] Tedizolid, approved for adults and now being investigated in children, appears to have a better safety profile compared with linezolid.

Sulfonamides and Trimethoprim. The most common adverse reaction to sulfonamides is a hypersensitivity rash. Stevens-Johnson syndrome, a life-threatening systemic reaction characterized by immune-mediated injury to the skin and mucous membranes, occurs in approximately 3 of 100,000 exposed people. Neutropenia, anemia, and thrombocytopenia occur occasionally. Sulfa drugs can precipitate hemolysis in patients with glucose-6-phosphate dehydrogenase deficiency. Drug fever and serum sickness are infrequent hypersensitivity reactions. Hepatitis with focal or diffuse necrosis is rare. A rare idiosyncratic reaction to sulfa drugs is acute aseptic meningitis.

Tetracyclines. Tetracyclines are used infrequently in pediatric patients because the major indications are uncommon diseases (rickettsial infections, brucellosis, Lyme disease), with the exception of acne. Tetracyclines are deposited in growing bones and teeth, with depression of linear bone growth, dental staining, and defects in enamel formation in deciduous and permanent teeth. This effect is dose related, and the risk extends up to 8 years of age. A single treatment course of tetracyclines has not been found to cause dental staining, leading to the recommendation for tetracyclines as the drugs of choice in children for a number of uncommon pathogens. **Doxycycline produces less dental staining than tetracycline.** A parenteral tetracycline approved for adults in 2005, tigecycline, produces the same "staining" of bones in experimental animals as seen with other tetracyclines and, therefore, did not undergo clinical investigation in children.

Side effects include minor gastrointestinal disturbances, photosensitization, angioedema, glossitis, pruritus ani, and exfoliative dermatitis. Potential adverse drug reactions from tetracyclines involve virtually every organ system. Hepatic and pancreatic injuries have occurred with accidental overdosage and in patients with renal failure. (Pregnant women are particularly at risk for hepatic injury.)

Vancomycin. Vancomycin can cause phlebitis if the drug is injected rapidly or in concentrated form. Vancomycin has the potential for ototoxicity and nephrotoxicity, and serum concentrations should be monitored for children on more than a few days of therapy. Hepatic toxicity is rare. Neutropenia has been reported. If the drug is infused too rapidly, a transient rash of the upper body with itching may occur from histamine release (red man syndrome). It is not a contraindication to continued use and the rash is less likely to occur if the infusion period is increased to 60 to 120 minutes and children are pretreated with oral or IV antihistamines.

Daptomycin. This antibiotic is now FDA approved in children down to 1 year of age (due to concerns for neurologic toxicity in a neonatal animal model, daptomycin was not studied in infants younger than 1 year, although small clinical series in younger infants have been published with no obvious safety concerns). Published data do not indicate adverse events that occur in children that have not been reported in adults. Specifically, no significant drug-attributable muscle toxicity or elevated creatine kinase concentrations have been reported. No neurologic toxicity was noted in global studies of skin infections or in global studies of pediatric osteomyelitis. The full safety profile is available on the current FDA-approved package label (https://dailymed.nlm.nih.gov/dailymed/index.cfm, accessed October 3, 2017). Daptomycin should be used with caution in infants younger than 1 year.

Antituberculous Drugs

Isoniazid (INH) is generally well tolerated and hypersensitivity reactions are rare. Peripheral neuritis (preventable or reversed by pyridoxine administration) and mental aberrations from euphoria to psychosis occur more often in adults than in children. Mild elevations of alanine transaminase in the first weeks of therapy, which disappear or remain stable with continued administration, are common. Rarely, hepatitis develops but is reversible if INH is stopped; if INH is not stopped, liver failure may develop in these children. Monitoring of liver functions is not routinely required in children receiving INH single drug therapy for latent tuberculosis as long as the children can be followed closely and liver functions can be drawn if the children develop symptoms of hepatitis.

Rifampin can also cause hepatitis; it is more common in patients with preexisting liver disease or in those taking large dosages. The risk of hepatic damage increases when rifampin and INH are taken together in dosages of more than 15 mg/kg/day of each. Gastrointestinal, hematologic, and neurologic side effects of various types have been observed on occasion. Hypersensitivity reactions are rare.

Pyrazinamide also can cause hepatic damage, which again seems to be dosage related. Ethambutol has the potential for optic neuritis, but this toxicity seems to be rare in children at currently prescribed dosages. Young children who cannot comment to examiners about color blindness or other signs of optic neuritis should be considered for an ophthalmologic examination every few months on therapy. Optic neuritis is usually reversible.

Adverse Reactions to Antimicrobial Agents

15

Antifungal Drugs

Amphotericin B (deoxycholate) causes chills, fever, flushing, and headaches, the most common of the many adverse reactions. Some degree of decreased renal function occurs in virtually all patients given amphotericin B. Anemia is common and, rarely, hepatic toxicity and neutropenia occur. Patients should be monitored for hyponatremia, hypomagnesemia, and hypokalemia. However, much better tolerated (but costlier) lipid formulations of amphotericin B are now commonly used (see Chapter 2). For reasons of safety and tolerability, the lipid formulations should be used whenever possible, except in neonates, who appear to tolerate amphotericin better than older children.

Fluconazole is usually very well tolerated from clinical and laboratory standpoints. Gastrointestinal symptoms, rash, and headache occur occasionally. Transient, asymptomatic elevations of hepatic enzymes have been reported but are rare.

Voriconazole may interfere with metabolism of other drugs the child may be receiving due to hepatic P450 metabolism. However, a poorly understood visual field abnormality has been described, usually at the beginning of a course of therapy and uniformly self-resolving, in which objects appear to the child to glow. There is no pain and no known anatomic or biochemical correlate of this side effect; lasting effects on vision have been sought, but none have yet been reported. Hepatic toxicity has also been reported but is not so common as to preclude the use of voriconazole for serious fungal infections. Phototoxic skin reaction with chronic use that has been reported to develop into carcinoma is another common reason for discontinuation.[16,17]

Caspofungin, micafungin, and anidulafungin (echinocandins) are very well tolerated as a class. Fever, rash, headache, and phlebitis at the site of infection have been reported in adults. Uncommon hepatic side effects have also been reported.

Flucytosine (5-FC) is seldom used due to the availability of safer, equally effective therapy. The major toxicity is bone marrow depression, which is dosage related, especially in patients treated concomitantly with amphotericin B. Flucytosine serum concentrations and renal function should be monitored.

Antiviral Drugs

After extensive clinical use, acyclovir has proved to be an extremely safe drug with only rare serious adverse effects. Renal dysfunction with IV acyclovir has occurred mainly with too rapid infusion of the drug. Neutropenia has been associated with administration of parenteral and oral acyclovir but is responsive to granulocyte colony-stimulating factor use and resolves spontaneously when the drug is stopped. At very high doses, parenteral acyclovir can cause neurologic irritation, including seizures. Rash, headache, and gastrointestinal side effects are uncommon. There has been little controlled experience in children with famciclovir and valacyclovir.

Ganciclovir causes hematologic toxicity that is dependent on the dosage and duration of therapy. Gastrointestinal disturbances and neurologic damage are rarely encountered. Oral valganciclovir can have these same toxicities as parenteral ganciclovir, but neutropenia is seen much less frequently following oral valganciclovir compared with IV ganciclovir. In preclinical test systems, ganciclovir (and, therefore, valganciclovir) is mutagenic, carcinogenic, and teratogenic. Additionally, it causes irreversible reproductive toxicity in animals.

Oseltamivir is well tolerated except for nausea with or without vomiting, which may be more likely to occur with the first few doses but usually resolves within a few days while still on therapy. Neuropsychiatric events have been reported, primarily from Japan, in patients with influenza treated with oseltamivir (a rate of approximately 1:50,000) but also are seen in patients on all the other influenza antivirals and in patients with influenza receiving no antiviral therapy. It seems that these spontaneously reported side effects may be a function of influenza itself and/or, possibly, a genetic predisposition to this clinical event.

Experience with peramivir in pediatric patients is limited. Adverse events associated with the administration of peramivir are diarrhea, nausea, vomiting, and decreased neutrophil count. Other, less common adverse events observed in studies to date include dizziness, headache, somnolence, nervousness, insomnia, agitation, depression, nightmares, hyperglycemia, hyperbilirubinemia, elevated blood pressure, cystitis, anorexia, and proteinuria.

Foscarnet can cause renal dysfunction, anemia, and cardiac rhythm disturbances. Alterations in plasma minerals and electrolytes occur, and any clinically significant metabolic changes should be corrected. Patients who experience mild (eg, perioral numbness or paresthesia) or severe (eg, seizures) symptoms of electrolyte abnormalities should have serum electrolyte and mineral levels assessed as close in time to the event as possible.

The primary adverse event with cidofovir is nephrotoxicity. Cidofovir concentrates in renal cells in amounts 100 times greater than in other tissues, producing severe nephrotoxicity involving the proximal convoluted tubule when concomitant hydration and administration of probenecid are not employed. Renal toxicity manifests as proteinuria and glycosuria. To decrease the potential for nephrotoxicity, aggressive IV prehydration and coadministration of probenecid are required with each cidofovir dose. In animal studies, cidofovir has been shown to be carcinogenic and teratogenic and to cause hypospermia. Intravitreal administration has been associated with ocular hypotony.

Experience with the newer hepatitis C antiviral agents is limited in the pediatric population. What is known to date is from use in adults. More common adverse events with dasabuvir co-packaged with ombitasvir/paritaprevir/ritonavir are fatigue, nausea, pruritus, other skin reactions, insomnia, and asthenia. Dasabuvir co-packaged with ombitasvir/paritaprevir/ritonavir has numerous medication contraindications, primarily because of the potent ritonavir inhibition of the cytochrome P450 (CYP) 3A4 enzyme. The most common adverse effects attributable to simeprevir are rash (including a potentially serious photosensitivity reaction), pruritus, and nausea; the photosensitivity reaction will usually start within the first 4 weeks of therapy but can

Adverse Reactions to Antimicrobial Agents

15

develop at any time during treatment. If a photosensitivity rash does occur while taking simeprevir, discontinuation of simeprevir should be considered, and the patient should have close monitoring until the rash has resolved. Due to its metabolism via CYP3A enzymes, administering simeprevir with medications that have moderate or strong induction of CYP3A, such as rifampin, St John's wort, and most anticonvulsants, may significantly reduce levels of simeprevir. In contrast, medications that have moderate or strong inhibition of CYP3A enzymes, such as clarithromycin, ketoconazole, and ritonavir, may significantly increase levels of simeprevir. Common adverse events with sofosbuvir treatment are fatigue (when used with ribavirin) and anemia, neutropenia, insomnia, headache, and nausea (when used with peg interferon and ribavirin). Increases in bilirubin, creatinine kinase, and lipase can occur. With ledipasvir, headache and fatigue are common adverse events, and elevated bilirubin and lipase can occur. Sofosbuvir/ledipasvir has significant drug-drug interactions with P-glycoprotein inducers (eg, St John's wort, rifampin), causing decreases in ledipasvir and sofosbuvir plasma concentrations.

Appendix

Nomogram for Determining Body Surface Area

Based on the nomogram shown below, a straight line joining the patient's height and weight will intersect the center column at the calculated body surface area (BSA). For children of normal height and weight, the child's weight in pounds is used, and then the examiner reads across to the corresponding BSA in meters. Alternatively, Mosteller's formula can be used.

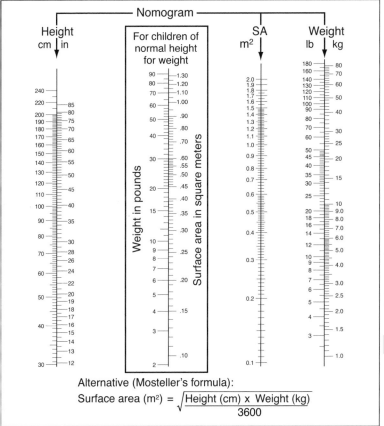

Alternative (Mosteller's formula):

$$\text{Surface area (m}^2\text{)} = \sqrt{\frac{\text{Height (cm)} \times \text{Weight (kg)}}{3600}}$$

Nomogram and equation to determine body surface area. (From Engorn B, Flerlage J, eds. *The Harriet Lane Handbook*. 20th ed. Philadelphia, PA: Elsevier Mosby; 2015. Reprinted with permission from Elsevier.)

Appendix: Nomogram for Determining Body Surface Area

References

Chapter 1

1. Cannavino CR, et al. *Pediatr Infect Dis J.* 2016;35(7):752–759 PMID: 27093162
2. Smyth AR, et al. *Cochrane Database Syst Rev.* 2017;3:CD002009 PMID: 28349527
3. Jackson MA, et al. *Pediatrics.* 2016;138(5):e20162706 PMID: 27940800
4. Bradley JS, et al. *Pediatrics.* 2014;134(1):e146–e153 PMID: 24918220

Chapter 2

1. Cornely OA, et al. *Clin Infect Dis.* 2007;44(10):1289–1297 PMID: 17443465
2. Lestner JM, et al. *Antimicrob Agents Chemother.* 2016;60(12):7340–7346 PMID: 27697762
3. Seibel NL, et al. *Antimicrob Agents Chemother.* 2017;61(2):e01477–16 PMID: 27855062
4. Azoulay E, et al. *PLoS One.* 2017;12(5):e0177093 PMID: 28531175
5. Ascher SB, et al. *Pediatr Infect Dis J.* 2012;31(5):439–443 PMID: 22189522
6. Piper L, et al. *Pediatr Infect Dis J.* 2011;30(5):375–378 PMID: 21085048
7. Watt KM, et al. *Antimicrob Agents Chemother.* 2015;59(7):3935–3943 PMID: 25896706
8. Friberg LE, et al. *Antimicrob Agents Chemother.* 2012;56(6):3032–3042 PMID: 22430956
9. Zembles TN, et al. *Pharmacotherapy.* 2016;36(10):1102–1108 PMID: 27548272
10. Moriyama B, et al. *Clin Pharmacol Ther.* 2016 PMID: 27981572
11. Maertens JA, et al. *Lancet.* 2016;387(10020):760–769 PMID: 26684607
12. Marty FM, et al. *Lancet Infect Dis.* 2016;16(7):828–837 PMID: 26969258
13. Smith PB, et al. *Pediatr Infect Dis J.* 2009;28(5):412–415 PMID: 19319022
14. Hope WW, et al. *Antimicrob Agents Chemother.* 2010;54(6):2633–2637 PMID: 20308367
15. Benjamin DK Jr, et al. *Clin Pharmacol Ther.* 2010;87(1):93–99 PMID: 19890251
16. Cohen-Wolkowiez M, et al. *Clin Pharmacol Ther.* 2011;89(5):702–707 PMID: 21412233

Chapter 4

1. Liu C, et al. *Clin Infect Dis.* 2011;52(3):e18–e55 PMID: 21208910
2. Le J, et al. *Pediatr Infect Dis J.* 2013;32(4):e155–e163 PMID: 23340565
3. McNeil JC, et al. *Pediatr Infect Dis J.* 2016;35(3):263–268 PMID: 26646549
4. Sader HS, et al. *Antimicrob Agents Chemother.* 2017;61(9):e01043-17 PMID: 28630196
5. Depardieu F, et al. *Clin Microbiol Rev.* 2007;20(1):79–114 PMID: 17223624
6. Miller LG, et al. *N Engl J Med.* 2015;372(12):1093–1103 PMID: 25785967
7. Bradley J, et al. *Pediatrics.* 2017;139(3):e20162477 PMID: 28202770
8. Korczowski B, et al. *Pediatr Infect Dis J.* 2016;35(8):e239–e247 PMID: 27164462
9. Cannavino CR, et al. *Pediatr Infect Dis J.* 2016;35(7):752–759 PMID: 27093162
10. Blumer JL, et al. *Pediatr Infect Dis J.* 2016;35(7):760–766 PMID: 27078119
11. Huang JT, et al. *Pediatrics.* 2009;123(5):808–814 PMID: 19403473
12. Finnell SM, et al. *Clin Pediatr (Phila).* 2015;54(5):445–450 PMID: 25385929
13. Creech CB, et al. *Infect Dis Clin North Am.* 2015;29(3):429–464 PMID: 26311356

Chapter 5

1. Fox E, et al. Drug therapy in neonates and pediatric patients. In: Atkinson AJ, et al, eds. *Principles of Clinical Pharmacology.* 2007:359–373
2. Wagner CL, et al. *J Perinatol.* 2000;20(6):346–350 PMID: 11002871
3. Bradley JS, et al. *Pediatrics.* 2009;123(4):e609–e613 PMID: 19289450
4. Martin E, et al. *Eur J Pediatr.* 1993;152(6):530–534 PMID: 8335024
5. Rours IG, et al. *Pediatrics.* 2008;121(2):e321–e326 PMID: 18245405
6. American Academy of Pediatrics. Chlamydial infections. In: Kimberlin DW, et al, eds. *Red Book: 2018 Report of the Committee on Infectious Diseases.* In press

7. Hammerschlag MR, et al. *Pediatr Infect Dis J.* 1998;17(11):1049–1050 PMID: 9849993

8. Zar HJ. *Paediatr Drugs.* 2005;7(2):103–110 PMID: 15871630

9. Honein MA, et al. *Lancet.* 1999;354(9196):2101–2105 PMID: 10609814

10. Laga M, et al. *N Engl J Med.* 1986;315(22):1382–1385 PMID: 3095641

11. Workowski KA, et al. *MMWR Recomm Rep.* 2015;64(RR-3):1–137 PMID: 26042815

12. Newman LM, et al. *Clin Infect Dis.* 2007;44(S3):S84–S101 PMID: 17342672

13. MacDonald N, et al. *Adv Exp Med Biol.* 2008;609:108–130 PMID: 18193661

14. American Academy of Pediatrics. Gonococcal infections. In: Kimberlin DW, et al, eds. *Red Book: 2018 Report of the Committee on Infectious Diseases.* In press

15. Cimolai N. *Am J Ophthalmol.* 2006;142(1):183–184 PMID: 16815280

16. Marangon FB, et al. *Am J Ophthalmol.* 2004;137(3):453–458 PMID: 15013867

17. American Academy of Pediatrics. Staphylococcal infections. In: Kimberlin DW, et al, eds. *Red Book: 2018 Report of the Committee on Infectious Diseases.* In press

18. Brito DV, et al. *Braz J Infect Dis.* 2003;7(4):234–235 PMID: 14533982

19. Chen CJ, et al. *Am J Ophthalmol.* 2008;145(6):966–970 PMID: 18378213

20. Shah SS, et al. *J Perinatol.* 1999;19(6pt1):462–465 PMID: 10685281

21. Kimberlin DW, et al. *J Pediatr.* 2003;143(1):16–25 PMID: 12915819

22. Kimberlin DW, et al. *J Infect Dis.* 2008;197(6):836–845 PMID: 18279073

23. American Academy of Pediatrics. Cytomegalovirus infection. In: Kimberlin DW, et al, eds. *Red Book: 2018 Report of the Committee on Infectious Diseases.* In press

24. Kimberlin DW, et al. *N Engl J Med.* 2015;372(10):933–943 PMID: 25738669

25. Rawlinson WD, et al. *Lancet Infect Dis.* 2017;17(6):e177–e188 PMID: 28291720

26. American Academy of Pediatrics. Candidiasis. In: Kimberlin DW, et al, eds. *Red Book: 2018 Report of the Committee on Infectious Diseases.* In press

27. Hundalani S, et al. *Expert Rev Anti Infect Ther.* 2013;11(7):709–721 PMID: 23829639

28. Saez-Llorens X, et al. *Antimicrob Agents Chemother.* 2009;53(3):869–875 PMID: 19075070

29. Ericson JE, et al. *Clin Infect Dis.* 2016;63(5):604–610 PMID: 27298330

30. Smith PB, et al. *Pediatr Infect Dis J.* 2009;28(5):412–415 PMID: 19319022

31. Wurthwein G, et al. *Antimicrob Agents Chemother.* 2005;49(12):5092–5098 PMID: 16304177

32. Heresi GP, et al. *Pediatr Infect Dis J.* 2006;25(12):1110–1115 PMID: 17133155

33. Kawaguchi C, et al. *Pediatr Int.* 2009;51(2):220–224 PMID: 19405920

34. Hsieh E, et al. *Early Hum Dev.* 2012;88(S2):S6–S10 PMID: 22633516

35. Swanson JR, et al. *Pediatr Infect Dis J.* 2016;35(5):519–523 PMID: 26835970

36. Santos RP, et al. *Pediatr Infect Dis J.* 2007;26(4):364–366 PMID: 17414408

37. Frankenbusch K, et al. *J Perinatol.* 2006;26(8):511–514 PMID: 16871222

38. Thomas L, et al. *Expert Rev Anti Infect Ther.* 2009;7(4):461–472 PMID: 19400765

39. Verweij PE, et al. *Drug Resist Updat.* 2015;21–22:30–40 PMID: 26282594

40. Shah D, et al. *Cochrane Database Syst Rev.* 2012;8:CD007448 PMID: 22895960

41. Brook I. *Am J Perinatol.* 2008;25(2):111–118 PMID: 18236362

42. Denkel LA, et al. *PLoS One.* 2016;11(6):e0158136 PMID: 27332554

43. Cohen-Wolkowiez M, et al. *Clin Infect Dis.* 2012;55(11):1495–1502 PMID: 22955430

44. Jost T, et al. *PLoS One.* 2012;7(8):e44595 PMID: 22957008

45. Dilli D, et al. *J Pediatr.* 2015;166(3):545–551 PMID: 25596096

46. American Academy of Pediatrics. *Salmonella* infections. In: Kimberlin DW, et al, eds. *Red Book: 2018 Report of the Committee on Infectious Diseases.* In press

47. Pinninti SG, et al. *Pediatr Clin North Am.* 2013;60(2):351–365 PMID: 23481105

48. American Academy of Pediatrics. Herpes simplex. In: Kimberlin DW, et al, eds. *Red Book: 2018 Report of the Committee on Infectious Diseases.* In press

49. Jones CA, et al. *Cochrane Database Syst Rev.* 2009;(3):CD004206 PMID: 19588350

50. Sampson MR, et al. *Pediatr Infect Dis J.* 2014;33(1):42–49 PMID: 24346595

51. Kimberlin DW, et al. *N Engl J Med.* 2011;365(14):1284–1292 PMID: 21991950

52. Panel on Antiretroviral Therapy and Medical Management of HIV-Infected Children. Guidelines for the use of antiretroviral agents in pediatric HIV infection. http://aidsinfo.nih.gov/ContentFiles/PediatricGuidelines.pdf. Updated April 27, 2017. Accessed October 11, 2017

53. Panel on Treatment of HIV-Infected Pregnant Women and Prevention of Perinatal Transmission. Recommendations for use of antiretroviral drugs in pregnant HIV-1-infected women for maternal health and interventions to reduce perinatal HIV transmission in the United States. http://aidsinfo.nih.gov/guidelines/html/3/perinatal-guidelines/0. Updated October 5, 2017. Accessed October 11, 2017

54. Luzuriaga K, et al. *N Engl J Med.* 2015;372(8):786–788 PMID: 25693029

55. Nielsen-Saines K, et al. *N Engl J Med.* 2012;366(25):2368–2379 PMID: 22716975

56. American Academy of Academy Committee on Infectious Diseases. *Pediatrics.* 2015;136(4):792–808 PMID: 26347430

57. Acosta EP, et al. *J Infect Dis.* 2010;202(4):563–566 PMID: 20594104

58. McPherson C, et al. *J Infect Dis.* 2012;206(6):847–850 PMID: 22807525

59. Kamal MA, et al. *Clin Pharmacol Ther.* 2014;96(3):380–389 PMID: 24865390

60. Kimberlin DW, et al. *J Infect Dis.* 2013;207(5):709–720 PMID: 23230059

61. Bradley JS, et al. *Pediatrics.* 2017;140(5):e20162727 PMID: 29051331

62. Fraser N, et al. *Acta Paediatr.* 2006;95(5):519–522 PMID: 16825129

63. Ulloa-Gutierrez R, et al. *Pediatr Emerg Care.* 2005;21(9):600–602 PMID: 16160666

64. Sawardekar KP. *Pediatr Infect Dis J.* 2004;23(1):22–26 PMID: 14743041

65. Bingol-Kologlu M, et al. *J Pediatr Surg.* 2007;42(11):1892–1897 PMID: 18022442

66. Brook I. *J Perinat Med.* 2002;30(3):197–208 PMID: 12122901

67. Kaplan SL. *Adv Exp Med Biol.* 2009;634:111–120 PMID: 19280383

68. Korakaki E, et al. *Jpn J Infect Dis.* 2007;60(2-3):129–131 PMID: 17515648

69. Dessi A, et al. *J Chemother.* 2008;20(5):542–550 PMID: 19028615

70. Berkun Y, et al. *Arch Dis Child.* 2008;93(8):690–694 PMID: 18337275

71. Greenberg D, et al. *Paediatr Drugs.* 2008;10(2):75–83 PMID: 18345717

72. Ismail EA, et al. *Pediatr Int.* 2013;55(1):60–64 PMID: 23039834

73. Engle WD, et al. *J Perinatol.* 2000;20(7):421–426 PMID: 11076325

74. Brook I. *Microbes Infect.* 2002;4(12):1271–1280 PMID: 12467770

75. Darville T. *Semin Pediatr Infect Dis.* 2005;16(4):235–244 PMID: 16210104

76. Eberly MD, et al. *Pediatrics.* 2015;135(3):483–488 PMID: 25687145

77. Waites KB, et al. *Semin Fetal Neonatal Med.* 2009;14(4):190–199 PMID: 19109084

78. Morrison W. *Pediatr Infect Dis J.* 2007;26(2):186–188 PMID: 17259889

79. American Academy of Pediatrics. Pertussis (whooping cough). In: Kimberlin DW, et al, eds. *Red Book: 2018 Report of the Committee on Infectious Diseases.* In press

80. Foca MD. *Semin Perinatol.* 2002;26(5):332–339 PMID: 12452505

81. American Academy of Pediatrics Committee on Infectious Diseases and Bronchiolitis Guidelines Committee. *Pediatrics.* 2014;134(2):e620–e638 PMID: 25070304

82. Banerji A, et al. *CMAJ Open.* 2016;4(4):E623–E633 PMID: 28443266

83. Borse RH, et al. *J Pediatric Infec Dis Soc.* 2014;3(3):201–212 PMID: 26625383

84. Vergnano S, et al. *Pediatr Infect Dis J.* 2011;30(10):850–854 PMID: 21654546

85. Nelson MU, et al. *Semin Perinatol.* 2012;36(6):424–430 PMID: 23177801

86. Lyseng-Williamson KA, et al. *Paediatr Drugs.* 2003;5(6):419–431 PMID: 12765493

87. American Academy of Pediatrics. Group B streptococcal infections. In: Kimberlin DW, et al, eds. *Red Book: 2018 Report of the Committee on Infectious Diseases.* In press

88. Schrag S, et al. *MMWR Recomm Rep.* 2002;51(RR-11):1–22 PMID: 12211284

89. American Academy of Pediatrics. *Ureaplasma urealyticum* and *Ureaplasma parvum* infections. In: Kimberlin DW, et al, eds. *Red Book: 2018 Report of the Committee on Infectious Diseases.* In press

90. Merchan LM, et al. *Antimicrob Agents Chemother.* 2015;59(1):570–578 PMID: 25385115

91. American Academy of Pediatrics. *Escherichia coli* and other gram-negative bacilli. In: Kimberlin DW, et al, eds. *Red Book: 2018 Report of the Committee on Infectious Diseases.* In press

92. Venkatesh MP, et al. *Expert Rev Anti Infect Ther.* 2008;6(6):929–938 PMID: 19053905

93. Abzug MJ, et al. *J Pediatric Infect Dis Soc.* 2016;5(1):53–62 PMID: 26407253

94. American Academy of Pediatrics. *Listeria monocytogenes* infections. In: Kimberlin DW, et al, eds. *Red Book: 2018 Report of the Committee on Infectious Diseases.* In press

95. Fortunov RM, et al. *Pediatrics.* 2006;118(3):874–881 PMID: 16950976

96. Fortunov RM, et al. *Pediatrics.* 2007;120(5):937–945 PMID: 17974729

References

97. van der Lugt NM, et al. *BMC Pediatr.* 2010;10:84 PMID: 21092087
98. Stauffer WM, et al. *Pediatr Emerg Care.* 2003;19(3):165–166 PMID: 12813301
99. Kaufman DA, et al. *Clin Infect Dis.* 2017;64(10):1387–1395 PMID: 28158439
100. Dehority W, et al. *Pediatr Infect Dis J.* 2006;25(11):1080–1081 PMID: 17072137
101. American Academy of Pediatrics. Syphilis. In: Kimberlin DW, et al, eds. *Red Book: 2018 Report of the Committee on Infectious Diseases.* In press
102. American Academy of Pediatrics. Tetanus. In: Kimberlin DW, et al, eds. *Red Book: 2018 Report of the Committee on Infectious Diseases.* In press
103. American Academy of Pediatrics. *Toxoplasma gondii* infections. In: Kimberlin DW, et al, eds. *Red Book: 2018 Report of the Committee on Infectious Diseases.* In press
104. Petersen E. Toxoplasmosis. *Semin Fetal Neonatal Med.* 2007;12(3):214–223 PMID: 17321812
105. Beetz R. *Curr Opin Pediatr.* 2012;24(2):205–211 PMID: 22227782
106. RIVUR Trial Investigators, et al. *N Engl J Med.* 2014;370(25):2367–2376 PMID: 24795142
107. Sahin L, et al. *Clin Pharmacol Ther.* 2016;100(1):23–25 PMID: 27082701
108. Roberts SW, et al. Placental transmission of antibiotics. In: *Glob Libr Women's Med.* DOI 10.3843/GLOWM.10174
109. Nanovskaya TN, et al. *J Matern Fetal Neonatal Med.* 2012;25(11):2312–2315 PMID: 22590979
110. Nanovskaya T, et al. *Am J Obstet Gynecol.* 2012;207(4):331.e1–331.e6 PMID: 22867688
111. Sachs HC, et al. *Pediatrics.* 2013;132(3):e796–e809 PMID: 23979084
112. Hale TW. *Medication and Mothers' Milk: A Manual of Lactational Pharmacology.* 16th ed. 2014

Chapter 6

1. Stevens DL, et al. *Clin Infect Dis.* 2014;59(2):147–159 PMID: 24947530
2. Liu C, et al. *Clin Infect Dis.* 2011;52(3):e18–e55 PMID: 21208910
3. Elliott DJ, et al. *Pediatrics.* 2009;123(6):e959–e966 PMID: 19470505
4. Walker PC, et al. *Laryngoscope.* 2013;123(1):249–252 PMID: 22952027
5. Martinez-Aguilar G, et al. *Pediatr Infect Dis J.* 2003;22(7):593–598 PMID: 12867833
6. American Academy of Pediatrics. Staphylococcal infections. In: Kimberlin DW, et al, eds. *Red Book: 2018 Report of the Committee on Infectious Diseases.* In press
7. American Academy of Pediatrics. Group A streptococcal infections. In: Kimberlin DW, et al, eds. *Red Book: 2018 Report of the Committee on Infectious Diseases.* In press
8. Bass JW, et al. *Pediatr Infect Dis J.* 1998;17(6):447–452 PMID: 9655532
9. Hatzenbuehler LA, et al. *Pediatr Infect Dis J.* 2014;33(1):89–91 PMID: 24346597
10. Lindeboom JA. *J Oral Maxillofac Surg.* 2012;70(2):345–348 PMID: 21741739
11. Wallace RJ Jr, et al. *Chest.* 2014;146(2):276–282 PMID: 24457542
12. Lindeboom JA. *Clin Infect Dis.* 2011;52(2):180–184 PMID: 21288841
13. Nahid P, et al. *Clin Infect Dis.* 2016;63(7):e147–e195 PMID: 27516382
14. American Academy of Pediatrics. Tuberculosis. In: Kimberlin DW, et al, eds. *Red Book: 2018 Report of the Committee on Infectious Diseases.* In press
15. Bradley JS, et al. *Pediatrics.* 2014;133(5):e1411–e1436 PMID: 24777226
16. Oehler RL, et al. *Lancet Infect Dis.* 2009;9(7):439–447 PMID: 19555903
17. Thomas N, et al. *Expert Rev Anti Infect Ther.* 2011;9(2):215–226 PMID: 21342069
18. Lion C, et al. *Int J Antimicrob Agents.* 2006;27(4):290–293 PMID: 16564680
19. Aziz H, et al. *J Trauma Acute Care Surg.* 2015;78(3):641–648 PMID: 25710440
20. Talan DA, et al. *N Engl J Med.* 1999;340(2):85–92 PMID: 9887159
21. Goldstein EJ, et al. *Antimicrob Agents Chemother.* 2012;56(12):6319–6323 PMID: 23027193
22. American Academy of Pediatrics. Rabies. In: Kimberlin DW, et al, eds. *Red Book: 2018 Report of the Committee on Infectious Diseases.* In press
23. Talan DA, et al. *Clin Infect Dis.* 2003;37(11):1481–1489 PMID: 14614671
24. Miller LG, et al. *N Engl J Med.* 2015;372(12):1093–1103 PMID: 25785967
25. Talan DA, et al. *N Engl J Med.* 2016;374(9):823–832 PMID: 26962903
26. Moran GJ, et al. *JAMA.* 2017;317(20):2088–2096 PMID: 28535235
27. American Academy of Pediatrics. *Haemophilus influenzae* infections. In: Kimberlin DW, et al, eds. *Red Book: 2018 Report of the Committee on Infectious Diseases.* In press

28. Ferreira A, et al. *Infection*. 2016;44(5):607–615 PMID: 27085865
29. Koning S, et al. *Cochrane Database Syst Rev*. 2012;1:CD003261 PMID: 22258953
30. Bass JW, et al. *Pediatr Infect Dis J*. 1997;16(7):708–710 PMID: 9239775
31. Lin HW, et al. *Clin Pediatr (Phila)*. 2009;48(6):583–587 PMID: 19286617
32. Pannaraj PS, et al. *Clin Infect Dis*. 2006;43(8):953–960 PMID: 16983604
33. Smith-Slatas CL, et al. *Pediatrics*. 2006;117(4):e796–e805 PMID: 16567392
34. Jamal N, et al. *Pediatr Emerg Care*. 2011;27(12):1195–1199 PMID: 22158285
35. Stevens DL. *Annu Rev Med*. 2000;51:271–288 PMID: 10774464
36. Abuhammour W, et al. *Pediatr Emerg Care*. 2006;22(1):48–51 PMID: 16418613
37. Levett D, et al. *Cochrane Database Syst Rev*. 2015;1:CD007937 PMID: 25879088
38. Daum RS. *N Engl J Med*. 2007;357(4):380–390 PMID: 17652503
39. Lee MC, et al. *Pediatr Infect Dis J*. 2004;23(2):123–127 PMID: 14872177
40. Karamatsu ML, et al. *Pediatr Emerg Care*. 2012;28(2):131–135 PMID: 22270497
41. Creech CB, et al. *Infect Dis Clin North Am*. 2015;29(3):429–464 PMID: 26311356
42. Elliott SP. *Clin Microbiol Rev*. 2007;20(1):13–22 PMID: 17223620
43. Berk DR, et al. *Pediatr Ann*. 2010;39(10):627–633 PMID: 20954609
44. Braunstein I, et al. *Pediatr Dermatol*. 2014;31(3):305–308 PMID: 24033633
45. Kaplan SL. *Adv Exp Med Biol*. 2009;634:111–120 PMID: 19280853
46. Branson J, et al. *Pediatr Infect Dis J*. 2017;36(3):267–273 PMID: 27870814
47. Keren R, et al. *JAMA Pediatr*. 2015;169(2):120–128 PMID: 25506733
48. Saphyakhajon P, et al. *Pediatr Infect Dis J*. 2008;27(8):765–767 PMID: 18600193
49. Pääkkönen M, et al. *Expert Rev Anti Infect Ther*. 2011;9(12):1125–1131 PMID: 22114963
50. Montgomery NI, et al. *Orthop Clin North Am*. 2017;48(2):209–216 PMID: 28336043
51. Arnold JC, et al. *Pediatrics*. 2012;130(4):e821–e828 PMID: 22966033
52. Chou AC, et al. *J Pediatr Orthop*. 2016;36(2):173–177 PMID: 25929777
53. Fogel I, et al. *Pediatrics*. 2015;136(4):e776–e782 PMID: 26347429
54. Farrow L. *BMC Musculoskelet Disord*. 2015;16:241 PMID: 26342736
55. Workowski KA, et al. *MMWR Recomm Rep*. 2015;64(RR-03):1–137 PMID: 26042815
56. American Academy of Pediatrics. Gonococcal infections. In: Kimberlin DW, et al, eds. *Red Book: 2018 Report of the Committee on Infectious Diseases*. In press
57. Pääkkönen M, et al. *N Engl J Med*. 2014;370(14):1365–1366 PMID: 24693913
58. Funk SS, et al. *Orthop Clin North Am*. 2017;48(2):199–208 PMID: 28336042
59. Messina AF, et al. *Pediatr Infect Dis J*. 2011;30(12):1019–1021 PMID: 21817950
60. Howard-Jones AR, et al. *J Paediatr Child Health*. 2013;49(9):760–768 PMID: 23745943
61. Jacqueline C, et al. *J Antimicrob Chemother*. 2014;69(Suppl1):i37–i40 PMID: 25135088
62. Ceroni D, et al. *J Pediatr Orthop*. 2010;30(3):301–304 PMID: 20357599
63. Chen CJ, et al. *Pediatr Infect Dis J*. 2007;26(11):985–988 PMID: 17984803
64. Chachad S, et al. *Clin Pediatr (Phila)*. 2004;43(3):213–216 PMID: 15094944
65. Volk A, et al. *Pediatr Emerg Care*. 2016 PMID: 26785095
66. Bradley JS, et al. *Pediatrics*. 2011;128(4):e1034–e1045 PMID: 21949152
67. Vaska VL, et al. *Pediatr Infect Dis J*. 2011;30(11):1003–1006 PMID: 21681121
68. Seltz LB, et al. *Pediatrics*. 2011;127(3):e566–e572 PMID: 21321025
69. Peña MT, et al. *JAMA Otolaryngol Head Neck Surg*. 2013;139(3):223–227 PMID: 23429877
70. Smith JM, et al. *Am J Ophthalmol*. 2014;158(2):387–394 PMID: 24794092
71. Wald ER. *Pediatr Rev*. 2004;25(9):312–320 PMID: 15342822
72. Sheikh A, et al. *Cochrane Database Syst Rev*. 2012;9:CD001211 PMID: 22972049
73. Williams L, et al. *J Pediatr*. 2013;162(4):857–861 PMID: 23092529
74. Pichichero ME. *Clin Pediatr (Phila)*. 2011;50(1):7–13 PMID: 20724317
75. Wilhelmus KR. *Cochrane Database Syst Rev*. 2015;1:CD002898 PMID: 25879115
76. Liu S, et al. *Ophthalmology*. 2012;119(10):2003–2008 PMID: 22796308
77. Young RC, et al. *Arch Ophthalmol*. 2010;128(9):1178–1183 PMID: 20837803
78. Azher TN, et al. *Clin Opthalmol*. 2017;11:185–191 PMID: 28176902
79. Khan S, et al. *J Pediatr Ophthalmol Strabismus*. 2014;51(3):140–153 PMID: 24877526
80. Soheilian M, et al. *Arch Ophthalmol*. 2007;125(4):460–465 PMID: 17420365

81. Pappas PG, et al. *Clin Infect Dis.* 2016;62(4):e1–e50 PMID: 26679628
82. Vishnevskia-Dai V, et al. *Ophthalmology.* 2015;122(4):866–868.e3 PMID: 25556113
83. Nassetta L, et al. *J Antimicrob Chemother.* 2009;63(5):862–867 PMID: 19287011
84. James SH, et al. *Curr Opin Pediatr.* 2016;28(1):81–85 PMID: 26709686
85. Groth A, et al. *Int J Pediatr Otorhinolaryngol.* 2012;76(10):1494–1500 PMID: 22832239
86. Stahelin-Massik J, et al. *Eur J Pediatr.* 2008;167(5):541–548 PMID: 17668240
87. Laulajainen-Hongisto A, et al. *Int J Pediatr Otorhinolaryngol.* 2014;78(12):2072–2078 PMID: 25281339
88. Rosenfeld RM, et al. *Otolaryngol Head Neck Surg.* 2014;150(1Suppl):S1–S24 PMID: 24491310
89. Kaushik V, et al. *Cochrane Database Syst Rev.* 2010;(1):CD004740 PMID: 20091565
90. Carfrae MJ, et al. *Otolaryngol Clin North Am.* 2008;41(3):537–549 PMID: 18435997
91. Hoberman A, et al. *N Engl J Med.* 2011;364(2):105–115 PMID: 21226576
92. Tähtinen PA, et al. *N Engl J Med.* 2011;364(2):116–126 PMID: 21226577
93. Lieberthal AS, et al. *Pediatrics.* 2013;131(3):e964–e999 PMID: 23439909
94. Venekamp RP, et al. *Cochrane Database Syst Rev.* 2015;(6):CD000219 PMID: 26099233
95. Hoberman A, et al. *N Engl J Med.* 2016;375(25):2446–2456 PMID: 28002709
96. Van Dyke MK, et al. *Pediatr Infect Dis J.* 2017;36(3):274–281 PMID: 27918383
97. Pichichero ME. *Pediatr Clin North Am.* 2013;60(2):391–407 PMID: 23481107
98. Olarte L, et al. *J Clin Microbiol.* 2017;55(3):724–734 PMID: 27847379
99. Macfadyen CA, et al. *Cochrane Database Syst Rev.* 2006;(1):CD005608 PMID: 16437533
100. Kutz JW Jr, et al. *Expert Opin Pharmacother.* 2013;14(17):2399–2405 PMID: 24093464
101. Haynes DS, et al. *Otolaryngol Clin North Am.* 2007;40(3):669–683 PMID: 17544701
102. Wald ER, et al. *Pediatrics.* 2009;124(1):9–15 PMID: 19564277
103. Wald ER, et al. *Pediatrics.* 2013;132(1):e262–e280 PMID: 23796742
104. Shaikh N, et al. *Cochrane Database Syst Rev.* 2014;(10):CD007909 PMID: 25347280
105. Chow AW, et al. *Clin Infect Dis.* 2012;54(8):e72–e112 PMID: 22438350
106. Brook I. *Int J Pediatr Otorhinolaryngol.* 2016;84:21–26 PMID: 27063747
107. Ellison SJ. *Br Dent J.* 2009;206(7):357–362 PMID: 19357666
108. Robertson DP. *BMJ.* 2015;350:h1300 PMID: 25804417
109. American Academy of Pediatrics. Diphtheria. In: Kimberlin DW, et al, eds. *Red Book: 2018 Report of the Committee on Infectious Diseases.* In press
110. Wheeler DS, et al. *Pediatr Emerg Care.* 2008;24(1):46–49 PMID: 18212612
111. Sobol SE, et al. *Otolaryngol Clin North Am.* 2008;41(3):551–566 PMID: 18435998
112. Nasser M, et al. *Cochrane Database Syst Rev.* 2008;(4):CD006700 PMID: 18843726
113. Amir J, et al. *BMJ.* 1997;314(7097):1800–1803 PMID: 9224082
114. Kimberlin DW, et al. *Clin Infect Dis.* 2010;50(2):221–228 PMID: 20014952
115. Riordan T. *Clin Microbiol Rev.* 2007;20(4):622–659 PMID: 17934077
116. Kizhner V, et al. *J Laryngol Otol.* 2013;127(7):721–723 PMID: 23701713
117. Ridgway JM, et al. *Am J Otolaryngol.* 2010;31(1):38–45 PMID: 19944898
118. Goldenberg NA, et al. *Pediatrics.* 2005;116(4):e543–e548 PMID: 16147971
119. Agrafiotis M, et al. *Am J Emerg Med.* 2015;33(5):733.e3–733.e4 PMID: 25455045
120. Baldassari CM, et al. *Otolaryngol Head Neck Surg.* 2011;144(4):592–595 PMID: 21493241
121. Hur K, et al. *Laryngoscope.* 2017 PMID: 28561258
122. Shulman ST, et al. *Clin Infect Dis.* 2012;55(10):e86–e102 PMID: 22965026
123. Lennon DR, et al. *Arch Dis Child.* 2008;93(6):474–478 PMID: 18337284
124. American Academy of Pediatrics. Group A streptococcal infections. In: Kimberlin DW, et al, eds. *Red Book: 2018 Report of the Committee on Infectious Diseases.* In press
125. Casey JR, et al. *Diagn Microbiol Infect Dis.* 2007;57(3Suppl):39S–45S PMID: 17292576
126. Altamimi S, et al. *Cochrane Database Syst Rev.* 2012;8:CD004872 PMID: 22895944
127. Abdel-Haq N, et al. *Pediatr Infect Dis J.* 2012;31(7):696–699 PMID: 22481424
128. Cheng J, et al. *Otolaryngol Head Neck Surg.* 2013;148(6):1037–1042 PMID: 23520072
129. Brown NK, et al. *Pediatr Infect Dis J.* 2015;34(4):454–456 PMID: 25760568
130. Shargorodsky J, et al. *Laryngoscope.* 2010;120(12):2498–2501 PMID: 21108480
131. Kuo CY, et al. *Pediatr Rev.* 2014;35(11):497–499 PMID: 25361911

132. Lemaître C, et al. *Pediatr Infect Dis J.* 2013;32(10):1146–1149 PMID: 23722529

133. Bender JM, et al. *Clin Infect Dis.* 2008;46(9):1346–1352 PMID: 18419434

134. Blumer JL, et al. *Pediatr Infect Dis J.* 2016;35(7):760–766 PMID: 27078119

135. Brook I. *Adv Exp Med Biol.* 2011;697:117–152 PMID: 21120724

136. Agarwal R, et al. *Future Microbiol.* 2013;8(11):1463–1474 PMID: 24199804

137. Meissner HC. *N Engl J Med.* 2016;374(1):62–72 PMID: 26735994

138. Zobell JT, et al. *Pediatr Pulmonol.* 2013;48(6):525–537 PMID: 23359557

139. Chmiel JF, et al. *Ann Am Thorac Soc.* 2014;11(7):1120–1129 PMID: 25102221

140. Flume PA, et al. *Am J Respir Crit Care Med.* 2009;180(9):802–808 PMID: 19729669

141. Cogen JD, et al. *Pediatrics.* 2017;139(2):e20162642 PMID: 28126911

142. Mayer-Hamblett N, et al. *Pediatr Pulmonol.* 2013;48(10):943–953 PMID: 23818295

143. Chmiel JF, et al. *Ann Am Thorac Soc.* 2014;11(8):1298–1306 PMID: 25167882

144. Waters V, et al. *Cochrane Database Syst Rev.* 2016;12:CD010004 PMID: 28000919

145. Ryan G, et al. *Cochrane Database Syst Rev.* 2012;12:CD008319 PMID: 23235659

146. Lahiri T, et al. *Pediatrics.* 2016;137(4):e20151784 PMID: 27009033

147. Waters V, et al. *Cochrane Database Syst Rev.* 2008;(3):CD006961 PMID: 18646176

148. Langton Hewer SC, et al. *Cochrane Database Syst Rev.* 2017;4:CD004197 PMID: 28440853

149. Cheer SM, et al. *Drugs.* 2003;63(22):2501–2520 PMID: 14609360

150. Hutchinson D, et al. *Expert Opin Pharmacother.* 2013;14(15):2115–2124 PMID: 23992352

151. Mogayzel PJ Jr, et al. *Am J Respir Crit Care Med.* 2013;187(7):680–689 PMID: 23540878

152. Southern KW, et al. *Cochrane Database Syst Rev.* 2012;11:CD002203 PMID: 23152214

153. Conole D, et al. *Drugs.* 2014;74(3):377–387 PMID: 24510624

154. American Academy of Pediatrics. Pertussis (whooping cough). In: Kimberlin DW, et al, eds. *Red Book: 2018 Report of the Committee on Infectious Diseases.* In press

155. Altunaiji S, et al. *Cochrane Database Syst Rev.* 2007;(3):CD004404 PMID: 17636756

156. Kilgore PE, et al. *Clin Microbiol Rev.* 2016;29(3):449–486 PMID: 27029594

157. Wang K, et al. *Cochrane Database Syst Rev.* 2014;(9):CD003257 PMID: 25243777

158. Jain S, et al. *N Engl J Med.* 2015;372(9):835–845 PMID: 25714161

159. Bradley JS, et al. *Clin Infect Dis.* 2011;53(7):e25–e76 PMID: 21880587

160. Esposito S, et al. *Pediatr Infect Dis J.* 2012;31(6):e78–e85 PMID: 22466326

161. Queen MA, et al. *Pediatrics.* 2014;133(1):e23–e29 PMID: 24324001

162. Ambroggio L, et al. *Pediatr Pulmonol.* 2016;51(5):541–548 PMID: 26367389

163. Leyenaar JK, et al. *Pediatr Infect Dis J.* 2014;33(4):387–392 PMID: 24168982

164. Bradley JS, et al. *Pediatr Infect Dis J.* 2007;26(10):868–878 PMID: 17901791

165. Hidron AI, et al. *Lancet Infect Dis.* 2009;9(6):384–392 PMID: 19467478

166. Wunderink RG, et al. *Clin Infect Dis.* 2012;54(5):621–629 PMID: 22247123

167. Freifeld AG, et al. *Clin Infect Dis.* 2011;52(4):e56–e93 PMID: 21258094

168. Kalil AC, et al. *Clin Infect Dis.* 2016;63(5):e61–e111 PMID: 27418577

169. Foglia E, et al. *Clin Microbiol Rev.* 2007;20(3):409–425 PMID: 17630332

170. Srinivasan R, et al. *Pediatrics.* 2009;123(4):1108–1115 PMID: 19336369

171. Kollef MH, et al. *Curr Opin Infect Dis.* 2013;26(6):538–544 PMID: 24126716

172. St Peter SD, et al. *J Pediatr Surg.* 2009;44(1):106–111 PMID: 19159726

173. Islam S, et al. *J Pediatr Surg.* 2012;47(11):2101–2110 PMID: 23164006

174. Redden MD, et al. *Cochrane Database Syst Rev.* 2017;3:CD010651 PMID: 28304084

175. Marhuenda C, et al. *Pediatrics.* 2014;134(5):e1301–e1307 PMID: 25349313

176. American Academy of Pediatrics. Chlamydial infections. In: Kimberlin DW, et al, eds. *Red Book: 2018 Report of the Committee on Infectious Diseases.* In press

177. American Academy of Pediatrics. Cytomegalovirus infection. In: Kimberlin DW, et al, eds. *Red Book: 2018 Report of the Committee on Infectious Diseases.* In press

178. Kotton CN, et al. *Transplantation.* 2013;96(4):333–360 PMID: 23896556

179. Erard V, et al. *Clin Infect Dis.* 2015;61(1):31–39 PMID: 25778751

180. American Academy of Pediatrics. Tularemia. In: Kimberlin DW, et al, eds. *Red Book: 2018 Report of the Committee on Infectious Diseases.* 2018:839–841

181. Galgiani JN, et al. *Clin Infect Dis.* 2016;63(6):e112–e146 PMID: 27470238
182. American Academy of Pediatrics. Coccidioidomycosis. In: Kimberlin DW, et al, eds. *Red Book: 2018 Report of the Committee on Infectious Diseases.* In press
183. American Academy of Pediatrics. Histoplasmosis. In: Kimberlin DW, et al, eds. *Red Book: 2018 Report of the Committee on Infectious Diseases.* In press
184. Wheat LJ, et al. *Clin Infect Dis.* 2007;45(7):807–825 PMID: 17806045
185. Harper SA, et al. *Clin Infect Dis.* 2009;48(8):1003–1032 PMID: 19281331
186. American Academy Pediatrics Committee on Infectious Diseases. *Pediatrics.* 2016;138(4):e20162527 PMID: 27600320
187. Kimberlin DW, et al. *J Infect Dis.* 2013;207(5):709–720 PMID: 23230059
188. Ng TM, et al. *PLoS One.* 2016;11(4):e0153696 PMID: 27104951
189. Badal RE, et al. *Pediatr Infect Dis J.* 2013;32(6):636–640 PMID: 23838732
190. Johnson MM, et al. *J Thorac Dis.* 2014;6(3):210–220 PMID: 24624285
191. Biondi E, et al. *Pediatrics.* 2014;133(6):1081–1090 PMID: 24864174
192. Cardinale F, et al. *J Clin Microbiol.* 2013;51(2):723–724 PMID: 23224091
193. Aidsinfo.gov. https://aidsinfo.nih.gov/contentfiles/lvguidelines/oi_guidelines_pediatrics.pdf. Accessed October 11, 2017
194. Caselli D, et al. *J Pediatr.* 2014;164(2):389–392.e1 PMID: 24252793
195. Rafailidis PI, et al. *Curr Opin Infect Dis.* 2014;27(6):479–483 PMID: 25259809
196. Micek ST, et al. *Medicine (Baltimore).* 2011;90(6):390–395 PMID: 22033455
197. Micek ST, et al. *Crit Care.* 2015;19:219 PMID: 25944081
198. American Academy of Pediatrics. Respiratory syncytial virus. In: Kimberlin DW, et al, eds. *Red Book: 2018 Report of the Committee on Infectious Diseases.* In press
199. Villarino ME, et al. *JAMA Pediatr.* 2015;169(3):247–255 PMID: 25580725
200. Meehan WP III, et al. *Pediatr Emerg Care.* 2010;26(12):875–880 PMID: 21088637
201. Biondi E, et al. *Pediatrics.* 2013;132(6):990–996 PMID: 24218461
202. Byington CL, et al. *Pediatrics.* 2003;111(5pt1):964–968 PMID: 12728072
203. Mischler M, et al. *Hosp Pediatr.* 2015;5(6):293–300 PMID: 26034160
204. Ishimine P. *Emerg Med Clin North Am.* 2013;31(3):601–626 PMID: 23915596
205. Greenhow TL, et al. *Pediatr Infect Dis J.* 2014;33(6):595–599 PMID: 24326416
206. McMullan BJ, et al. *JAMA Pediatr.* 2016;170(10):979–986 PMID: 27533601
207. Luthander J, et al. *Acta Paediatr.* 2013;102(2):182–186 PMID: 23121094
208. Russell CD, et al. *J Med Microbiol.* 2014;63(Pt6):841–848 PMID: 24623637
209. Ligon J, et al. *Pediatr Infect Dis J.* 2014;33(5):e132–e134 PMID: 24732394
210. Baddour LM, et al. *Circulation.* 2015;132(15):1435–1486. [Erratum: *Circulation.* 2015;132(17):e215. Erratum: *Circulation.* 2016;134(8):e113] PMID: 26373316
211. Baltimore RS, et al. *Circulation.* 2015;132(15):1487–1515 PMID: 26373317
212. Johnson JA, et al. *Mayo Clin Proc.* 2012;87(7):629–635 PMID: 22766082
213. Russell HM, et al. *Ann Thorac Surg.* 2013;96(1):171–174 PMID: 23602067
214. Baddour LM, et al. *Circulation.* 2015;132(15):1435–1486 PMID: 26373316
215. Tacke D, et al. *Curr Opin Infect Dis.* 2013;26(6):501–507 PMID: 24126720
216. Wilson W, et al. *Circulation.* 2007;116(15):1736–1754 PMID: 17446442
217. Sakai Bizmark R, et al. *Am Heart J.* 2017;189:110–119 PMID: 28625367
218. Lutmer JE, et al. *Ann Am Thorac Soc.* 2013;10(3):235–238 PMID: 23802820
219. Demmler GJ. *Pediatr Infect Dis J.* 2006;25(2):165–166 PMID: 16462296
220. Denno DM, et al. *Clin Infect Dis.* 2012;55(7):897–904 PMID: 22700832
221. Riddle MS, et al. *Am J Gastroenterol.* 2016;111(5):602–622 PMID: 27068718
222. Butler T. *Trans R Soc Trop Med Hyg.* 2012;106(7):395–399 PMID: 22579556
223. Wong CS, et al. *Clin Infect Dis.* 2012;55(1):33–41 PMID: 22431799
224. Bennish ML, et al. *Clin Infect Dis.* 2006;42(3):356–362 PMID: 16392080
225. Smith KE, et al. *Pediatr Infect Dis J.* 2012;31(1):37–41 PMID: 21892124
226. Safdar N, et al. *JAMA.* 2008;288(8):996–1001 PMID: 12190370
227. Tribble DR, et al. *Clin Infect Dis.* 2007;44(3):338–346 PMID: 17205438
228. Steffen R, et al. *JAMA.* 2015;313(1):71–80 PMID: 25562268

229. Paredes-Paredes M, et al. *Curr Gastroenterol Rep.* 2011;13(5):402–407 PMID: 21773708
230. Riddle MS, et al. *J Travel Med.* 2017;24(Suppl1):S57–S74 PMID: 28521004
231. Ouyang-Latimer J, et al. *Antimicrob Agents Chemother.* 2011;55(2):874–878 PMID: 21115800
232. O'Ryan M, et al. *Expert Rev Anti Infect Ther.* 2010;8(6):671–682 PMID: 20521895
233. Koo HL, et al. *Curr Opin Gastroenterol.* 2010;26(1):17–25 PMID: 19881343
234. Advice for travelers. *Med Lett Drugs Ther.* 2015;57(1466):52–58 PMID: 25853663
235. Kantele A, et al. *Clin Infect Dis.* 2015;60(6):837–846 PMID: 25613287
236. Riddle MS, et al. *Clin Infect Dis.* 2008;47(8):1007–1014 PMID: 18781873
237. Butler T. *Clin Infect Dis.* 2008;47(8):1015–1016 PMID: 18781871
238. Janda JM, et al. *Clin Microbiol Rev.* 2010;23(1):35–73 PMID: 20065325
239. American Academy of Pediatrics. *Campylobacter* infections. In: Kimberlin DW, et al, eds. *Red Book: 2018 Report of the Committee on Infectious Diseases.* In press
240. Fullerton KE, et al. *Pediatr Infect Dis J.* 2007;26(1):19–24 PMID: 17195700
241. Kirkpatrick BD, et al. *Curr Opin Gastroenterol.* 2011;27(1):1–7 PMID: 21124212
242. Leibovici-Weissman Y, et al. *Cochrane Database Syst Rev.* 2014;6:CD008625 PMID: 24944120
243. Pant C, et al. *Curr Med Res Opin.* 2013;29(8):967–984 PMID: 23659563
244. American Academy of Pediatrics. *Clostridium difficile.* In: Kimberlin DW, et al, eds. *Red Book: 2018 Report of the Committee on Infectious Diseases.* In press
245. Kelly CP, et al. *N Engl J Med.* 2008;359(18):1932–1940 PMID: 18971494
246. Adams DJ, et al. *J Pediatr.* 2017;186:105–109 PMID: 28396027
247. O'Gorman MA, et al. *J Pediatric Infect Dis Soc.* 2017 PMID: 28575523
248. Khanna S, et al. *Clin Infect Dis.* 2013;56(10):1401–1406 PMID: 23408679
249. Jones NL, et al. *J Pediatr Gastroenterol Nutr.* 2017;64(6):991–1003 PMID: 28541262
250. McColl KE. *N Engl J Med.* 2010;362(17):1597–1604 PMID: 20427808
251. Kalach N, et al. *Ann Gastroenterol.* 2015;28(1):10–18 PMID: 25608573
252. American Academy of Pediatrics. *Helicobacter pylori* infections. In: Kimberlin DW, et al, eds. *Red Book: 2018 Report of the Committee on Infectious Diseases.* In press
253. Fallone CA, et al. *Gastroenterology.* 2016;151(1):51–69.e14 PMID: 27102658
254. Kalach N, et al. *Ann Gastroenterol.* 2015;28(1):10–18 PMID: 25608573
255. American Academy of Pediatrics. *Giardia intestinalis* (formerly *Giardia lamblia* and *Giardia duodenalis*) infections. In: Kimberlin DW, et al, eds. *Red Book: 2018 Report of the Committee on Infectious Diseases.* In press
256. Bula-Rudas FJ, et al. *Adv Pediatr.* 2015;62(1):29–58 PMID: 26205108
257. Wen SC, et al. *J Paediatr Child Health.* 2017;53(10):936–941 PMID: 28556448
258. American Academy of Pediatrics. *Shigella* infections. In: Kimberlin DW, et al, eds. *Red Book: 2018 Report of the Committee on Infectious Diseases.* In press
259. Frenck RW Jr, et al. *Clin Infect Dis.* 2004;38(7):951–957 PMID: 15034826
260. Effa EE, et al. *Cochrane Database Syst Rev.* 2008;(4):CD006083 PMID: 18843701
261. Effa EE, et al. *Cochrane Database Syst Rev.* 2011;(10):CD004530 PMID: 21975746
262. Begum B, et al. *Mymensingh Med J.* 2014;23(3):441–448 PMID: 25178594
263. National Antimicrobial Resistance Monitoring System, Centers for Diseases Control and Prevention. http://www.cdc.gov/narms/reports/index.html. Updated August 26, 2016. Accessed October 11, 2017
264. Basualdo W, et al. *Pediatr Infect Dis J.* 2003;22(4):374–377 PMID: 12712971
265. American Academy of Pediatrics. *Shigella* infections. In: Kimberlin DW, et al, eds. *Red Book: 2018 Report of the Committee on Infectious Diseases.* In press
266. Abdel-Haq NM, et al. *Pediatr Infect Dis J.* 2000;19(10):954–958 PMID: 11055595
267. Abdel-Haq NM, et al. *Int J Antimicrob Agents.* 2006;27(5):449–452 PMID: 16621458
268. El Qouqa IA, et al. *Int J Infect Dis.* 2011;15(1):e48–e53 PMID: 21131221
269. Fallon SC, et al. *J Surg Res.* 2013;185(1):273–277 PMID: 23835072
270. Lee SL, et al. *J Pediatr Surg.* 2010;45(11):2181–2185 PMID: 21034941
271. Chen CY, et al. *Surg Infect (Larchmt).* 2012;13(6):383–390 PMID: 23231389
272. Solomkin JS, et al. *Clin Infect Dis.* 2010;50(2):133–164 PMID: 20034345
273. Sawyer RG, et al. *N Engl J Med.* 2015;372(21):1996–2005 PMID: 25992746
274. Fraser JD, et al. *J Pediatr Surg.* 2010;45(6):1198–1202 PMID: 20620320

275. Bradley JS, et al. *Pediatr Infect Dis J.* 2001;20(1):19–24 PMID: 11176562
276. Lee JY, et al. *J Pediatr Pharmacol Ther.* 2016;21(2):140–145 PMID: 27199621
277. St Peter SD, et al. *J Pediatr Surg.* 2008;43(6):981–985 PMID: 18558169
278. Kronman MP, et al. *Pediatrics.* 2016;138(1):e20154547 PMID: 27354453
279. Cruz AT, et al. *Int J Tuberc Lung Dis.* 2013;17(2):169–174 PMID: 23317951
280. Hlavsa MC, et al. *Clin Infect Dis.* 2008;47(2):168–175 PMID: 18532886
281. Alrajhi AA, et al. *Clin Infect Dis.* 1998;27(1):52–56 PMID: 9675450
282. Arditi M, et al. *Pediatr Infect Dis J.* 1990;9(6):411–415 PMID: 2367163
283. Ballinger AE, et al. *Cochrane Database Syst Rev.* 2014;4:CD005284 PMID: 24771351
284. Warady BA, et al. *Perit Dial Int.* 2012;32(Suppl2):S32–S86 PMID: 22851742
285. Preece ER, et al. *ANZ J Surg.* 2012;82(4):283–284 PMID: 22510192
286. Workowski K. *Ann Intern Med.* 2013;158(3):ITC2–1 PMID: 23381058
287. Santillanes G, et al. *Pediatr Emerg Care.* 2011;27(3):174–178 PMID: 21346680
288. Klin B, et al. *Isr Med Assoc J.* 2001;3(11):833–835 PMID: 11729579
289. Smith JC, et al. *Adv Exp Med Biol.* 2013;764:219–239 PMID: 23654071
290. Centers for Disease Control and Prevention. *MMWR Morb Mortal Wkly Rep.* 2012;61(31):590–594 PMID: 22874837
291. Kirkcaldy RD, et al. *MMWR Surveill Summ.* 2016;65(7):1–19 PMID: 27414503
292. James SH, et al. *Clin Pharmacol Ther.* 2010;88(5):720–724 PMID: 20881952
293. Fife KH, et al. *Sex Transm Dis.* 2008;35(7):668–673 PMID: 18461016
294. Stephenson-Famy A, et al. *Obstet Gynecol Clin North Am.* 2014;41(4):601–614 PMID: 25454993
295. Mitchell C, et al. *Infect Dis Clin North Am.* 2013;27(4):793–809 PMID: 24275271
296. Cohen SE, et al. *Infect Dis Clin North Am.* 2013;27(4):705–722 PMID: 24275265
297. Manhart LE, et al. *Clin Infect Dis.* 2015;61(Suppl8):S802–S817 PMID: 26602619
298. O'Brien G. *Pediatr Rev.* 2008;29(6):209–211 PMID: 18515339
299. das Neves J, et al. *Drugs.* 2008;68(13):1787–1802 PMID: 18729533
300. Bumbuliene Ž, et al. *Postgrad Med J.* 2014;90(1059):8–12 PMID: 24191064
301. Jasper JM, et al. *Pediatr Emerg Care.* 2006;22(8):585–586 PMID: 16912629
302. Hansen MT, et al. *J Pediatr Adolesc Gynecol.* 2007;20(5):315–317 PMID: 17868900
303. Yogev R, et al. *Pediatr Infect Dis J.* 2004;23(2):157–159 PMID: 14872183
304. Bonfield CM, et al. *J Infect.* 2015;71(Suppl1):S42–S46 PMID: 25917804
305. Bitnun A, et al. *Can J Infect Dis Med Microbiol.* 2015;26(2):69–72 PMID: 26015788
306. Abzug MJ, et al. *J Pediatr Infect Dis Soc.* 2016;5(1):53–62 PMID: 26407253
307. Abzug MJ, et al. *Pediatr Infect Dis J.* 2003;22(4):335–341 PMID: 12690273
308. Doja A, et al. *J Child Neurol.* 2006;21(5):384–391 PMID: 16901443
309. Gnann JW Jr, et al. *Curr Infect Dis Rep.* 2017;19(3):13 PMID: 28251511
310. Brouwer MC, et al. *Cochrane Database Syst Rev.* 2015;(9):CD004405 PMID: 26362566
311. Fritz D, et al. *Neurology.* 2012;79(22):2177–2179 PMID: 23152589
312. Tunkel AR, et al. *Clin Infect Dis.* 2004;39(9):1267–1284 PMID: 15494903
313. Prasad K, et al. *Cochrane Database Syst Rev.* 2008;(1):CD002244 PMID: 18254003
314. Kandasamy J, et al. *Childs Nerv Syst.* 2011;27(4):575–581 PMID: 20953871
315. Tunkel AR, et al. *Clin Infect Dis.* 2017 PMID: 28203777
316. National Institute for Health and Care Excellence. Urinary tract infection in under 16s: diagnosis and management. http://www.nice.org.uk/guidance/CG54. Updated September 2017. Accessed October 11, 2017
317. Montini G, et al. *N Engl J Med.* 2011;365(3):239–250 PMID: 21774712
318. Conley SP, et al. *J Emerg Med.* 2014;46(5):624–626 PMID: 24286715
319. Chen WL, et al. *Pediatr Neonatal.* 2015;56(3):176–182 PMID: 25459491
320. Strohmeier Y, et al. *Cochrane Database Syst Rev.* 2014;7:CD003772 PMID: 25066627
321. Perez F, et al. *Clin Infect Dis.* 2015;60(9):1326–1329 PMID: 25586684
322. Bocquet N, et al. *Pediatrics.* 2012;129(2):e269–e275 PMID: 22291112
323. American Academy of Pediatrics Subcommittee on Urinary Tract Infection, Steering Committee on Quality Improvement and Management. *Pediatrics.* 2011;128(3):595–610 PMID: 21873693

324. Craig JC, et al. *N Engl J Med.* 2009;361(18):1748–1759 PMID: 19864673

325. Williams GJ, et al. *Adv Exp Med Biol.* 2013;764:211–218 PMID: 23654070

326. Hoberman A, et al. *N Engl J Med.* 2014;370(25):2367–2376 PMID: 24795142

327. Craig JC. *J Pediatr.* 2015;166(3):778 PMID: 25722276

328. American Academy of Pediatrics. Actinomycosis. In: Kimberlin DW, et al, eds. *Red Book: 2018 Report of the Committee on Infectious Diseases.* In press

329. Brook I. *South Med J.* 2008;101(10):1019–1023 PMID: 18791528

330. Wacharachaisurapol N, et al. *Pediatr Infect Dis J.* 2017;36(3):e76–e79 PMID: 27870811

331. Thomas RJ, et al. *Expert Rev Anti Infect Ther.* 2009;7(6):709–722 PMID: 19681699

332. Dahlgren FS, et al. *Am J Trop Med Hyg.* 2015;93(1):66–72 PMID: 25870428

333. American Academy of Pediatrics. Brucellosis. In: Kimberlin DW, et al, eds. *Red Book: 2018 Report of the Committee on Infectious Diseases.* In press

334. Shen MW. *Pediatrics.* 2008;121(5):e1178–e1183 PMID: 18450861

335. Mile B, et al. *Trop Doct.* 2012;42(1):13–17 PMID: 22290107

336. Yagupsky P. *Adv Exp Med Biol.* 2011;719:123–132 PMID: 22125040

337. Florin TA, et al. *Pediatrics.* 2008;121(5):e1413–e1425 PMID: 18443019

338. Zangwill KM. *Adv Exp Med Biol.* 2013;764:159–166 PMID: 23654065

339. Chang CC, et al. *Paediatr Int Child Health.* 2016;1–3 PMID: 27077606

340. Nichols Heitman K, et al. *Am J Trop Med Hyg.* 2016;94(1):52–60 PMID: 26621561

341. Schutze GE, et al. *Pediatr Infect Dis J.* 2007;26(6):475–479 PMID: 17529862

342. Sanchez E, et al. *JAMA.* 2016;315(16):1767–1777 PMID: 27115378

343. Averbuch D, et al. *Haematologica.* 2013;98(12):1826–1835 [Erratum: *Haematologica.* 2014;99(2):400] PMID: 24323983

344. Freifeld AG, et al. *Clin Infect Dis.* 2011;52(4):e56–e93 PMID: 21258094

345. Miedema KG, et al. *Eur J Cancer.* 2016;53:16–24 PMID: 26700076

346. Arnon SS. *Pediatrics.* 2007;119(4):785–789 PMID: 17403850

347. Newburger JW. *Congenit Heart Dis.* 2017;12(5):641–643 PMID: 28580631

348. Kobayashi T, et al. *Lancet.* 2012;379(9826):1613–1620 PMID: 22405251

349. Son MB, et al. *J Pediatr.* 2011;158(4):644–649 PMID: 21129756

350. McCrindle BW, et al. *Circulation.* 2017;135(17):e927–e999 PMID: 28356445

351. American Academy of Pediatrics. Leprosy. In: Kimberlin DW, et al, eds. *Red Book: 2018 Report of the Committee on Infectious Diseases.* In press

352. Griffith ME, et al. *Curr Opin Infect Dis.* 2006;19(6):533–537 PMID: 17075327

353. American Academy of Pediatrics. Leptospirosis. In: Kimberlin DW, et al, eds. *Red Book: 2018 Report of the Committee on Infectious Diseases.* In press

354. American Academy of Pediatrics. Lyme disease. In: Kimberlin DW, et al, eds. *Red Book: 2018 Report of the Committee on Infectious Diseases.* In press

355. Shapiro ED. *N Engl J Med.* 2014;370(18):1724–1731 PMID: 24785207

356. Sood SK. *Infect Dis Clin North Am.* 2015;29(2):281–294 PMID: 25999224

357. Wiersinga WJ, et al. *N Engl J Med.* 2012;367(11):1035–1044 PMID: 22970946

358. Chetchotisakd P, et al. *Lancet.* 2014;383(9919):807–814 PMID: 24284287

359. Griffith DE, et al. *Am J Respir Crit Care Med.* 2007;175(4):367–416 [Erratum: *Am J Respir Crit Care Med.* 2007;175(7):744–745] PMID: 17277290

360. Philley JV, et al. *Semin Respir Crit Care Med.* 2013;34(1):135–142 PMID: 23460013

361. Kasperbauer SH, et al. *Clin Chest Med.* 2015;36(1):67–78 PMID: 25676520

362. Henkle E, et al. *Clin Chest Med.* 2015;36(1):91–99 PMID 25676522

363. Wilson JW. *Mayo Clin Proc.* 2012;87(4):403–407 PMID: 22469352

364. American Academy of Pediatrics. Nocardiosis. In: Kimberlin DW, et al, eds. *Red Book: 2018 Report of the Committee on Infectious Diseases.* In press

365. Butler T. *Clin Infect Dis.* 2009;49(5):736–742 PMID: 19606935

366. Stenseth NC, et al. *PLoS Med.* 2008;5(1):e3 PMID: 18198939

367. American Academy of Pediatrics. Plague. In: Kimberlin DW, et al, eds. *Red Book: 2018 Report of the Committee on Infectious Diseases.* In press

368. Kersh GJ. *Expert Rev Anti Infect Ther.* 2013;11(11):1207–1214 PMID: 24073941
369. Anderson A, et al. *MMWR Recomm Rep.* 2013;62(RR-03):1–30 PMID: 23535757
370. Woods CR. *Pediatr Clin North Am.* 2013;60(2):455–470 PMID: 23481111
371. American Academy of Pediatrics. Rocky Mountain spotted fever. In: Kimberlin DW, et al, eds. *Red Book: 2085 Report of the Committee on Infectious Diseases.* In press
372. American Academy of Pediatrics. Tetanus. In: Kimberlin DW, et al, eds. *Red Book: 2018 Report of the Committee on Infectious Diseases.* In press
373. Brook I. *Expert Rev Anti Infect Ther.* 2008;6(3):327–336 PMID: 18588497
374. Curtis N. *Arch Dis Child.* 2014;99(12):1062–1064 PMID: 25395586
375. Dellinger RP, et al. *Crit Care Med.* 2013;41(2):580–637 PMID: 23353941
376. Harik NS. *Pediatr Ann.* 2013;42(7):288–292 PMID: 23805970

Chapter 7

1. Qureshi ZA, et al. *Clin Infect Dis.* 2015;60(9):1295–1303 PMID: 25632010
2. Fishbain J, et al. *Clin Infect Dis.* 2010;51(1):79–84 PMID: 20504234
3. Hsu AJ, et al. *Clin Infect Dis.* 2014;58(10):1439–1448 PMID: 24501388
4. Bonnin RA, et al. *Expert Rev Anti Infect Ther.* 2013;11(6):571–583 PMID: 23750729
5. Brook I. *South Med J.* 2008;101(10):1019–1023 PMID: 18791528
6. Janda JM, et al. *Clin Microbiol Rev.* 2010;23(1):35–73 PMID: 20065325
7. Sharma K, et al. *Ann Clin Microbiol Antimicrob.* 2017;16(1):12 PMID: 28288638
8. Thomas RJ, et al. *Expert Rev Anti Infect Ther.* 2009;7(6):709–722 PMID: 19681699
9. Ismail N, et al. *Clin Lab Med.* 2010;30(1):261–292 PMID: 20513551
10. Therriault BL, et al. *Ann Pharmacother.* 2008;42(11):1697–1702 PMID: 18812563
11. Bradley JS, et al. *Pediatrics.* 2014;133(5):e1411–e1436 PMID: 24777226
12. American Academy of Pediatrics. *Bacillus cereus* infections. In: Kimberlin DW, et al, eds. *Red Book: 2018 Report of the Committee on Infectious Diseases.* In press
13. Bottone EJ. *Clin Microbiol Rev.* 2010;23(2):382–398 PMID: 20375358
14. Wexler HM. *Clin Microbiol Rev.* 2007;20(4):593–621 PMID: 17934076
15. Brook I. *J Infect Chemother.* 2016;22(1):1–13 PMID: 26620376
16. Florin TA, et al. *Pediatrics.* 2008;121(5):e1413–e1425 PMID: 18443019
17. Zangwill KM. *Adv Exp Med Biol.* 2013;764:159–166 PMID: 23654065
18. Foucault C, et al. *Emerg Infect Dis.* 2006;12(2):217–223 PMID: 16494745
19. Tiwari T, et al. *MMWR Recomm Rep.* 2005;54(RR-14):1–16 PMID: 16340941
20. American Academy of Pediatrics. Pertussis (whooping cough). In: Kimberlin DW, et al, eds. *Red Book: 2018 Report of the Committee on Infectious Diseases.* In press
21. Shapiro ED. *N Engl J Med.* 2014;370(18):1724–1731 PMID: 24785207
22. American Academy of Pediatrics. Lyme disease. In: Kimberlin DW, et al, eds. *Red Book: 2018 Report of the Committee on Infectious Diseases.* In press
23. Wormser GP, et al. *Clin Infect Dis.* 2006;43(9):1089–1134 PMID: 17029130
24. American Academy of Pediatrics. *Borrelia* infections other than Lyme Disease. In: Kimberlin DW, et al, eds. *Red Book: 2018 Report of the Committee on Infectious Diseases.* In press
25. Dworkin MS, et al. *Infect Dis Clin North Am.* 2008;22(3):449–468 PMID: 18755384
26. American Academy of Pediatrics. Brucellosis. In: Kimberlin DW, et al, eds. *Red Book: 2018 Report of the Committee on Infectious Diseases.* In press
27. Shen MW. *Pediatrics.* 2008;121(5):e1178–e1183 PMID: 18450861
28. Yagupsky P. *Adv Exp Med Biol.* 2011;719:123–132 PMID: 22125040
29. American Academy of Pediatrics. *Burkholderia* infections. In: Kimberlin DW, et al, eds. *Red Book: 2018 Report of the Committee on Infectious Diseases.* In press
30. Waters V. *Curr Pharm Des.* 2012;18(5):696–725 PMID: 22229574
31. King P, et al. *Antimicrob Agents Chemother.* 2010;54(1):143–148 PMID: 19805554
32. Horsley A, et al. *Cochrane Database Syst Rev.* 2016;(1):CD009529 PMID: 26789750
33. Wiersinga WJ, et al. *N Engl J Med.* 2012;367(11):1035–1044 PMID: 22970946
34. Cheng AC, et al. *Am J Trop Med Hyg.* 2008;78(2):208–209 PMID: 18256414
35. Chetchotisakd P, et al. *Lancet.* 2014;383(9919):807–814 PMID: 24284287

36. Fujihara N, et al. *J Infect.* 2006;53(5):e199–e202 PMID: 16542730
37. Wagenaar JA, et al. *Clin Infect Dis.* 2014;58(11):1579–1586 PMID: 24550377
38. American Academy of Pediatrics. *Campylobacter* infections. In: Kimberlin DW, et al, eds. *Red Book: 2018 Report of the Committee on Infectious Diseases.* In press
39. Kirkpatrick BD, et al. *Curr Opin Gastroenterol.* 2011;27(1):1–7 PMID: 21124212
40. Oehler RL, et al. *Lancet Infect Dis.* 2009;9(7):439–447 PMID: 19555903
41. Jolivet-Gougeon A, et al. *Int J Antimicrob Agents.* 2007;29(4):367–373 PMID: 17250994
42. Wang HK, et al. *J Clin Microbiol.* 2007;45(2):645–647 PMID: 17135428
43. Kohlhoff SA, et al. *Expert Opin Pharmacother.* 2015;16(2):205–212 PMID: 25579069
44. American Academy of Pediatrics. Chlamydial infections. In: Kimberlin DW, et al, eds. *Red Book: 2018 Report of the Committee on Infectious Diseases.* In press
45. Workowski KA, et al. *MMWR Recomm Rep.* 2015;64(RR-03):1–137 PMID: 26042815
46. Blasi F, et al. *Clin Microbiol Infect.* 2009;15(1):29–35 PMID: 19220337
47. Burillo A, et al. *Infect Dis Clin North Am.* 2010;24(1):61–71 PMID: 20171546
48. Knittler MR, et al. *Pathog Dis.* 2015;73(1):1–15 PMID: 25853998
49. Campbell JI, et al. *BMC Infect Dis.* 2013;13:4 PMID: 23286235
50. Sirinavin S, et al. *Pediatr Infect Dis J.* 2005;24(6):559–561 PMID: 15933571
51. Nuñez Cuadros E, et al. *J Med Microbiol.* 2014;63(Pt1):144–147 PMID: 24243285
52. Jacoby GA. *Clin Microbiol Rev.* 2009;22(1):161–182 PMID: 19136439
53. Carrillo-Marquez MA. *Pediatr Rev.* 2016;37(5):183–192 PMID: 27139326
54. American Academy of Pediatrics. Botulism and infant botulism. In: Kimberlin DW, et al, eds. *Red Book: 2018 Report of the Committee on Infectious Diseases.* In press
55. Hill SE, et al. *Ann Pharmacother.* 2013;47(2):e12 PMID: 23362041
56. Sammons JS, et al. *JAMA Pediatr.* 2013;167(6):567–573 PMID: 23460123
57. American Academy of Pediatrics. *Clostridium difficile.* In: Kimberlin DW, et al, eds. *Red Book: 2018 Report of the Committee on Infectious Diseases.* In press
58. Cohen SH, et al. *Infect Control Hosp Epidemiol.* 2010;31(5):431–455 PMID: 20307191
59. O'Gorman MA. *J Pediatric Infect Dis Soc.* 2017 PMID: 28575523
60. American Academy of Pediatrics. Clostridial myonecrosis. In: Kimberlin DW, et al, eds. *Red Book: 2018 Report of the Committee on Infectious Diseases.* In press
61. American Academy of Pediatrics. *Clostridium perfringens* food poisoning. In: Kimberlin DW, et al, eds. *Red Book: 2018 Report of the Committee on Infectious Diseases.* In press
62. American Academy of Pediatrics. Tetanus. In: Kimberlin DW, et al, eds. *Red Book: 2018 Report of the Committee on Infectious Diseases.* In press
63. Brook I. *Expert Rev Anti Infect Ther.* 2008;6(3):327–336 PMID: 18588497
64. American Academy of Pediatrics. Diphtheria. In: Kimberlin DW, et al, eds. *Red Book: 2018 Report of the Committee on Infectious Diseases.* In press
65. Fernandez-Roblas R, et al. *Int J Antimicrob Agents.* 2009;33(5):453–455 PMID: 19153032
66. Mookadam F, et al. *Eur J Clin Microbiol Infect Dis.* 2006;25(6):349–353 PMID: 16767481
67. Holdiness MR. *Drugs.* 2002;62(8):1131–1141 PMID: 12010076
68. Dalal A, et al. *J Infect.* 2008;56(1):77–79 PMID: 18036665
69. Anderson A, et al. *MMWR Recomm Rep.* 2013;62(RR-03):1–30 PMID: 23535757
70. Kersh GJ. *Expert Rev Anti Infect Ther.* 2013;11(11):1207–1214 PMID: 24073941
71. Pritt BS, et al. *N Engl J Med.* 2011;365(5):422–429 PMID: 21812671
72. Paul K, et al. *Clin Infect Dis.* 2001;33(1):54–61 PMID: 11389495
73. Ceyhan M, et al. *Int J Pediatr.* 2011;2011:215–237 PMID: 22046191
74. Hsu MS, et al. *Eur J Clin Microbiol Infect Dis.* 2011;30(10):1271–1278 PMID: 21461847
75. Siedner MJ, et al. *Clin Infect Dis.* 2014;58(11):1554–1563 PMID: 24647022
76. Harris PN, et al. *Int J Antimicrob Agents.* 2012;40(4):297–305 PMID: 22824371
77. Doi Y, et al. *Semin Respir Crit Care Med.* 2015;36(1):74–84 PMID: 25643272
78. Arias CA, et al. *Nat Rev Microbiol.* 2012;10(4):266–278 PMID: 22421879
79. American Academy of Pediatrics. Non-group A or B streptococcal and enterococcal infections. In: Kimberlin DW, et al, eds. *Red Book: 2018 Report of the Committee on Infectious Diseases.* In press
80. Hollenbeck BL, et al. *Virulence.* 2012;3(5):421–433 PMID: 23076243

81. Veraldi S, et al. *Clin Exp Dermatol.* 2009;34(8):859–862 PMID: 19663854
82. Principe L, et al. *Infect Dis Rep.* 2016;8(1):6368 PMID: 27103974
83. American Academy of Pediatrics. Tularemia. In: Kimberlin DW, et al, eds. *Red Book: 2018 Report of the Committee on Infectious Diseases.* In press
84. Hepburn MJ, et al. *Expert Rev Anti Infect Ther.* 2008;6(2):231–240 PMID: 18380605
85. Huggan PJ, et al. *J Infect.* 2008;57(4):283–289 PMID: 18805588
86. Riordan T. *Clin Microbiol Rev.* 2007;20(4):622–659 PMID: 17934077
87. Donders G. *Obstet Gynecol Surv.* 2010;65(7):462–473 PMID: 20723268
88. Maraki S, et al. *J Microbiol Immunol Infect.* 2016;49(1):119–122 PMID: 24529567
89. Agrawal A, et al. *J Clin Microbiol.* 2011;49(11):3728–3732 PMID: 21900515
90. American Academy of Pediatrics. *Helicobacter pylori* infections. In: Kimberlin DW, et al, eds. *Red Book: 2018 Report of the Committee on Infectious Diseases.* In press
91. Jones NL, et al. *J Pediatr Gastroenterol Nutr.* 2017;64(6):991–1003 PMID: 28541262
92. Kalach N, et al. *Ann Gastroenterol.* 2015;28(1):10–18 PMID: 25608573
93. Yagupsky P. *Clin Microbiol Rev.* 2015;28(1):54–79 PMID: 25567222
94. Weiss-Salz I, et al. *Adv Exp Med Biol.* 2011;719:67–80 PMID: 22125036
95. Petrosillo N, et al. *Expert Rev Anti Infect Ther.* 2013;11(2):159–177 PMID: 23409822
96. Doi Y, et al. *Semin Respir Crit Care Med.* 2015;36(1):74–84 PMID: 25643272
97. Bergen PJ, et al. *Curr Opin Infect Dis.* 2012;25(6):626–633 PMID: 23041772
98. Viasus D, et al. *Medicine (Baltimore).* 2013;92(1):51–60 PMID: 23266795
99. American Academy of Pediatrics. Leptospirosis. In: Kimberlin DW, et al, eds. *Red Book: 2018 Report of the Committee on Infectious Diseases.* In press
100. Florescu D, et al. *Pediatr Infect Dis J.* 2008;27(11):1013–1019 PMID: 18833028
101. Bortolussi R. *CMAJ.* 2008;179(8):795–797 PMID: 18787096
102. Murphy TF, et al. *Clin Infect Dis.* 2009;49(1):124–131 PMID: 19480579
103. Liu H, et al. *Int J Infect Dis.* 2016;50:10–17 PMID: 27421818
104. Milligan KL, et al. *Clin Pediatr (Phila).* 2013;52(5):462–464 PMID: 22267858
105. American Academy of Pediatrics. Diseases caused by nontuberculous mycobacteria. In: Kimberlin DW, et al, eds. *Red Book: 2018 Report of the Committee on Infectious Diseases.* In press
106. Nessar R, et al. *J Antimicrob Chemother.* 2012;67(4):810–818 PMID: 22290346
107. Koh WJ, et al. *Int J Tuberc Lung Dis.* 2014;18(10):1141–1148 PMID: 25216826
108. Griffith DE, et al. *Am J Respir Crit Care Med.* 2007;175(4):367–416 PMID: 17277290
109. Philley JV, et al. *Curr Treat Options Infect Dis.* 2016;8(4):275–296 PMID: 28529461
110. American Academy of Pediatrics. Tuberculosis. In: Kimberlin DW, et al, eds. *Red Book: 2018 Report of the Committee on Infectious Diseases.* In press
111. Hlavsa MC, et al. *Clin Infect Dis.* 2008;47(2):168–175 PMID: 18532886
112. Hay RJ. *Curr Opin Infect Dis.* 2009;22(2):99–101 PMID: 19276876
113. Colombo RE, et al. *Semin Respir Crit Care Med.* 2008;29(5):577–588 PMID: 18810691
114. American Academy of Pediatrics. Leprosy. In: Kimberlin DW, et al, eds. *Red Book: 2018 Report of the Committee on Infectious Diseases.* In press
115. Doedens RA, et al. *Pediatr Infect Dis J.* 2008;27(1):81–83 PMID: 18162949
116. Nahid P, et al. *Clin Infect Dis.* 2016;63(7):e147–e195 PMID: 27516382
117. Waites KB, et al. *Semin Fetal Neonatal Med.* 2009;14(4):190–199 PMID: 19109084
118. Watt KM, et al. *Pediatr Infect Dis J.* 2012;31(2):197–199 PMID: 22016080
119. Pereyre S, et al. *Front Microbiol.* 2016;7:974 PMID: 27446015
120. Gardiner SJ, et al. *Cochrane Database Syst Rev.* 2015;1:CD004875 PMID: 25566754
121. Akaike H, et al. *Jpn J Infect Dis.* 2012;65(6):535–538 PMID: 23183207
122. Centers for Disease Control and Prevention. *MMWR Morb Mortal Wkly Rep.* 2012;61(31):590–594 PMID: 22874837
123. American Academy of Pediatrics. Meningococcal infections. In: Kimberlin DW, et al, eds. *Red Book: 2018 Report of the Committee on Infectious Diseases.* In press
124. Wu HM, et al. *N Engl J Med.* 2009;360(9):886–892 PMID: 19246360
125. Wilson JW. *Mayo Clin Proc.* 2012;87(4):403–407 PMID: 22469352

126. American Academy of Pediatrics. Nocardiosis. In: Kimberlin DW, et al, eds. *Red Book: 2018 Report of the Committee on Infectious Diseases.* In press

127. Casanova-Román M, et al. *Infection.* 2010;38(4):321–323 PMID: 20376528

128. Goldstein EJ, et al. *Antimicrob Agents Chemother.* 2012;56(12):6319–6323 PMID: 23027193

129. Murphy EC, et al. *FEMS Microbiol Rev.* 2013;37(4):520–553 PMID: 23030831

130. Ozdemir O, et al. *J Microbiol Immunol Infect.* 2010;43(4):344–346 PMID: 20688296

131. Stock I, Wiedemann B. *J Antimicrob Chemother.* 2001;48(6):803–811 PMID: 11733464

132. Brook I, et al. *Clin Microbiol Rev.* 2013;26(3):526–546 PMID: 23824372

133. Perry A, et al. *Expert Rev Anti Infect Ther.* 2011;9(12):1149–1156 PMID: 22114965

134. Tunkel AR, et al. *Clin Infect Dis.* 2017 PMID: 28203777

135. Schaffer JN, et al. *Microbiol Spectr.* 2015;3(5) PMID: 26542036

136. Tumbarello M, et al. *J Antimicrob Chemother.* 2004;53(2):277–282 PMID: 14688041

137. Fish DN, et al. *Pharmacotherapy.* 2013;33(10):1022–1034 PMID: 23744833

138. Kalil AC, et al. *Clin Infect Dis.* 2016;63(5):e61–e111 PMID: 27418577

139. Tam VH, et al. *Antimicrob Agents Chemother.* 2010;54(3):1160–1164 PMID: 20086165

140. Freifeld AG, et al. *Clin Infect Dis.* 2011;52(4):e56–e93 PMID: 21258094

141. Velkov T, et al. *Future Microbiol.* 2013;8(6):711–724 PMID: 23701329

142. Döring G, et al. *J Cyst Fibros.* 2012;11(6):461–479 PMID: 23137712

143. Mogayzel PJ Jr, et al. *Am J Respir Crit Care Med.* 2013;187(7):680–689 PMID: 23540878

144. Saiman L. *Paediatr Respir Rev.* 2007;8(3):249–255 PMID: 17868923

145. Mogayzel PJ Jr, et al. *Ann Am Thorac Soc.* 2014;11(10):1640–1650 PMID: 25549030

146. Yamshchikov AV, et al. *Lancet Infect Dis.* 2010;10(5):350–359 PMID: 20417417

147. American Academy of Pediatrics. Rickettsial diseases. In: Kimberlin DW, et al, eds. *Red Book: 2018 Report of the Committee on Infectious Diseases.* In press

148. Woods CR. *Pediatr Clin North Am.* 2013;60(2):455–470 PMID: 23481111

149. American Academy of Pediatrics. *Salmonella* infections. In: Kimberlin DW, et al, eds. *Red Book: 2018 Report of the Committee on Infectious Diseases.* In press

150. Haeusler GM, et al. *Adv Exp Med Biol.* 2013;764:13–26 PMID: 23654054

151. Onwuezobe IA, et al. *Cochrane Database Syst Rev.* 2012;11:CD001167 PMID: 23152205

152. Effa EE, et al. *Cochrane Database Syst Rev.* 2008;(4):CD006083 PMID: 18843701

153. Yousfi K, et al. *Eur J Clin Microbiol Infect Dis.* 2017;36(8):1353–1362 PMID: 28299457

154. Klontz KC, et al. *Expert Rev Anti Infect Ther.* 2015;13(1):69–80 PMID: 25399653

155. American Academy of Pediatrics. *Shigella* infections. In: Kimberlin DW, et al, eds. *Red Book: 2018 Report of the Committee on Infectious Diseases.* In press

156. Sjölund Karlsson M, et al. *Antimicrob Agents Chemother.* 2013;57(3):1559–1560 PMID: 23274665

157. Holmes LC. *Pediatr Rev.* 2014;35(6):261–262 PMID: 24891600

158. Gaastra W, et al. *Vet Microbiol.* 2009;133(3):211–228 PMID: 19008054

159. American Academy of Pediatrics. Rat-bite fever. In: Kimberlin DW, et al, eds. *Red Book: 2018 Report of the Committee on Infectious Diseases.* In press

160. Liu C, et al. *Clin Infect Dis.* 2011;52(3):e18–e55 PMID: 21208910

161. Long CB, et al. *Expert Rev Anti Infect Ther.* 2010;8(2):183–195 PMID: 20109048

162. Korczowski B, et al. *Pediatr Infect Dis J.* 2016;35(8):e239–e247 PMID: 27164462

163. Bradley J, et al. *Pediatrics.* 2017;139(3):e20162477 PMID: 28202770

164. Blanchard AC, et al. *Clin Perinatol.* 2015;42(1):119–132 PMID: 25678000

165. Marchant EA, et al. *Clin Dev Immunol.* 2013;2013:586076 PMID: 23762094

166. Samonis G, et al. *PLoS One.* 2012;7(5):e37375 PMID: 22624022

167. Church D, et al. *Scand J Infect Dis.* 2013;45(4):265–270 PMID: 23113657

168. American Academy of Pediatrics. Group A streptococcal infections. In: Kimberlin DW, et al, eds. *Red Book: 2018 Report of the Committee on Infectious Diseases.* In press

169. American Academy of Pediatrics. Group B streptococcal infections. In: Kimberlin DW, et al, eds. *Red Book: 2018 Report of the Committee on Infectious Diseases.* In press

170. Faden H, et al. *Pediatr Infect Dis J.* 2017 PMID: 28640003

171. Broyles LN, et al. *Clin Infect Dis.* 2009;48(6):706–712 PMID: 19187026

172. Stelzmueller I, et al. *Eur J Pediatr Surg.* 2009;19(1):21–24 PMID: 19221948
173. Deutschmann MW, et al. *JAMA Otolaryngol Head Neck Surg.* 2013;139(2):157–160 PMID: 23429946
174. Pichichero ME. *Pediatr Clin North Am.* 2013;60(2):391–407 PMID: 23481107
175. American Academy of Pediatrics. Pneumococcal infections. In: Kimberlin DW, et al, eds. *Red Book: 2018 Report of the Committee on Infectious Diseases.* In press
176. Mendes RE, et al. *Diagn Microbiol Infect Dis.* 2014;80(1):19–25 PMID: 24974272
177. Olarte L, et al. *Clin Infect Dis.* 2017;64(12):1699–1704 PMID: 28199482
178. Baltimore RS, et al. *Circulation.* 2015;132(13):1487–1515 PMID: 26373317
179. American Academy of Pediatrics. Syphilis. In: Kimberlin DW, et al, eds. *Red Book: 2018 Report of the Committee on Infectious Diseases.* In press
180. Merchan LM, et al. *Antimicrob Agents Chemother.* 2015;59(1):570–578 PMID: 25385115
181. American Academy of Pediatrics. Cholera. In: Kimberlin DW, et al, eds. *Red Book: 2018 Report of the Committee on Infectious Diseases.* In press
182. Clemens JD, et al. *Lancet.* 2017;S0140–S6736 PMID: 28302312
183. Heng SP, et al. *Front Microbiol.* 2017;8:997 PMID: 28620366
184. Daniels NA. *Clin Infect Dis.* 2011;52(6):788–792 PMID: 21367733
185. American Academy of Pediatrics. *Yersinia enterocolitica* and *Yersinia pseudotuberculosis* infections. In: Kimberlin DW, et al, eds. *Red Book: 2018 Report of the Committee on Infectious Diseases.* In press
186. Kato H, et al. *Medicine (Baltimore).* 2016;95(26):e3988 PMID: 27368001
187. American Academy of Pediatrics. Plague. In: Kimberlin DW, et al, eds. *Red Book: 2018 Report of the Committee on Infectious Diseases.* In press
188. Butler T. *Clin Infect Dis.* 2009;49(5):736–742 PMID: 19606935
189. Bertelli L, et al. *J Pediatr.* 2014;165(2):411 PMID: 24793203

Chapter 8

1. Groll AH, et al. *Lancet Oncol.* 2014;15(8):e327–e340 PMID: 24988936
2. Wingard JR, et al. *Blood.* 2010;116(24):5111–5118 PMID: 20826719
3. Van Burik JA, et al. *Clin Infect Dis.* 2004;39(10):1407–1416 PMID: 15546073
4. Cornely OA, et al. *N Engl J Med.* 2007;356(4):348–359 PMID: 17251531
5. Kung HC, et al. *Cancer Med.* 2014;3(3):667–673 PMID: 24644249
6. Science M, et al. *Pediatr Blood Cancer.* 2014;61(3):393–400 PMID: 24424789
7. Bow EJ, et al. *BMC Infect Dis.* 2015;15:128 PMID: 25887385
8. Tacke D, et al. *Ann Hematol.* 2014;93(9):1449–1456 PMID: 24951122
9. Almyroudis NG, et al. *Curr Opin Infect Dis.* 2009;22(4):385–393 PMID: 19506476
10. Maschmeyer G. *J Antimicrob Chemother.* 2009;63(Suppl1):i27–i30 PMID: 19372178
11. Freifeld AG, et al. *Clin Infect Dis.* 2011;52(4):e56–e93 PMID: 21258094
12. De Pauw BE, et al. *N Engl J Med.* 2007;356(4):409–411 PMID: 17251538
13. Salavert M. *Int J Antimicrob Agents.* 2008;32(Suppl2):S149–S153 PMID: 19013340
14. Eschenauer GA, et al. *Liver Transpl.* 2009;15(8):842–858 PMID: 19642130
15. Winston DJ, et al. *Am J Transplant.* 2014;14(12):2758–2764 PMID: 25376267
16. Sun HY, et al. *Transplantation.* 2013;96(6):573–578 PMID: 23842191
17. Radack KP, et al. *Curr Infect Dis Rep.* 2009;11(6):427–434 PMID: 19857381
18. Patterson TF, et al. *Clin Infect Dis.* 2016;63(4):e1–e60 PMID: 27365388
19. Thomas L, et al. *Expert Rev Anti Infect Ther.* 2009;7(4):461–472 PMID: 19400765
20. Friberg LE, et al. *Antimicrob Agents Chemother.* 2012;56(6):3032–3042 PMID: 22430956
21. Burgos A, et al. *Pediatrics.* 2008;121(5):e1286–e1294 PMID: 18450871
22. Herbrecht R, et al. *N Engl J Med.* 2002;347(6):408–415 PMID: 12167683
23. Mousset S, et al. *Ann Hematol.* 2014;93(1):13–32 PMID: 24026426
24. Blyth CC, et al. *Intern Med J.* 2014;44(12b):1333–1349 PMID: 25482744
25. Denning DW, et al. *Eur Respir J.* 2016;47(1):45–68 PMID: 26699723
26. Cornely OA, et al. *Clin Infect Dis.* 2007;44(10):1289–1297 PMID: 17443465
27. Maertens JA, et al. *Lancet.* 2016;387(10020):760–769 PMID: 26684607
28. Tissot F, et al. *Haematologica.* 2017;102(3):433–444 PMID: 28011902
29. Walsh TJ, et al. *Antimicrob Agents Chemother.* 2010;54(10):4116–4123 PMID: 20660687

30. Bartelink IH, et al. *Antimicrob Agents Chemother.* 2013;57(1):235–240 PMID: 23114771
31. Marr KA, et al. *Ann Intern Med.* 2015;162(2):81–89 PMID: 25599346
32. Verweij PE, et al. *Drug Resist Updat.* 2015;21–22:30–40 PMID: 26282594
33. Kohno S, et al. *Eur J Clin Microbiol Infect Dis.* 2013;32(3):387–397 PMID: 23052987
34. Naggie S, et al. *Clin Chest Med.* 2009;30(2):337–353 PMID: 19375639
35. Revankar SG, et al. *Clin Microbiol Rev.* 2010;23(4):884–928 PMID: 20930077
36. Wong EH, et al. *Infect Dis Clin North Am.* 2016;30(1):165–178 PMID: 26897066
37. Revankar SG, et al. *Clin Infect Dis.* 2004;38(2):206–216 PMID: 14699452
38. Li DM, et al. *Lancet Infect Dis.* 2009;9(6):376–383 PMID: 19467477
39. Chowdhary A, et al. *Clin Microbiol Infect.* 2014;20(Suppl3):47–75 PMID: 24483780
40. McCarty TP, et al. *Med Mycol.* 2015;53(5):440–446 PMID: 25908651
41. Schieffelin JS, et al. *Transplant Infect Dis.* 2014;16(2):270–278 PMID: 24628809
42. Chapman SW, et al. *Clin Infect Dis.* 2008;46(12):1801–1812 PMID: 18462107
43. McKinnell JA, et al. *Clin Chest Med.* 2009;30(2):227–239 PMID: 19375630
44. Walsh CM, et al. *Pediatr Infect Dis J.* 2006;25(7):656–658 PMID: 16804444
45. Fanella S, et al. *Med Mycol.* 2011;49(6):627–632 PMID: 21208027
46. Smith JA, et al. *Proc Am Thorac Soc.* 2010;7(3):173–180 PMID: 20463245
47. Bariola JR, et al. *Clin Infect Dis.* 2010;50(6):797–804 PMID: 20166817
48. Limper AH, et al. *Am J Respir Crit Care Med.* 2011;183(1):96–128 PMID: 21193785
49. Pappas PG, et al. *Clin Infect Dis.* 2016;62(4):e1–e50 PMID: 26679628
50. Lortholary O, et al. *Clin Microbiol Infect.* 2012;18(Suppl7):68–77 PMID: 23137138
51. Ullman AJ, et al. *Clin Microbiol Infect.* 2012;18(Suppl7):53–67 PMID: 23137137
52. Hope WW, et al. *Clin Microbiol Infect.* 2012;18(Suppl7):38–52 PMID: 23137136
53. Cornely OA, et al. *Clin Microbiol Infect.* 2012;18(Suppl7):19–37 PMID: 23137135
54. Hope WW, et al. *Antimicrob Agents Chemother.* 2015;59(2):905–913 PMID: 25421470
55. Piper L, et al. *Pediatr Infect Dis J.* 2011;30(5):375–378 PMID: 21085048
56. Watt KM, et al. *Antimicrob Agents Chemother.* 2015;59(7):3935–3943 PMID: 25896706
57. Ascher SB, et al. *Pediatr Infect Dis J.* 2012;31(5):439–443 PMID 22189522
58. Sobel JD. *Lancet.* 2007;369(9577):1961–1971 PMID: 17560449
59. Lopez Martinez R, et al. *Clin Dermatol.* 2007;25(2):188–194 PMID: 17350498
60. Ameen M. *Clin Exp Dermatol.* 2009;34(8):849–854 PMID: 19575735
61. Chowdhary A, et al. *Clin Microbiol Infect.* 2014;20(Suppl3):47–75 PMID: 24483780
62. Queiroz-Telles F. *Rev Inst Med Trop Sao Paulo.* 2015;57(Suppl19):46–50 PMID: 26465369
63. Queiroz-Telles F, et al. *Clin Microbiol Rev.* 2017;30(1):233–276 PMID: 27856522
64. Galgiani JN, et al. *Clin Infect Dis.* 2016;63(6):717–722 PMID: 27559032
65. Anstead GM, et al. *Infect Dis Clin North Am.* 2006;20(3):621–643 PMID: 16984872
66. Williams PL. *Ann N Y Acad Sci.* 2007;1111:377–384 PMID: 17363442
67. Homans JD, et al. *Pediatr Infect Dis J.* 2010;29(1):65–67 PMID: 19884875
68. Kauffman CA, et al. *Transplant Infectious Diseases.* 2014;16(2):213–224 PMID: 24589027
69. McCarty JM, et al. *Clin Infect Dis.* 2013;56(11):1579–1585 PMID: 23463637
70. Bravo R, et al. *J Pediatr Hematol Oncol.* 2012;34(5):389–394 PMID: 22510771
71. Catanzaro A, et al. *Clin Infect Dis.* 2007;45(5):562–568 PMID: 17682989
72. Thompson GR, et al. *Clin Infect Dis.* 2016;63(3):356–362 PMID: 27169478
73. Thompson GR 3rd, et al. *Clin Infect Dis.* 2017;65(2):338–341 PMID: 28419259
74. Chayakulkeeree M, et al. *Infect Dis Clin North Am.* 2006;20(3):507–544 PMID: 16984867
75. Jarvis JN, et al. *Semin Respir Crit Care Med.* 2008;29(2):141–150 PMID: 18365996
76. Perfect JR, et al. *Clin Infect Dis.* 2010;50(3):291–322 PMID: 20047480
77. Joshi NS, et al. *Pediatr Infect Dis J.* 2010;29(12):e91–e95 PMID: 20935590
78. Day JN, et al. *N Engl J Med.* 2013;368(14):1291–1302 PMID: 23550668
79. Cortez KJ, et al. *Clin Microbiol Rev.* 2008;21(1):157–197 PMID: 18202441
80. Tortorano AM, et al. *Clin Microbiol Infect.* 2014;20(Suppl3):27–46 PMID: 24548001
81. Horn DL, et al. *Mycoses.* 2014;57(11):652–658 PMID: 24943384
82. Muhammed M, et al. *Medicine (Baltimore).* 2013;92(6):305–316 PMID: 24145697
83. Rodriguez-Tudela JL, et al. *Med Mycol.* 2009;47(4):359–370 PMID: 19031336

84. Wheat LJ, et al. *Clin Infect Dis.* 2007;45(7):807–825 PMID: 17806045
85. Myint T, et al. *Medicine (Baltimore).* 2014;93(1):11–18 PMID: 24378739
86. Assi M, et al. *Clin Infect Dis.* 2013;57(11):1542–1549 PMID: 24046304
87. Chayakulkeeree M, et al. *Eur J Clin Microbiol Infect Dis.* 2006;25(4):215–229 PMID: 16568297
88. Spellberg B, et al. *Clin Infect Dis.* 2009;48(12):1743–1751 PMID: 19435437
89. Reed C, et al. *Clin Infect Dis.* 2008;47(3):364–371 PMID: 18558882
90. Cornely OA, et al. *Clin Microbiol Infect.* 2014;20(Suppl3):5–26 PMID: 24479848
91. Spellberg B, et al. *Clin Infect Dis.* 2012;54(Suppl1):S73–S78 PMID: 22247449
92. Chitasombat MN, et al. *Curr Opin Infect Dis.* 2016;29(4):340–345 PMID: 27191199
93. Pana ZD, et al. *BMC Infect Dis.* 2016;16(1):667 PMID: 27832748
94. Kyvernitakis A, et al. *Clin Microbiol Infect.* 2016;22(9):811.e1–811.e8 PMID: 27085727
95. Marty FM, et al. *Lancet Infect Dis.* 2016;16(7):828–837 PMID: 26969258
96. Queiroz-Telles F, et al. *Clin Infect Dis.* 2007;45(11):1462–1469 PMID: 17990229
97. Menezes VM, et al. *Cochrane Database Syst Rev.* 2006;(2):CD004967 PMID: 16625617
98. Marques SA. *An Bras Dermatol.* 2013;88(5):700–711 PMID: 24173174
99. Borges SR, et al. *Med Mycol.* 2014;52(3):303–310 PMID: 24577007
100. Panel on Opportunistic Infections in HIV-Exposed and HIV-Infected Children. Guidelines for the prevention and treatment of opportunistic infections in HIV-exposed and HIV-infected children. http://aidsinfo.nih.gov/contentfiles/lvguidelines/oi_guidelines_pediatrics.pdf. Updated December 15, 2016. Accessed October 11, 2017
101. Siberry GK, et al. *Pediatr Infect Dis J.* 2013;32(Suppl2):i–KK4 PMID: 24569199
102. Kauffman CA, et al. *Clin Infect Dis.* 2007;45(10):1255–1265 PMID: 17968818
103. Aung AK, et al. *Med Mycol.* 2013;51(5):534–544 PMID: 23286352
104. Ali S, et al. *Pediatr Emerg Care.* 2007;23(9):662–668 PMID: 17876261
105. Shy R. *Pediatr Rev.* 2007;28(5):164–174 PMID: 17473121
106. Andrews MD, et al. *Am Fam Physician.* 2008;77(10):1415–1420 PMID: 18533375
107. Kakourou T, et al. *Pediatr Dermatol.* 2010;27(3):226–228 PMID: 20609140
108. Gupta AK, et al. *Pediatr Dermatol.* 2013;30(1):1–6 PMID: 22994156
109. Chen X, et al. *J Am Acad Dermatol.* 2017;76(2):368–374 PMID: 27816294
110. de Berker D. *N Engl J Med.* 2009;360(20):2108–2116 PMID: 19439745
111. Ameen M, et al. *Br J Dermatol.* 2014;171(5):937–958 PMID: 25409999
112. Pantazidou A, et al. *Arch Dis Child.* 2007;92(11):1040–1042 PMID: 17954488
113. Gupta AK, et al. *J Cutan Med Surg.* 2014;18(2):79–90 PMID: 24636433

Chapter 9

1. Terrault NA, et al. *Hepatology.* 2016;63(1):261–283 PMID: 26566064
2. Lenaerts L, et al. *Rev Med Virol.* 2008;18(6):357–374 PMID: 18655013
3. Michaels MG. *Expert Rev Anti Infect Ther.* 2007;5(3):441–448 PMID: 17547508
4. Biron KK. *Antiviral Res.* 2006;71(2–3):154–163 PMID: 16765457
5. Boeckh M, et al. *Blood.* 2009;113(23):5711–5719 PMID: 19299333
6. Vaudry W, et al. *Am J Transplant.* 2009;9(3):636–643 PMID: 19260840
7. Emanuel D, et al. *Ann Intern Med.* 1988;109(10):777–782 PMID: 2847609
8. Reed EC, et al. *Ann Intern Med.* 1988;109(10):783–788 PMID: 2847610
9. *Ophthalmology.* 1994;101(7):1250–1261 PMID: 8035989
10. Musch DC, et al. *N Engl J Med.* 1997;337(2):83–90 PMID: 9211677
11. Martin DF, et al. *N Engl J Med.* 2002;346(15):1119–1126 PMID: 11948271
12. Kempen JH, et al. *Arch Ophthalmol.* 2003;121(4):466–476 PMID: 12695243
13. Studies of Ocular Complications of AIDS Research Group. The AIDS Clinical Trials Group. *Am J Ophthalmol.* 2001;131(4):457–467 PMID: 11292409
14. Dieterich DT, et al. *J Infect Dis.* 1993;167(2):278–282 PMID: 8380610
15. Gerna G, et al. *Antiviral Res.* 1997;34(1):39–50 PMID: 9107384
16. Markham A, et al. *Drugs.* 1994;48(3):455–484 PMID: 7527763
17. Kimberlin DW, et al. *J Infect Dis.* 2008;197(6):836–845 PMID: 18279073
18. Kimberlin DW, et al. *N Engl J Med.* 2015;372(10):933–943 PMID: 25738669

19. Griffiths P, et al. *Herpes.* 2008;15(1):4–12 PMID: 18983762
20. Panel on Opportunistic Infections in HIV-Exposed and HIV-Infected Children. Guidelines for the prevention and treatment of opportunistic infections in HIV-exposed and HIV-infected children. http://aidsinfo.nih.gov/contentfiles/lvguidelines/oi_guidelines_pediatrics.pdf. Updated December 15, 2016. Accessed October 11, 2017
21. Abzug MJ, et al. *J Pediatr Infect Dis Soc.* 2016;5(1):53–62 PMID: 26407253
22. Biebl A, et al. *Nat Clin Pract Neurol.* 2009;5(3):171–174 PMID: 19262593
23. Chadaide Z, et al. *J Med Virol.* 2008;80(11):1930–1932 PMID: 18814244
24. American Academy of Pediatrics. Epstein-Barr virus infections. In: Kimberlin DW, et al, eds. *Red Book: 2018 Report of the Committee on Infectious Diseases.* In press
25. Gross TG. *Herpes.* 2009;15(3):64–67 PMID: 19306606
26. Styczynski J, et al. *Bone Marrow Transplant.* 2009;43(10):757–770 PMID: 19043458
27. Jonas MM, et al. *Hepatology.* 2016;63(2):377–387 PMID: 26223345
28. Marcellin P, et al. *Gastroenterology.* 2016;150(1):134–144.e10 PMID: 26453773
29. Chen HL, et al. *Hepatology.* 2015;62(2):375–386 PMID: 25851052
30. Wu Q, et al. *Clin Gastroenterol Hepatol.* 2015;13(6):1170–1176 PMID: 25251571
31. Hou JL, et al. *J Viral Hepat.* 2015;22(2):85–93 PMID: 25243325
32. Kurbegov AC, et al. *Expert Rev Gastroenterol Hepatol.* 2009;3(1):39–49 PMID: 19210112
33. Jonas MM, et al. *Hepatology.* 2008;47(6):1863–1871 PMID: 18433023
34. Lai CL, et al. *Gastroenterology.* 2002;123(6):1831–1838 PMID: 12454840
35. Honkoop P, et al. *Expert Opin Investig Drugs.* 2003;12(4):683–688 PMID: 12665423
36. Shaw T, et al. *Expert Rev Anti Infect Ther.* 2004;2(6):853–871 PMID: 15566330
37. Elisofon SA, et al. *Clin Liver Dis.* 2006;10(1):133–148 PMID: 16376798
38. Jonas MM, et al. *Hepatology.* 2010;52(6):2192–2205 PMID: 20890947
39. Haber BA, et al. *Pediatrics.* 2009;124(5):e1007–e1013 PMID: 19805457
40. Shneider BL, et al. *Hepatology.* 2006;44(5):1344–1354 PMID: 17058223
41. Jain MK, et al. *J Viral Hepat.* 2007;14(3):176–182 PMID: 17305883
42. Sokal EM, et al. *Gastroenterology.* 1998;114(5):988–995 PMID: 9558288
43. Jonas MM, et al. *N Engl J Med.* 2002;346(22):1706–1713 PMID: 12037150
44. Chang TT, et al. *N Engl J Med.* 2006;354(10):1001–1010 PMID: 16525137
45. Liaw YF, et al. *Gastroenterology.* 2009;136(2):486–495 PMID: 19027013
46. Keam SJ, et al. *Drugs.* 2008;68(9):1273–1317 PMID: 18547135
47. Marcellin P, et al. *Gastroenterology.* 2011;140(2):459–468 PMID: 21034744
48. Poordad F, et al. *N Engl J Med.* 2011;364(13):1195–1206 PMID: 21449783
49. Schwarz KB, et al. *Gastroenterology.* 2011;140(2):450–458 PMID: 21036173
50. Nelson DR. *Liver Int.* 2011;31(Suppl1):53–57 PMID: 21205138
51. Strader DB, et al. *Hepatology.* 2004;39(4):1147–1171 PMID: 15057920
52. Soriano V, et al. *AIDS.* 2007;21(9):1073–1089 PMID: 17502718
53. Feld JJ, et al. *N Engl J Med.* 2014;370(17):1594–1603 PMID: 24720703
54. Zeuzem S, et al. *N Engl J Med.* 2014;370(17):1604–1614 PMID: 24720679
55. Andreone P, et al. *Gastroenterology.* 2014;147(2):359–365.e1 PMID: 24818763
56. Ferenci P, et al. *N Engl J Med.* 2014;370(21):1983–1992 PMID: 24795200
57. Poordad F, et al. *N Engl J Med.* 2014;370(21):1973–1982 PMID: 24725237
58. Jacobson IM, et al. *Lancet.* 2014;384(9941):403–413 PMID: 24907225
59. Manns M, et al. *Lancet.* 2014;384(9941):414–426 PMID: 24907224
60. Forns X, et al. *Gastroenterology.* 2014;146(7):1669–1679.e3 PMID: 24602923
61. Zeuzem S, et al. *Gastroenterology.* 2014;146(2):430–441.e6 PMID: 24184810
62. Lawitz E, et al. *Lancet.* 2014;384(9956):1756–1765 PMID: 25078309
63. Afdhal N, et al. *N Engl J Med.* 2014;370(20):1889–1898 PMID: 24725239
64. Afdhal N, et al. *N Engl J Med.* 2014;370(16):1483–1493 PMID: 24725238
65. Kowdley KV, et al. *N Engl J Med.* 2014;370(20):1879–1888 PMID: 24720702
66. Lawitz E, et al. *N Engl J Med.* 2013;368(20):1878–1887 PMID: 23607594
67. Jacobson IM, et al. *N Engl J Med.* 2013;368(20):1867–1877 PMID: 23607593
68. Zeuzem S, et al. *N Engl J Med.* 2014;370(21):1993–2001 PMID: 24795201

69. Hollier LM, et al. *Cochrane Database Syst Rev.* 2008;(1):CD004946 PMID: 18254066
70. Pinninti SG, et al. *J Pediatr.* 2012;161(1):134–138 PMID: 22336576
71. Kimberlin DW, et al. *Clin Infect Dis.* 2010;50(2):221–228 PMID: 20014952
72. Abdel Massih RC, et al. *World J Gastroenterol.* 2009;15(21):2561–2569 PMID: 19496184
73. Mofenson LM, et al. *MMWR Recomm Rep.* 2009;58(RR-11):1–166 PMID: 19730409
74. Kuhar DT, et al. *Infect Control Hosp Epidemiol.* 2013;34(9):875–892 PMID: 23917901
75. Acosta EP, et al. *J Infect Dis.* 2010;202(4):563–566 PMID: 20594104
76. Kimberlin DW, et al. *J Infect Dis.* 2013;207(5):709–720 PMID: 23230059
77. McPherson C, et al. *J Infect Dis.* 2012;206(6):847–850 PMID: 22807525
78. Bradley JS, et al. *Pediatrics.* 2017;140(5):e20162727 PMID: 29051331
79. American Academy of Pediatrics. Measles. In: Kimberlin DW, et al, eds. *Red Book: 2018 Report of the Committee on Infectious Diseases.* In press
80. American Academy of Pediatrics Committee on Infectious Diseases and Bronchiolitis Guidelines Committee. *Pediatrics.* 2014;134(2):415–420 PMID: 25070315
81. American Academy of Pediatrics Committee on Infectious Diseases and Bronchiolitis Guidelines Committee. *Pediatrics.* 2014;134(2):e620–e638 PMID: 25070304
82. Whitley RJ. *Adv Exp Med Biol.* 2008;609:216–232 PMID: 18193668

Chapter 10

1. Blessmann J, et al. *J Clin Microbiol.* 2003;41(10):4745–4750 PMID: 14532214
2. Haque R, et al. *N Engl J Med.* 2003;348(16):1565–1573 PMID: 1270037
3. Rossignol JF, et al. *Trans R Soc Trop Med Hyg.* 2007;101(10):1025–1031 PMID: 17658567
4. Mackey-Lawrence NM, et al. *BMJ Clin Evid.* 2011;pii:0918 PMID: 21477391
5. Fox LM, et al. *Clin Infect Dis.* 2005;40(8):1173–1180 PMID: 15791519
6. Cope JR, et al. *Clin Infect Dis.* 2016;62(6):774–776 PMID: 26679626
7. Vargas-Zepeda J, et al. *Arch Med Res.* 2005;36(1):83–86 PMID: 15900627
8. Linam WM, et al. *Pediatrics.* 2015;135(3):e744–e748 PMID: 25667249
9. Visvesvara GS, et al. *FEMS Immunol Med Microbiol.* 2007;50(1):1–26 PMID: 17428307
10. Deetz TR, et al. *Clin Infect Dis.* 2003;37(10):1304–1312 PMID: 14583863
11. Chotmongkol V, et al. *Am J Trop Med Hyg.* 2009;81(3):443–445 PMID: 19706911
12. Lo Re V III, et al. *Am J Med.* 2003;114(3):217–223 PMID: 12637136
13. Jitpimolmard S, et al. *Parasitol Res.* 2007;100(6):1293–1296 PMID: 17177056
14. Checkley AM, et al. *J Infect.* 2010;60(1):1–20 PMID: 19931558
15. Bethony J, et al. *Lancet.* 2006;367(9521):1521–1532 PMID: 16679166
16. Krause PJ, et al. *N Engl J Med.* 2000;343(20):1454–1458 PMID: 11078770
17. Vannier E, et al. *Infect Dis Clin North Am.* 2008;22(3):469–488 PMID: 18755385
18. Wormser GP, et al. *Clin Infect Dis.* 2006;43(9):1089–1134 PMID: 17029130
19. Fisk T, et al. In: Mandell GL, et al, eds. *Principles and Practice of Infectious Diseases.* 2005:3228–3237
20. Murray WJ, et al. *Clin Infect Dis.* 2004;39(10):1484–1492 PMID: 15546085
21. Sircar AD, et al. *MMWR Morb Mortal Wkly Rep.* 2016;65(35):930–933 PMID: 27608169
22. Shlim DR, et al. *Clin Infect Dis.* 1995;21(1):97–101 PMID: 7578767
23. Udkow MP, et al. *J Infect Dis.* 1993;168(1):242–244 PMID: 8515120
24. Bern C, et al. *JAMA.* 2007;298(18):2171–2181 PMID: 18000201
25. Maguire JH. Trypanosoma. In: Gorbach SL, Bartlett JG, Blacklow NR, eds. *Infectious Diseases.* 3rd ed. 2004:2327–2334
26. Miller DA, et al. *Clin Infect Dis.* 2015;60(8):1237–1240 PMID: 25601454
27. Smith HV, et al. *Curr Opin Infect Dis.* 2004;17(6):557–564 PMID: 15640710
28. Davies AP, et al. *BMJ.* 2009;339:b4168 PMID: 19841008
29. Krause I, et al. *Pediatr Infect Dis J.* 2012;31(11):1135–1138 PMID: 22810017
30. Abubakar I, et al. *Cochrane Database Syst Rev.* 2007;(1):CD004932 PMID: 17253532
31. Jelinek T, et al. *Clin Infect Dis.* 1994;19(6):1062–1066 PMID: 7534125
32. Schuster A, et al. *Clin Infect Dis.* 2013;57(8):1155–1157 PMID: 23811416
33. Hoge CW, et al. *Lancet.* 1995;345(8951):691–693 PMID: 7885125
34. Ortega YR, et al. *Clin Microbiol Rev.* 2010;23(1):218–234 PMID: 20065331

35. Nash TE, et al. *Neurology.* 2006;67(7):1120–1127 PMID: 17030744
36. Garcia HH, et al. *Lancet Neurol.* 2014;13(12):1202–1215 PMID: 25453460
37. Lillie P, et al. *J Infect.* 2010;60(5):403–404 PMID: 20153773
38. Mitchell WG, et al. *Pediatrics.* 1988;82(1):76–82 PMID: 3288959
39. Stark DJ, et al. *Trends Parasitol.* 2006;22(2):92–96 PMID: 16380293
40. Johnson EH, et al. *Clin Microbiol Rev.* 2004;17(3):553–570 PMID: 15258093
41. Smego RA Jr, et al. *Clin Infect Dis.* 2003;37(8):1073–1083 PMID: 14523772
42. Brunetti E, et al. *Acta Trop.* 2010;114(1):1–16 PMID: 19931502
43. Fernando SD, et al. *J Trop Med.* 2011;2011:175941 PMID: 21234244
44. Tisch DJ, et al. *Lancet Infect Dis.* 2005;5(8):514–523 PMID: 16048720
45. Mand S, et al. *Clin Infect Dis.* 2012;55(5):621–630 PMID: 22610930
46. Ottesen EA, et al. *Annu Rev Med.* 1992;43:417–424 PMID: 1580599
47. Jong EC, et al. *J Infect Dis.* 1985;152(3):637–640 PMID: 3897401
48. Sayasone S, et al. *Clin Infect Dis.* 2017;64(4):451–458 PMID: 28174906
49. Calvopina M, et al. *Trans R Soc Trop Med Hyg.* 1998;92(5):566–569 PMID: 9861383
50. Johnson RJ, et al. *Rev Infect Dis.* 1985;7(2):200–206 PMID: 4001715
51. Graham CS, et al. *Clin Infect Dis.* 2001;33(1):1–5 PMID: 11389487
52. Granados CE, et al. *Cochrane Database Syst Rev.* 2012;12:CD007787 PMID: 23235648
53. Ross AG, et al. *N Engl J Med.* 2013;368(19):1817–1825 PMID: 23656647
54. Abboud P, et al. *Clin Infect Dis.* 2001;32(12):1792–1794 PMID: 11360222
55. Hotez PJ, et al. *N Engl J Med.* 2004;351(8):799–807 PMID: 15317893
56. Keiser J, et al. *JAMA.* 2008;299(16):1937–1948 PMID: 18430913
57. Steinmann P, et al. *PLoS One.* 2011;6(9):e25003 PMID: 21980373
58. Aronson N, et al. *Clin Infect Dis.* 2016;63(12):e202–e264 PMID: 27941151
59. World Health Organization, Technical Report Series 949. Control of the leishmaniases. Report of a meeting of the WHO Expert Committee on the Control of Leishmaniases, Geneva, 22–26 March 2010
60. Alrajhi AA, et al. *N Engl J Med.* 2002;346(12):891–895 PMID: 11907288
61. Bern C, et al. *Clin Infect Dis.* 2006;43(7):917–924 PMID: 16941377
62. Ritmeijer K, et al. *Clin Infect Dis.* 2006;43(3):357–364 PMID: 16804852
63. Monge-Maillo B, et al. *Clin Infect Dis.* 2015;60(9):1398–1404 PMID: 25601455
64. Sundar S, et al. *N Engl J Med.* 2002;347(22):1739–1746 PMID: 12456849
65. Sundar S, et al. *N Engl J Med.* 2007;356(25):2571–2581 PMID: 17582067
66. Drugs for head lice. *JAMA.* 2017;317(19):2010–2011
67. Foucault C, et al. *J Infect Dis.* 2006;193(3):474–476 PMID: 16388498
68. Fischer PR, et al. *Clin Infect Dis.* 2002;34(4):493–498 PMID: 11797176
69. Freedman DO. *N Engl J Med.* 2008;359(6):603–612 PMID: 18687641
70. Overbosch D, et al. *Clin Infect Dis.* 2001;33(7):1015–1021 PMID: 11528574
71. Arguin PM, et al. Malaria. In: Brunette GW, ed. *CDC Health Information for International Travel 2018: The Yellow Book.* 2018. https://wwwnc.cdc.gov/travel/yellowbook/2018/infectious-diseases-related-to-travel/malaria. Updated June 12, 2017. Accessed October 11, 2017
72. Griffith KS, et al. *JAMA.* 2007;297(20):2264–2277 PMID: 17519416
73. Usha V, et al. *J Am Acad Dermatol.* 2000;42(2pt1):236–240 PMID: 10642678
74. Brodine SK, et al. *Am J Trop Med Hyg.* 2009;80(3):425–430 PMID: 19270293
75. Doenhoff MJ, et al. *Expert Rev Anti Infect Ther.* 2006;4(2):199–210 PMID: 16597202
76. Fenwick A, et al. *Curr Opin Infect Dis.* 2006;19(6):577–582 PMID: 17075334
77. Marti H, et al. *Am J Trop Med Hyg.* 1996;55(5):477–481 PMID: 8940976
78. Segarra-Newnham M. *Ann Pharmacother.* 2007;41(12):1992–2001 PMID: 17940124
79. Barisani-Asenbauer T, et al. *J Ocul Pharmacol Ther.* 2001;17(3):287–294 PMID: 11436948
80. McAuley JB. *Pediatr Infect Dis J.* 2008;27(2):161–162 PMID: 18227714
81. McLeod R, et al. *Clin Infect Dis.* 2006;42(10):1383–1394 PMID: 16619149
82. Petersen E. *Expert Rev Anti Infect Ther.* 2007;5(2):285–293 PMID: 17402843
83. Adachi JA, et al. *Clin Infect Dis.* 2003;37(9):1165–1171 PMID: 14557959
84. Diemert DJ. *Clin Microbiol Rev.* 2006;19(3):583–594 PMID: 16847088
85. DuPont HL. *Clin Infect Dis.* 2007;45(Suppl1):S78–S84 PMID: 17582576

86. Riddle MS, et al. *J Travel Med.* 2017;24(Suppl1):S57–S74 PMID: 28521004
87. Gottstein B, et al. *Clin Microbiol Rev.* 2009;22(1):127–145 PMID: 19136437
88. Workowski KA, et al. *MMWR Recomm Rep.* 2015;64(RR-03):1–137 PMID: 26042815
89. Fairlamb AH. *Trends Parasitol.* 2003;19(11):488–494 PMID: 14580959
90. Schmid C, et al. *Lancet.* 2004;364(9436):789–790 PMID: 15337407
91. Bisser S, et al. *J Infect Dis.* 2007;195(3):322–329 PMID: 17205469
92. Priotto G, et al. *Lancet.* 2009;374(9683):56–64 PMID: 19559476

Chapter 13

1. Nelson JD. *J Pediatr.* 1978;92(1):175–176 PMID: 619073
2. Nelson JD, et al. *J Pediatr.* 1978;92(1):131–134 PMID: 619055
3. Tetzlaff TR, et al. *J Pediatr.* 1978;92(3):485–490 PMID: 632997
4. Ballock RT, et al. *J Pediatr Orthop.* 2009;29(6):636–642 PMID: 19700997
5. Peltola H, et al. *N Engl J Med.* 2014;370(4):352–360 PMID: 24450893
6. Bradley JS, et al. *Pediatrics.* 2011;128(4):e1034–e1045 PMID: 21949152
7. Rice HE, et al. *Arch Surg.* 2001;136(12):1391–1395 PMID: 11735866
8. Fraser JD, et al. *J Pediatr Surg.* 2010;45(6):1198–1202 PMID: 20620320
9. Strohmeier Y, et al. *Cochrane Database Syst Rev.* 2014;7:CD003772 PMID: 25066627
10. Drusano GL, et al. *J Infect Dis.* 2014;210(8):1319–1324 PMID: 24760199
11. Arnold JC, et al. *Pediatrics.* 2012;130(4):e821–e828 PMID: 22966033
12. Zaoutis T, et al. *Pediatrics.* 2009;123(2):636–642 PMID: 19171632
13. Keren R, et al. *JAMA Pediatr.* 2015;169(2):120–128 PMID: 25506733
14. Liu C, et al. *Clin Infect Dis.* 2011;52(3):e18–e55 [Erratum: *Clin Infect Dis.* 2011;53(3):319] PMID: 21208910
15. Syrogiannopoulos GA, et al. *Lancet.* 1988;1(8575–8576):37–40 PMID: 2891899

Chapter 14

1. Oehler RL, et al. *Lancet Infect Dis.* 2009;9(7):439–447 PMID: 19555903
2. Wu PS, et al. *Pediatr Emerg Care.* 2011;27(9):801–803 PMID: 21878832
3. Stevens DL, et al. *Clin Infect Dis.* 2014;59(2):147–159 PMID: 24947530
4. Talan DA, et al. *Clin Infect Dis.* 2003;37(11):1481–1489 PMID: 14614671
5. Aziz H, et al. *J Trauma Acute Care Surg.* 2015;78(3):641–648 PMID: 25710440
6. American Academy of Pediatrics. Rabies. In: Kimberlin DW, et al, eds. *Red Book: 2018 Report of the Committee on Infectious Diseases.* In press
7. American Academy of Pediatrics. Tetanus. In: Kimberlin DW, et al, eds. *Red Book: 2018 Report of the Committee on Infectious Diseases.* In press
8. Wilson W, et al. *Circulation.* 2007;116(15):1736–1754 PMID: 17446442
9. Baltimore RS, et al. *Circulation.* 2015;132(15):1487–1515 PMID: 26373317
10. Pasquali SK, et al. *Am Heart J.* 2012;163(5):894–899 PMID: 22607869
11. Pant S, et al. *J Am Coll Cardiol.* 2015;65(19):2070–2076 PMID: 25975469
12. Dayer MJ, et al. *Lancet.* 2015;385(9974):1219–1228 PMID: 25467569
13. Toyoda N, et al. *JAMA.* 2017;317(16):1652–1660 PMID: 28444279
14. American Academy of Pediatrics. Lyme disease. In: Kimberlin DW, et al, eds. *Red Book: 2018 Report of the Committee on Infectious Diseases.* In press
15. Cohn AC, et al. *MMWR Recomm Rep.* 2013;62(RR-2):1–28 PMID: 23515099
16. American Academy of Pediatrics. Pertussis (whooping cough). In: Kimberlin DW, et al, eds. *Red Book: 2018 Report of the Committee on Infectious Diseases.* In press
17. Centers for Disease Control and Prevention. Pertussis (whooping cough). Postexposure antimicrobial prophylaxis. http://www.cdc.gov/pertussis/outbreaks/PEP.html. Updated August 7, 2017. Accessed October 11, 2017
18. Brook I. *Expert Rev Anti Infect Ther.* 2008;6(3):327–336 PMID: 18588497
19. American Academy of Pediatrics. Tetanus. In: Kimberlin DW, et al, eds. *Red Book: 2018 Report of the Committee on Infectious Diseases.* In press

20. Centers for Disease Control and Prevention. Tuberculosis (TB). Treatment regimens for latent TB infection (LBTI). http://www.cdc.gov/tb/topic/treatment/ltbi.htm. Updated June 29, 2017. Accessed October 11, 2017

21. American Academy of Pediatrics. Tuberculosis. In: Kimberlin DW, et al, eds. *Red Book: 2018 Report of the Committee on Infectious Diseases.* In press

22. Centers for Disease Control and Prevention. *MMWR Morb Mortal Wkly Rep.* 2011;60(48):1650–1653 PMID: 22157884

23. ACOG Committee on Practice Bulletins. *Obstet Gynecol.* 2007;109(6):1489–1498 PMID: 17569194

24. Pinninti SG, et al. *J. Pediatr.* 2012;161(1):134–138 PMID: 22336576

25. Kimberlin DW, et al. *Pediatrics.* 2013;131(2):e635–e646 PMID: 23359576

26. American Academy of Academy Committee on Infectious Diseases. *Pediatrics.* 2015;136(4):792–808 PMID: 26347430

27. Kimberlin DW, et al. *J Infect Dis.* 2013;207(5):709–720 PMID: 23230059

28. American Academy of Pediatrics. Rabies. In: Kimberlin DW, et al, eds. *Red Book: 2018 Report of the Committee on Infectious Diseases.* In press

29. American Academy of Pediatrics. *Pneumocystis jirovecii* infections. In: Kimberlin DW, et al, eds. *Red Book: 2018 Report of the Committee on Infectious Diseases.* In press

30. Siberry GK, et al. *Pediatr Infect Dis J.* 2013;32(Suppl2):i–KK4 PMID: 24569199

31. Leach AJ, et al. *Cochrane Database Syst Rev.* 2006;(4):CD004401 PMID: 17054203

32. McDonald S, et al. *Cochrane Database Syst Rev.* 2008;(4):CD004741 PMID: 18843668

33. Williams GJ, et al. *Adv Exp Med Biol.* 2013;764:211–218 PMID: 23654070

34. Craig JC, et al. *N Engl J Med.* 2009;361(18):1748–1759 PMID: 19864673

35. RIVUR Trial Investigators, et al. *N Engl J Med.* 2014;370(25):2367–2376 PMID: 24795142

36. American Academy of Pediatrics Subcommittee on Urinary Tract Infection and Steering Committee on Quality Improvement and Management. *Pediatrics.* 2011;128(3):595–610 PMID: 21873693

37. *Treat Guidel Med Lett.* 2012;10(122):73–80 PMID: 22996382

38. Mangram AJ, et al. *Infect Control Hosp Epidemiol.* 1999;20(4):250–280 PMID: 10219875

39. Edwards FH, et al. *Ann Thorac Surg.* 2006;81(1):397–404 PMID: 16368422

40. Engelman R, et al. *Ann Thorac Surg.* 2007;83(4):1569–1576 PMID: 17383396

41. Hansen E, et al. *J Orthop Res.* 2014;32(Suppl1):S31–S59 PMID: 24464896

42. Saleh A, et al. *Ann Surg.* 2015;261(1):72–80 PMID: 25119119

43. Haley RW, et al. *Am J Epidemiol.* 1985;121(2):206–215 PMID: 4014116

44. Dellinger EP. *Ann Surg.* 2008;247(6):927–928 PMID: 18520218

45. Shaffer WO, et al. *Spine J.* 2013;13(10):1387–1392 PMID: 23988461

Chapter 15

1. Best EJ, et al. *Pediatr Infect Dis J.* 2011;30(10):827–832 PMID: 21577177

2. Zakova M, et al. *Ther Drug Monit.* 2014;36(3):288–294 PMID: 24695354

3. Rao SC, et al. *Cochrane Database Syst Rev.* 2016;12:CD005091 PMID: 27921299

4. Smyth AR, et al. *Cochrane Database Syst Rev.* 2012;2:CD002009 PMID: 22336782

5. Workowski KA, et al. *MMWR Recomm Rep.* 2015;64(RR-3):1–137 PMID: 26042815

6. Gruchalla RS, et al. *N Engl J Med.* 2006;354(6):601–609 PMID: 16467547

7. Solensky R. *J Allergy Clin Immunol.* 2012;130(6):1442 PMID: 23195529

8. *Med Lett Drugs Ther.* 2012;54(1406):101 PMID: 23282790

9. Bradley JS, et al. *Pediatrics.* 2009;123(4):e609–e613 PMID: 19289450

10. Wong VK, et al. *Pediatr Infect Dis J.* 1991;10(2):122–125 PMID: 2062603

11. Bradley JS, et al. *Pediatrics.* 2014;134(1):e146–e153 PMID: 24918220

12. Bradley JS, et al. *Pediatrics.* 2011;128(4):e1034–e1045 PMID: 21949152

13. Jacobs RF, et al. *Pediatr Infect Dis J.* 2005;24(1):34–39 PMID: 15665708

14. American Academy of Pediatrics. Pertussis (whooping cough). In: Kimberlin DW, et al, eds. *Red Book: 2018 Report of the Committee on Infectious Diseases.* In press

15. Nambiar S, et al. *Pediatrics.* 2011;127(6):e1528–e1532 PMID: 21555496

16. Williams K, et al. *Clin Infect Dis.* 2014;58(7):997–1002 PMID: 24363331

17. Sheu J, et al. *J Am Acad Dermatol.* 2015;72(2):314–320 PMID: 25481710

Index